Latest Advances in Diagnosis and Management of Skin Cancer

Latest Advances in Diagnosis and Management of Skin Cancer

Guest Editor
Choon Chiat Oh

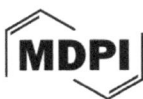

Basel • Beijing • Wuhan • Barcelona • Belgrade • Novi Sad • Cluj • Manchester

Guest Editor
Choon Chiat Oh
Department of Dermatology
Singapore General Hospital
Singapore
Singapore

Editorial Office
MDPI AG
Grosspeteranlage 5
4052 Basel, Switzerland

This is a reprint of the Special Issue, published open access by the journal *Diagnostics* (ISSN 2075-4418), freely accessible at: www.mdpi.com/journal/diagnostics/special_issues/D8F0MRQ3G4.

For citation purposes, cite each article independently as indicated on the article page online and as indicated below:

Lastname, A.A.; Lastname, B.B. Article Title. *Journal Name* **Year**, *Volume Number*, Page Range.

ISBN 978-3-7258-4251-3 (Hbk)
ISBN 978-3-7258-4252-0 (PDF)
https://doi.org/10.3390/books978-3-7258-4252-0

© 2025 by the authors. Articles in this book are Open Access and distributed under the Creative Commons Attribution (CC BY) license. The book as a whole is distributed by MDPI under the terms and conditions of the Creative Commons Attribution-NonCommercial-NoDerivs (CC BY-NC-ND) license (https://creativecommons.org/licenses/by-nc-nd/4.0/).

Contents

About the Editor vii

Preface ix

Shi Huan Tay and Choon Chiat Oh
Editorial for "Latest Advances in Diagnosis and Management of Skin Cancer"
Reprinted from: *Diagnostics* 2025, 15, 1196, https://doi.org/10.3390/diagnostics15101196 1

Simon Schwendinger, Wolfram Jaschke, Theresa Walder, Jürgen Hench, Verena Vogi, Stephan Frank, et al.
DNA Methylation Array Analysis Identifies Biological Subgroups of Cutaneous Melanoma and Reveals Extensive Differences with Benign Melanocytic Nevi
Reprinted from: *Diagnostics* 2025, 15, 531, https://doi.org/10.3390/diagnostics15050531 3

Martina D'Onghia, Francesca Falcinelli, Lorenzo Barbarossa, Alberto Pinto, Alessandra Cartocci, Linda Tognetti, et al.
Zoom-in Dermoscopy for Facial Tumors
Reprinted from: *Diagnostics* 2025, 15, 324, https://doi.org/10.3390/diagnostics15030324 19

Andrea Ronchi, Giuseppe D'Abbronzo, Emma Carraturo, Giuseppe Argenziano, Gabriella Brancaccio, Camila Scharf, et al.
High Incidence of Isolated Tumor Cells in Sentinel Node Biopsies of Thin Melanomas: A Potential Factor in the Paradoxical Prognosis of Stage IIIA Cutaneous Melanoma?
Reprinted from: *Diagnostics* 2025, 15, 69, https://doi.org/10.3390/diagnostics15010069 33

Iulia Zboraș, Loredana Ungureanu, Simona Șenilă, Bobe Petrushev, Paula Zamfir, Doinița Crișan, et al.
PRAME Immunohistochemistry in Thin Melanomas Compared to Melanocytic Nevi
Reprinted from: *Diagnostics* 2024, 14, 2015, https://doi.org/10.3390/diagnostics14182015 43

Agnes Yeok-Loo Lim, Jason Yongsheng Chan and Choon Chiat Oh
Cutaneous Adverse Reactions and Survival Outcomes of Advanced Melanoma Treated with Immune Checkpoint Inhibitors in an Academic Medical Centre in Singapore
Reprinted from: *Diagnostics* 2024, 14, 1601, https://doi.org/10.3390/diagnostics14151601 55

Carlo Metta, Andrea Beretta, Riccardo Guidotti, Yuan Yin, Patrick Gallinari, Salvatore Rinzivillo and Fosca Giannotti
Advancing Dermatological Diagnostics: Interpretable AI for Enhanced Skin Lesion Classification
Reprinted from: *Diagnostics* 2024, 14, 753, https://doi.org/10.3390/diagnostics14070753 66

Ibrahim Yel, Vitali Koch, Leon D. Gruenewald, Scherwin Mahmoudi, Leona S. Alizadeh, Aynur Goekduman, et al.
Advancing Differentiation of Hepatic Metastases in Malignant Melanoma through Dual-Energy Computed Tomography Rho/Z Maps
Reprinted from: *Diagnostics* 2024, 14, 742, https://doi.org/10.3390/diagnostics14070742 92

Linda Tognetti, Alessandra Cartocci, Aimilios Lallas, Elvira Moscarella, Ignazio Stanganelli, Gianluca Nazzaro, et al.
A European Multicentric Investigation of Atypical Melanocytic Skin Lesions of Palms and Soles: The *iDScore-PalmoPlantar* Database
Reprinted from: *Diagnostics* 2024, 14, 460, https://doi.org/10.3390/diagnostics14050460 106

Agnieszka Rydz, Jakub Żółkiewicz, Michał Kunc, Martyna Sławińska, Michał Sobjanek, Roman J. Nowicki and Magdalena Lange
Eruptive Syringoma—Clinical, Dermoscopic, and Reflectance Confocal Microscopy Features
Reprinted from: *Diagnostics* **2025**, *15*, 110, https://doi.org/10.3390/diagnostics15010110 . . . . . **123**

Adrian Vasile Dumitru, Dana Antonia Țăpoi, Mariana Costache, Ana Maria Ciongariu, Andreea Iuliana Ionescu, Horia Dan Liscu, et al.
Metastatic Nodular Melanoma with Angiosarcomatous Transdifferentiation—A Case Report and Review of the Literature
Reprinted from: *Diagnostics* **2024**, *14*, 1323, https://doi.org/10.3390/diagnostics14131323 . . . . **129**

Shi Huan Tay and Choon Chiat Oh
T Cell Immunity in Human Papillomavirus-Related Cutaneous Squamous Cell Carcinoma—A Systematic Review
Reprinted from: *Diagnostics* **2024**, *14*, 473, https://doi.org/10.3390/diagnostics14050473 . . . . . **143**

About the Editor

Choon Chiat Oh

Dr. Oh is a Senior Consultant at the Department of Dermatology, Singapore General Hospital (SGH), and has a keen interest in skin cancer surgery and research. He holds a Master of Clinical Investigation from the National University of Singapore (2018) and a Master of Science in Dermoscopy and Preventive Dermato-oncology from the Medical University of Graz, Austria (2020).

His research interests focus on skin care for organ transplant recipients, addressing unmet needs through epidemiological studies, systematic reviews, and investigations into viral oncogenic pathways and chemo-preventive strategies for skin cancer in immunosuppressed patients. His other research interests include the use of innovative medical devices and artificial intelligence for the treatment of skin cancers.

Preface

The global rise in skin cancer has made it a major public health concern. Recent technological advances enable more precise diagnoses and novel treatments for advanced disease. This Special Issue showcases 11 contributions, spanning rare case reports to key developments in diagnostics, therapy, and AI-assisted decision-making. Within this scope, the featured articles reflect a rapidly evolving field, covering topics such as explainable AI, advanced imaging, and innovations in immunotherapy and cellular approaches. Through this publication, we aim to highlight these breakthroughs, motivate further research, and improve patient outcomes. This issue is intended for clinicians, researchers, and healthcare professionals dedicated to advancing skin cancer care. The authors, a multidisciplinary group of experts, hope to foster collaboration and inspire ongoing progress in the understanding and management of skin cancer.

Choon Chiat Oh
Guest Editor

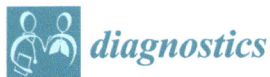

Editorial

Editorial for "Latest Advances in Diagnosis and Management of Skin Cancer"

Shi Huan Tay [1] and Choon Chiat Oh [2],*

[1] Department of Internal Medicine, Singapore General Hospital, Singapore 169608, Singapore; tay.shi.huan@mohh.com.sg
[2] Department of Dermatology, Singapore General Hospital, Singapore 169608, Singapore
* Correspondence: oh.choon.chiat@singhealth.com.sg

The rising global incidence of skin cancer has established this disease as a critical public health issue. In recent years, numerous technological innovations have enabled more precise and timely diagnoses, while novel treatments have emerged for advanced stages of the disease. To highlight these significant developments, this Special Issue presents 11 valuable contributions to the field—ranging from detailed observations of rare and atypical cases to crucial advancements in diagnostics, treatment, and artificial intelligence (AI)-assisted decision-making.

The future of skin cancer diagnoses is increasingly poised to incorporate AI-assisted technologies, as the field moves toward integrating multi-modality data from global sources [1]. One study in our Special Issue explored Explainable AI (XAI) using ABELE for skin lesion classification. The saliency maps generated by ABELE provided useful topographical information that enhanced physicians' confidence in their diagnoses. To realise ABELE's potential, the training dataset must be expanded to include a broader range of lesion types, disease stages, and patient demographics. Future international collaborations will be essential for advancing our knowledge amidst increasingly complex experimental designs and analytical methodologies.

Beyond the promise of AI, the field of cutaneous melanoma has also witnessed advances in bedside, histopathological, and molecular diagnostics [2,3]. In particular, novel imaging techniques have emerged to improve early melanoma diagnosis. D'Onghia et al. highlighted the strengths of high-magnification dermoscopy and fluorescence-assisted videodermatoscopy in a study involving 85 patients with facial skin lesions [4]. Alongside the advent of line-field confocal optical coherence tomography [5], we are one step closer to untangling this Gordian knot non-invasively, potentially reducing the need for biopsies.

The emergence of programmed cell death-1 (PD1) inhibitors has transformed the management of metastatic melanoma; however, clinicians must remain vigilant regarding immune-related adverse events [6]. Another study in our Special Issue contributes a Southeast Asian perspective to the growing body of evidence on anti-PD1 inhibitors. Consistent with findings from other parts of the world, these inhibitors were shown to increase overall median survival, although a subset of melanoma patients developed cutaneous adverse reactions. Interestingly, the development of such reactions may be associated with improved overall survival, underscoring the need for future mechanistic work to unravel the underlying intricacies.

Cellular therapy represents the next frontier in skin cancer treatment, offering tailored therapeutic potential for patients who are unresponsive to current standard-of-care treatment. Indeed, several landmark trials involving tumour-infiltrating lymphocytes (TILs) and personalised, neoantigen-specific autologous T cells have demonstrated significant efficacy and safety in advanced melanoma refractory to immune checkpoint inhibitors (ICIs) and BRAF/MEK inhibitors [7,8]. Additionally, T cell-based vaccines against commonly occurring β-human papillomaviruses (β-HPVs), along with β-HPV-specific T cell immunotherapy, are also promising strategies in the fight against HPV-related cutaneous squamous cell carcinoma (cSCC).

All in all, we are witnessing a paradigm shift in skin cancer, marked by multiple breakthroughs across diagnostics and therapeutics. We hope this Special Issue will inspire continued contributions to the scientific understanding and clinical management of skin cancer, ultimately advancing patient care worldwide.

Author Contributions: Writing—original draft preparation, S.H.T.; writing—review and editing, C.C.O. All authors have read and agreed to the published version of the manuscript.

Funding: This research received no external funding.

Conflicts of Interest: The authors declare no conflicts of interest.

References

1. Du-Harpur, X.; Watt, F.M.; Luscombe, N.M.; Lynch, M.D. What is AI? Applications of artificial intelligence to dermatology. *Br. J. Dermatol.* **2020**, *183*, 423–430. [CrossRef] [PubMed]
2. Merlino, G.; Herlyn, M.; Fisher, D.E.; Bastian, B.C.; Flaherty, K.T.; Davies, M.A.; Wargo, J.A.; Curiel-Lewandrowski, C.; Weber, M.J.; Leachman, S.A.; et al. The state of melanoma: Challenges and opportunities. *Pigment. Cell Melanoma Res.* **2016**, *29*, 404–416. [CrossRef] [PubMed]
3. Davis, L.E.; Shalin, S.C.; Tackett, A.J. Current state of melanoma diagnosis and treatment. *Cancer Biol. Ther.* **2019**, *20*, 1366–1379. [CrossRef] [PubMed]
4. D'Onghia, M.; Falcinelli, F.; Barbarossa, L.; Pinto, A.; Cartocci, A.; Tognetti, L.; Rubegni, G.; Batsikosta, A.; Rubegni, P.; Cinotti, E. Zoom-in Dermoscopy for Facial Tumors. *Diagnostics* **2025**, *15*, 324. [CrossRef] [PubMed]
5. Latriglia, F.; Ogien, J.; Tavernier, C.; Fischman, S.; Suppa, M.; Perrot, J.L.; Dubois, A. Line-Field Confocal Optical Coherence Tomography (LC-OCT) for Skin Imaging in Dermatology. *Life* **2023**, *13*, 2268. [CrossRef] [PubMed]
6. Bastacky, M.L.; Wang, H.; Fortman, D.; Rahman, Z.; Mascara, G.P.; Brenner, T.; Najjar, Y.G.; Luke, J.J.; Kirkwood, J.M.; Zarour, H.M.; et al. Immune-Related Adverse Events in PD-1 Treated Melanoma and Impact Upon Anti-Tumor Efficacy: A Real World Analysis. *Front. Oncol.* **2021**, *11*, 749064. [CrossRef] [PubMed]
7. Chesney, J.; Lewis, K.D.; Kluger, H.; Hamid, O.; Whitman, E.; Thomas, S.; Wermke, M.; Cusnir, M.; Domingo-Musibay, E.; Phan, G.Q.; et al. Efficacy and safety of lifileucel, a one-time autologous tumor-infiltrating lymphocyte (TIL) cell therapy, in patients with advanced melanoma after progression on immune checkpoint inhibitors and targeted therapies: Pooled analysis of consecutive cohorts of the C-144-01 study. *J. Immunother. Cancer* **2022**, *10*, e005755. [CrossRef] [PubMed]
8. Borgers, J.S.W.; Lenkala, D.; Kohler, V.; Jackson, E.K.; Linssen, M.D.; Hymson, S.; McCarthy, B.; O'Reilly Cosgrove, E.; Balogh, K.N.; Esaulova, E.; et al. Personalized, autologous neoantigen-specific T cell therapy in metastatic melanoma: A phase 1 trial. *Nat. Med.* **2025**, *31*, 881–893. [CrossRef] [PubMed]

Disclaimer/Publisher's Note: The statements, opinions and data contained in all publications are solely those of the individual author(s) and contributor(s) and not of MDPI and/or the editor(s). MDPI and/or the editor(s) disclaim responsibility for any injury to people or property resulting from any ideas, methods, instructions or products referred to in the content.

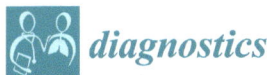

Article

DNA Methylation Array Analysis Identifies Biological Subgroups of Cutaneous Melanoma and Reveals Extensive Differences with Benign Melanocytic Nevi

Simon Schwendinger [1], Wolfram Jaschke [2], Theresa Walder [1], Jürgen Hench [3], Verena Vogi [1], Stephan Frank [3], Per Hoffmann [4], Stefan Herms [4], Johannes Zschocke [1], Van Anh Nguyen [2], Matthias Schmuth [2] and Emina Jukic [1,*]

[1] Institute of Human Genetics, Medical University Innsbruck, 6020 Innsbruck, Austria; simon.schwendinger@i-med.ac.at (S.S.)
[2] Department of Dermatology, Venereology and Allergy, Medical University Innsbruck, 6020 Innsbruck, Austria
[3] Institute of Medical Genetics and Pathology, University Hospital Basel, 4031 Basel, Switzerland
[4] Institute of Human Genetics, University Hospital Bonn, 53127 Bonn, Germany
* Correspondence: emina.jukic@i-med.ac.at; Tel.: +43-512-9003-70539

Abstract: Background/Objectives: Genetics and epigenetics play an important role in the pathogenesis of cutaneous melanoma. The majority of cases harbor mutations in genes associated with the MAPK signaling pathway, i.e., *BRAF*, *NRAS*, or *NF1*. The remaining neoplasms, often located on acral sites, are condensed as the triple-wildtype subtype and are characterized by other molecular drivers. This study aimed to elucidate genetic and epigenetic differences within cutaneous melanoma and to compare it with melanocytic nevi. **Methods**: DNA was extracted from archived tissue samples of cutaneous melanoma ($n = 19$), melanocytic nevi ($n = 11$), and skin controls ($n = 11$) and subsequently analyzed by massive parallel (next generation) gene panel sequencing and genome-wide DNA methylation array analysis. The sample size was increased by including repository data from an external study. **Results**: There were major differences in the genomic landscape of MAPK-altered and triple-wildtype cutaneous melanoma, the latter presenting with a lower number of mutations, a different pattern of copy number variants, and a low frequency of *TERT* promoter mutations. Dimensional reduction of DNA methylation array analysis clearly separated cutaneous melanoma from melanocytic nevi but revealed no major differences between classical cutaneous melanoma and the triple-wildtype cases. However, it identified a possible biological subgroup characterized by intermediately methylated CpGs. **Conclusions**: Dimensional reduction of methylation array data is a useful tool for the analysis of melanocytic tumors to differentiate between malignant and benign lesions and may be able to identify biologically distinct subtypes of cutaneous melanoma.

Keywords: cutaneous melanoma; melanocytic nevi; genetics; epigenetics

1. Introduction

Cutaneous melanoma (CM) is characterized by activating mutations in the MAPK signaling pathway, including *BRAF* mutations in 50% of cases, *RAS* alterations in about 30% of cases, and *NF1* deficiencies in 15% of the neoplasms [1,2]. CMs lacking these common mutations have been classified as the triple wildtype (TWT) subtype. This group of neoplasms is very heterogeneous, and different molecular drivers, such as *KIT* gene mutations, seem to play a role [2]. TWT-CMs are often located at acral sites. TWT-CMs, in general, and acral CM, in particular, are usually not associated with sun damage and have fewer genetic alterations than classical MAPK-activated CM [1]. The most common subtype of acral CM is acral lentiginous melanoma (ALM), which has a characteristic lentiginous growth pattern. Rarer manifestations at acral sites are nodular or superficial spreading CMs [3,4].

Epigenetic alterations play an important role in the development of CM. The DNA methylation pattern (methylome) of CM is characterized by global hypomethylation combined with local hypermethylation. Both mechanisms contribute to tumorigenesis by activation of oncogenic factors and suppression of tumor suppressor genes [5,6]. Various studies have found that the methylation status of CM changes during disease progression [7,8]. In particular, gene promoter hypermethylation increases with CM progression. A high degree of promoter methylation is referred to as CpG island hypermethylation phenotype (CIMP) and is associated with poor clinical outcomes [7–11].

Our present study aimed to investigate the genetic and epigenetic landscape of CM in comparison to melanocytic nevi (MN). Regarding methodology, the study is based on massive parallel sequencing (next-generation sequencing; NGS) and genome-wide DNA methylation array (DMA) analysis. Apart from CM with classical driver genes, a high number of TWT cases (many of them from acral sites) are included in the study to characterize the genetics and DNA methylation patterns in this rare CM subtype. We examine whether methylome analysis can distinguish CM from MN and identify differences between MAPK-altered CM and TWT-CM in relation to genetic markers. Additionally, we analyze epigenetic differences between MN and the two CM subgroups based on differentially methylated positions (DMPs) and regions (DMRs).

2. Materials and Methods

2.1. Patients and Samples

A cohort was generated from formalin-embedded paraffin (FFPE) blocks derived from primary CM tumors (n = 56) with a Breslow's thickness $\geq$ 1.8 mm. Additionally, MN (n = 56) with >3 mm diameter and healthy skin samples (n = 11) were included. CM patients from the time period between 2006 and 2021 were identified in the Tumor Registry Tyrol. Written informed consent was obtained under two protocols approved by the Ethics Committee of the Medical University of Innsbruck (No. 1182/2018 and 1170/2019). Clinical information, including sex, age at diagnosis, tumor location, tumor stage, the morphological classification of the primary tumor at diagnosis, as well as histological subtype and Breslow's thickness, were recorded. The cases were re-evaluated by a dermatopathologist to confirm the diagnosis and morphological classification. All cases were retrieved from residual tissue blocks from the dermatopathology archives of the Medical University of Innsbruck and cooperating institutes. Analyses were performed after de-identification of the specimen. Additional data for samples from an external study published by Pradhan et al., 2019 [4] were downloaded from the Gene Expression Omnibus [12]. This dataset includes CM samples (n = 40) and MN specimens (n = 3), most of them localized in acral skin.

2.2. Macrodissection and DNA Isolation

Serial sections were prepared from FFPE tissue blocks. A hematoxylin and eosin (H&E)-stained reference slide was prepared from the central section. This specimen was assessed by a dermatopathologist, and tumor areas were marked. The marks were transferred to adjacent unstained sections. A standard xylol–ethanol protocol was used to remove paraffin from the samples, and a manual macrodissection of the sections was performed. After incubation with proteinase K, genomic DNA was isolated using the QIAmp DNA FFPE tissue kit (Qiagen, Hilden, Germany) according to the manufacturer's instructions. The DNA was quantified using a micro-volume photometer and the Qubit 4 fluorometer with the dsDNA High Sensitivity or dsDNA Broad Range assay kits (Thermo Fisher Scientific, Waltham, MA, USA).

2.3. Methylation Array Analysis

2.3.1. Array Preparation and Scanning

For methylation array analysis, the Illumina Infinium MethylationEPIC BeadChip Array platform (Illumina, San Diego, CA, USA) was used. Depending on the available DNA quantity, between 150 and 250 ng of DNA was utilized per sample. The specimens were prepared with the standard protocol for FFPE materials according to the manufacturer's instructions and scanned on an iScan device (Illumina, San Diego, CA, USA).

2.3.2. Quality Control and Tumor Purity Estimation

For quality control and tumor purity estimation, the IDAT files containing the methylation data were loaded into R Studio (version 1.4.1717; R version: 4.1.0) using the minfi [13] package (version 1.40.0). For every probe on the array, the detection p-value (detp) was calculated. As the share of failed probes (i.e., a detp > 0.01) can be used as a surrogate marker for array data quality [14], all samples with more than 5% of failed probes were excluded from the dataset. To estimate the tumor cell content of the CM and the MN samples, the RFpurify [15] package (version 0.1.2) was used. In brief, this method uses the methylation status of 856 CpGs to estimate the ABSOLUTE and ESTIMATE values of a sample by random forest regression and, therefore, predicts the tumor purity of the sample [15]. A careful evaluation in synopsis with the subsequently described UMAP analysis showed that a predicted ABSOLUTE score of below 0.445 or a predicted ESTIMATE value of below 0.775 seemed to work best for excluding samples with low tumor purity to achieve clearly separated sample clusters. Samples that failed the prediction cutoffs but were still localized in one of the sample clusters were included again to increase the sample size.

2.3.3. Uniform Manifold Approximation and Projection (UMAP) Analysis

Methylome analysis was performed by uniform manifold approximation and projection (UMAP). This method reduces the highly dimensional methylation array datasets down to two dimensions. The EpiDiP server of the University Hospital, Basel, Switzerland (available from http://s1665.rootserver.io/, accessed on 15 April 2022) was utilized. The total dataset for dimensional reduction includes about 25,000 datasets from various cancer samples derived from publicly available data repositories such as The Cancer Genome Atlas [16] and the Gene Expression Omnibus [12], as well as thousands of samples derived from various contributors. UMAP reduction was performed using the 50,000 probes with the highest standard deviations among all samples. For the presented two-dimensional plots, only the coordinates from the samples of the current project were extracted.

2.3.4. Differential Methylation Analysis

For DMP and DMR analysis, a strategy based on a protocol published by Maksimovic et al., 2016 [14] was applied. Normalization was performed using the functional normalization method in minfi. Subsequently, all probes with a detp > 0.01 in at least one sample, probes containing a SNP in their sequence, and all probes mapping to sex chromosomes were excluded. Further, probes known to be cross-reactive were filtered using the maxprobes package (version 0.0.2; available from https://github.com/markgene/maxprobes, accessed on 28 April 2022). After filtering, 678,635 CpGs remained in this pipeline. DMP analysis between the methylation clusters was performed using a linear model design with group-wise comparisons and empirical Bayes statistics from the limma package (version 3.50.3) [17]. The same model was subsequently used for the identification of DMRs with the DMRcate package (version 2.8.5) [18]. Regions comprising at least five CpGs and a mean methylation difference of 0.25 were called. The top ten significant DMRs from all three comparisons were evaluated using the UCSC genome browser [19] with the tracks "RefSeq Transcripts" and GeneHancer [20] (double elite) promoters and enhancers displayed.

2.4. Copy Number Variant (CNV) Detection

Copy number variant (CNV) profiles were calculated using the methylation array data and the conumee package (version 1.9.0; available from http://bioconductor.org/packages/conumee, accessed on 30 April 2022) in R Studio. The method uses the total intensities (red and green) of every probe for calculation, segmentation, and calling of differences in copy numbers of chromosomal regions. The analysis was conducted according to the instructions in the package vignette. In short, samples were loaded and normalized using the quantile normalization method of the minfi package version 1.40.0 [13]. For the actual analysis, a minimum number of 30 probes per bin and a minimum bin size of 100,000 bp were chosen. Genes of interest were chosen according to several publications and our personal interests. Because of the limited data quality for CNV analysis from FFPE-derived DNA, automated CNV calling was not expedient (too many false positives or false negatives due to strong scattering of log2 ratio values). Instead, CNVs were identified by careful manual inspection of the genome plots produced by the package. For this, the plots were inspected for segments of chromosomes with deviations in the log2 ratio of at least 0.3–0.4.

2.5. Next Generation Sequencing

2.5.1. Library Preparation and Sequencing

Enriched sample libraries for sequencing were prepared using an in-house pipeline based on the Illumina DNA Prep with Enrichment kit and a custom-designed hybridization probe panel (Illumina, San Diego, CA, USA). A total of 100–250 ng of DNA was used per sample. The utilized probe panel includes selected exons or full coding regions of about 153 genes with a total covered region of 0.49 mbp. Detailed information about the covered regions is provided in Supplementary Table S1. Paired-end sequencing was performed on an Illumina NextSeq 500 device (Illumina, San Diego, CA, USA). The mean target coverage depth of the samples was 936 ± 451 SD reads, with a mean of $99.78\% \pm 0.32\%$ SD of the targeted regions covered at least 50-fold. For FASTQ generation and data processing, the Illumina BaseSpace Sequencing Hub (BSSH; European instance in Frankfurt, Germany; available from https://euc1.sh.basespace.illumina.com, accessed on 3 October 2021) was utilized. Alignment of raw reads and variant calling was performed with the DRAGEN Enrichment app v3.6.3, with hg19 as the reference genome. Variants with a variant allele frequency (VAF) of at least 10% and a quality score of 20 were called. Only CM and MN samples were analyzed; no sequencing was performed for the skin control samples.

2.5.2. Small Variant Evaluation

The called variants were annotated to RefSeq transcripts using the Illumina annotation engine (Illumina, San Diego, CA, USA) in BSSH Variant Interpreter (European instance in Frankfurt, Germany; available from https://variantinterpreter.euc1.vi.basespace.illumina.com, accessed on 3 October 2021). All datasets were filtered for coding variants and splice site variants. As no matched normal samples were available, the exclusion of probable germline variants was performed by filtering polymorphisms with a minor allele frequency of above 0.01 in the non-Finnish European population data in the Genome Aggregation Database (GnomAD) [21]. The remaining variants were verified by manual evaluation of alignments with the Integrative Genomics Viewer (IGV) [22]. Some variants were excluded during this process because they were identified as sequencing artifacts. As a last step, variants were carefully evaluated using the Catalogue of Somatic Mutations in Cancer (COSMIC) [23] as well as the ClinVar [24] and the My Cancer Genome [25] databases.

Variants with prevailing evidence of germline origin were excluded from the dataset; the other variants were classified as pathogenic, likely pathogenic, or unclear significance based on their database presence or predicted functionality using SIFT [26] and PolyPhen2 [27]. *TERT* promotor analysis was performed by manual evaluation of alignments using IGV. Variants were manually annotated to the RefSeq transcript NM_198253.3. According to Nagore et al., 2019 [28] and Hugdahl et al., 2018 [29], samples were scoured for the variants c.-57A>C, c.-124C>T, c.-124/-125CC>TT, c.-138/-139CC>TT, and c.-146C>T.

2.6. Data Evaluation and Statistics

All statistical analyses were performed using R. During differential methylation analysis, hundreds of thousands of parallel hypothesis tests are conducted; therefore, strategies to control for false positive results are routinely implemented for both DMP and DMR discovery. For DMP identification, the limma package uses a significance level of $\alpha = 0.05$ and adjusts all *p*-values using the Benjamini–Hochberg method [30], with an accepted false discovery rate of 5% [17]. DMRcate additionally uses a kernel smoothing approach to average test statistics across adjacent CpG sites, reducing variability in individual tests and improving the detection sensitivity of DMR identification [18].

During data evaluation, different statistical tests were performed to compare groups, depending on the specific hypothesis. In summary, the Wilcoxon rank-sum test, Fisher's exact test, or analysis of variance (ANOVA) followed by pairwise t-tests were applied. The non-parametric tests were chosen because sample sizes for the corresponding research questions were relatively small. When necessary (i.e., when two or more parallel tests were conducted within one comparison of groups), *p*-values were adjusted using the Benjamini–Hochberg method [30]. The test used for calculation is indicated with each individual *p*-value.

3. Results

In this study, FFPE tissue blocks of primary CM or MN were analyzed. For some samples, the absence of a *BRAF* or *NRAS* hotspot mutation was known from a preceding study [31] or from routine diagnostic testing. Such cases were preferably chosen to ensure a high proportion of cases with TWT status. All samples were manually macrodissected and DNA was isolated from the tumor fraction. In total, 56 samples from both groups were used; however, the majority of samples had to be excluded due to technical reasons or low tumor purity (i.e., low content of tumor cells). A complete list of all analyzed samples with additional metadata and (if applicable) exclusion reason is provided in the Supplementary Data File. Supplementary Figure S1 visualizes the age of FFPE blocks for included and excluded samples. The median block age of excluded samples was significantly higher than the included ones both for MN (Wilcoxon test *p*-value: <0.001) and CM (Wilcoxon test *p*-value: 0.005). Evaluation of biological parameters of CMs such as tumor area, Breslow's depth, and cell vitality did not reveal clear differences between included and excluded samples. However, the inclusion rate was much higher in tumors presenting ulceration, and all included samples were of tumor stage IIB or higher; these comparisons are visualized in Supplementary Figure S2.

The final cohort consisted of 19 CM and eleven MN specimens. As reference material, eleven skin samples from healthy donor skin were included. A list of the samples in the final cohort with all collected biological as well as clinical parameters is provided in the Supplementary Data File; an aggregated overview of the cohort can be seen in Table 1. In summary, the majority of the included CM samples were derived from acral or extremity localization and presented with nodular histology, advanced tumor stage, and a high Breslow's depth.

Table 1. General overview of the clinical characteristics of the samples included.

Variable	n (%) or Mean ± SD
Gender	
Cutaneous melanoma	
Female	10 (53%)
Male	9 (47%)
Melanocytic nevi	
Female	5 (45%)
Male	6 (55%)
Skin	
Female	6 (55%)
Male	5 (45%)
Age at diagnosis (years, mean ± SD)	
Cutaneous melanoma	59.8 ± 23.8 (31–96)
Melanocytic nevi	34.1 ± 11.9 (16–52)
Altitude of residence (cutaneous melanoma)	
<1000 m	16 (84%)
>1000 m	3 (16%)
Localization	
Cutaneous melanoma	
Head or neck	3 (15%)
Trunk	4 (21%)
Extremities	6 (32%)
Acral	6 (32%)
Melanocytic nevi	
Head or neck	3 (27%)
Trunk	6 (55%)
Extremities	2 (18%)
Histological subtype	
Cutaneous melanoma	
Desmoplastic melanoma	1 (5.25%)
Acral lentiginous melanoma	4 (21%)
Lentigo maligna melanoma	1 (5.25%)
Nodular melanoma	8 (42%)
Spindle cell melanoma	2 (11%)
Superficial spreading melanoma	3 (16%)
Melanocytic nevi	
Compound nevus	7 (64%)
Dermal nevus	4 (36%)
Tumor stage (cutaneous melanoma)	
IIA	1 (5.25%)
IIB	3 (16%)
IIC	4 (21%)
III	1 (5.25%)
IIIA	1 (5.25%)
IIIB	1 (5.25%)
IIIC	5 (26%)
IV	3 (16%)

3.1. Genetic Analysis Reveals Distinct Differences Between Cases with Alterations in the MAPK Signaling Pathway and TWT Status

Genetic analyses of CM samples by NGS of approximately 150 genes revealed—as expected due to the selection bias of specimens—that most of the cases (7/19; 37%) had a genetic TWT status (Figure 1a). *BRAF* mutations (exclusively p.V600E or p.V600K) were found in 5/19 samples (26%), *NF1* mutations were found in 4/19 (21%) samples, while

3/19 (16%) samples harbored an *NRAS* mutation (Figure 1a). In addition to the established driver mutations, the most common alterations classified as pathogenic or likely pathogenic were *TERT* promoter mutations in 12/19 (63%) cases, followed by mutations in *CDKN2A* in 4/19 (27%) cases, and *ARID2* and *PTEN* mutations in 3/19 (16%) cases.

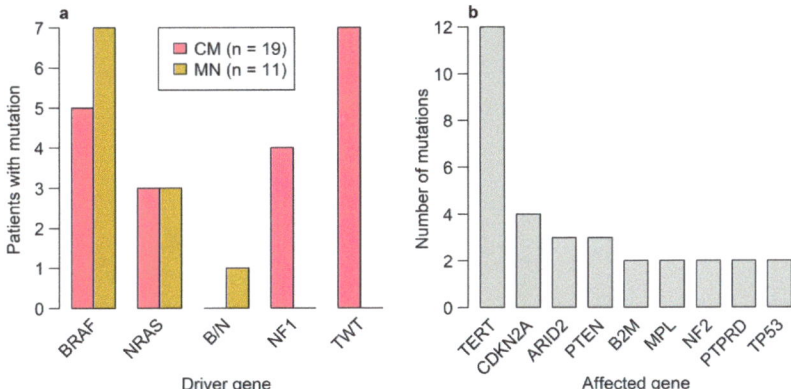

Figure 1. Driver mutations in CM and BN cases and mutational landscape of CM patients. (**a**) Bar plot depicting the proportion of patients with a MAPK-associated driver mutation (pink = CM, orange = MN; B/N = BRAF and NRAS mutations) for both CM and BN. (**b**) Bar plot showing the absolute frequencies of genes with a pathogenic or likely pathogenic mutation in the overall CM cohort. Only genes that were recurrently mutated (i.e., at least twice) are shown.

An overview of the most recurrently mutated genes is shown in Figure 1b. The complete list of all detected mutations, including information used for classification, is provided in the Supplementary Data File. The mean number of mutations per sample (including variants of unclear significance) was 5.3 ± 4.8 standard deviation (SD). Samples with one of the three driver mutations had a significantly higher mean mutation count of 5.3 ± 3.1 SD compared to 4 ± 3.2 SD in the TWT group (Wilcoxon test *p*-value: 0.005). *TERT* promoter mutations were found in 10/12 (83%) cases with a MAPK signaling pathway activating driver mutation but only in 2/7 (29%) of samples with TWT status (Fisher's exact test *p*-value: 0.009). In accordance with De Martino et al., 2020 [31], no apparent connection between genetics and altitude of residence of the patient was observed. In the remaining sample, both *BRAF* p.V600E and *NRAS* p.Q61K mutations were detected.

Apart from the driver mutations, only a few mutations were detected in MN cases, with a mean mutation count of 2.4 ± 1.3 SD. None of the MN samples harbored a *TERT* promoter mutation.

Data obtained from the DMA analysis were used for the analysis of CNVs. Due to the limited quality of FFPE-derived DNA, we generated CNV plots and identified extensive CNVs by manual inspection of the plots (see Section 2). The CNV plots of all samples and a list of the detected alterations, as well as a general assessment of the CNV pattern profile (i.e., widespread or more focal changes), are provided in the Supplementary Data File. Figure 2 summarizes CNVs in the two sample groups affecting certain genes considered relevant for CM development. For MAPK-CM, the CNV patterns showed mainly extensive abnormalities involving large parts of chromosomal arms or whole chromosomes, consistent with reports from the literature [32]. The most commonly deleted regions included 9p21 (*CDKN2A* locus) in 8/12 (67%) and 10q23 (*PTEN* locus) in 4/12 (33%) samples, whereas the most prevalent amplified region was 7q34 (*BRAF* locus) in 5/12 (42%) samples. Similar CNV patterns were observed in most TWT samples; however, these samples had a tendency for more focal amplifications or deletions. Loss of the *CDKN2A* locus appeared in 7/7 (100%) of the samples, and deletions including the *PTEN* locus were observed in 3/7 (33%) samples. Recurrently amplified regions were again the *BRAF* locus on 7q34 and the *TERT* region on 11q13 in 2/7 (33%) of cases. One TWT sample (in0597) presented a distinct, generally flat CNV profile with only a few but very complex focal abnormalities. The latter sample was derived from an acral desmoplastic melanoma and did not show any mutations except an in-frame deletion in a gene called *SOCS1*. None of the MN samples harbored CNVs.

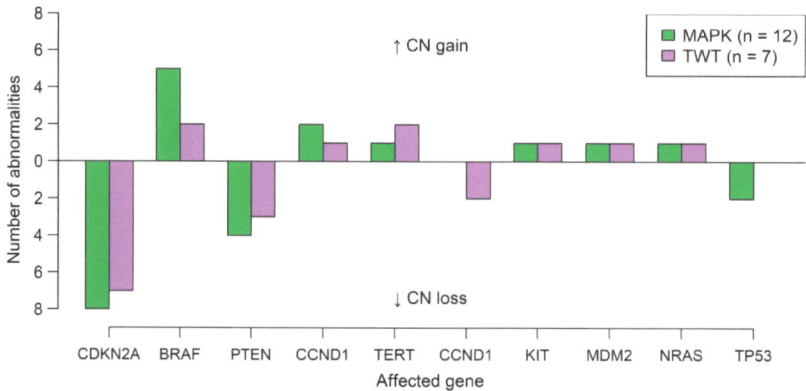

Figure 2. Cytogenomic landscape of CM samples. Frequencies of CNVs detected in MAKP-altered CM (green) and TWT (violet) cases. CNVs are shown as mirrored bar plots, with gains of chromosomal material oriented to the top and losses displayed on the bottom.

3.2. DNA Methylome Analysis Identifies Differences Between CM and MN and Indicates a Distinct Biological Subtype of CM

To assess the general differences in the methylome structures of CM, MN, and skin samples, a DMA analysis was performed and the dimensional reduction method UMAP was applied. This method reduces the highly complex datasets down to two dimensions, which can be plotted and viewed. Samples with a similar methylome are located near each other, whereas distinct samples are separated into individual clusters [33]. In the chosen approach, the samples are evaluated within a big data lake consisting of about 25,000 different tumor samples [34], and the coordinates of the relevant specimens are extracted afterward. A depiction of the reduction can be seen in Supplementary Figure S3. It resulted in three distinct groups of sample clusters (termed methylation clusters) comprising all but one of the CM specimens (termed melanoma methylation cluster 1; MMC1), MN samples (nevus methylation cluster; NMC), and healthy skin controls (skin methylation cluster; SMC). One CM sample (in0597) was localized separately from the other samples. This sample is of particular interest, as it shows a methylome structure different from all other CM cases. Intriguingly, this sample is also the one described before, harboring a distinct CNV pattern and TWT genetic status.

To see whether this result can be reproduced with additional samples, we searched the Gene Expression Omnibus [12] for publicly available methylation datasets and found a promising study published by Pradhan et al. in 2019 [4] focusing on the epigenetics of ALM and other acral CMs. We processed those samples with our quality control pipeline and analyzed the remaining 21 CM specimens and two MN samples with our cohort. As shown in Figure 3, 17 of those specimens clustered together with our in0597 sample and comprised a second methylation cluster (melanoma methylation cluster 2; MMC2) separated from the MMC1 cluster. The UMAP coordinates used to produce the plot, as well as the cluster designation of each individual sample, are provided in the Supplementary

Data File. According to the available metadata, most of the samples located in MMC2 were derived from primary ALM specimens; additionally, three samples classified as non-ALM acral CM and two samples classified as CM were located in this cluster. The dataset also added four samples of mixed histology to our MMC1 cluster and contained two acral MN samples that co-clustered with the NMC cluster.

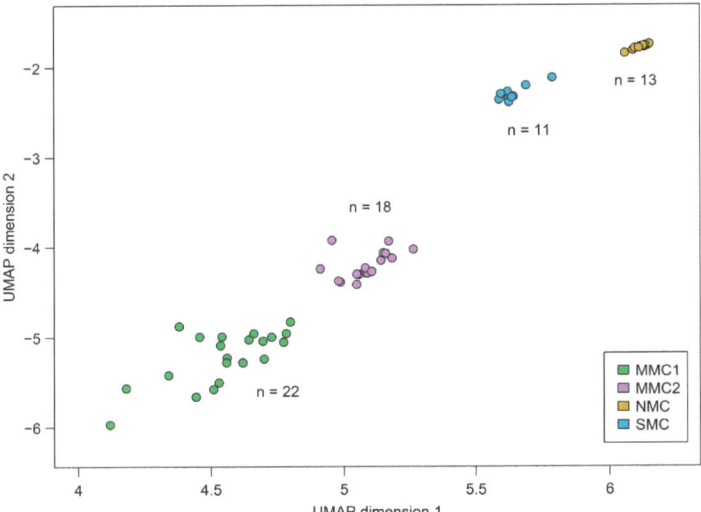

Figure 3. Methylation clusters determined by UMAP reduction analysis. Two-dimensional UMAP reduction plot of all samples from the internal and external cohorts. Each dot represents the overall methylome structure of one sample. UMAP reduction was performed on the EpiDip server together with approximately 25,000 other cancer and normal samples. The coordinates of the specimens in this study were subsequently extracted. The individual methylation clusters are classified as melanoma methylation cluster 1 (MMC1; green), melanoma methylation cluster 2 (MMC2; magenta), nevus methylation cluster (NMC; orange), and skin methylation cluster (SMC; blue).

We then used the data from both cohorts together to assess the DMPs and DMRs between MMC1, MMC2, and NMC. For this, we used an analysis pipeline with group-wise comparisons based on a protocol published by Maksimovic et al., 2016 [14]. This approach identified 25.3% CpGs as significantly differentially methylated between MMC1 and NMC, 27% for MMC2 vs. NMC, and 23.9% for MMC1 vs. MMC2. A list of the top 100 significant DMPs for all three comparisons, with appropriate metadata, is provided in the Supplementary Data File. While the comparison between MMC1 and NMC resulted in DMPs with a high difference in methylation status, both comparisons with MMC2 showed mainly CpGs with more or less intermediate (but nonetheless homogenous) methylation status in one of the groups. This can be seen in Supplementary Figures S4–S6, which show plots of the individual β-values of the top 10 significant CpGs in the two groups. The phenomenon was also statistically confirmed by comparing the mean difference (delta) of M-values for the top 100 CpGs from all contrasts by ANOVA and pairwise t-tests (adjusted p-value < 0.001 for all comparisons; Figure 4).

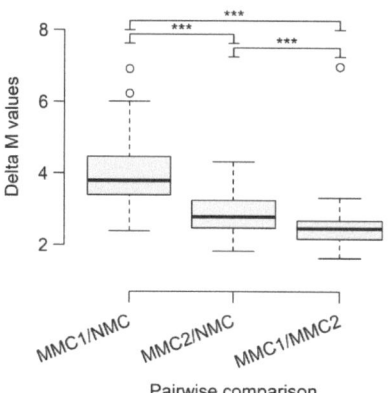

Figure 4. Median differences in M-values for pairwise DMA. The differences in the M-values of the top 100 significant CpGs from each of the three comparisons during DMP analysis were calculated. Their distributions are shown as Box-and-Whisker plots, with the box representing the median and interquartile range (IQR), whiskers extending to 1.5-times the IQR, and circles indicating outliers. Significance testing between the three comparisons was performed with ANOVA and pairwise t-tests, with p-values adjusted using the Benjamini–Hochberg method. The three stars (***) depict that for all three pairwise comparisons, the adjusted p-value was far below 0.001.

The comparison between MMC1 and NMC resulted in 597 significant DMRs, with a medium size of 1350 bp (99–10,750 bp). The comparison between MMC2 and NMC resulted in much fewer (63) DMRS, with a median size of 1307 bp (145–3026 bp). An intermediate number of 128 DMRs, with a median size of 1255 bp (199–7186 bp), was called when comparing MMC1 vs. MMC2. The top ten DMRs from each comparison were evaluated with the UCSC genome browser [15] to identify overlapping gene transcription start sites or regulatory DNA elements such as gene promoters or enhancers. The top DMRs of MMC1 compared with the other two groups were quite similar and mostly encompassed regulatory elements such as miRNA clusters (e.g., on chromosome 14), gene promoters, or the *PRAME* gene on chromosome 22 (Table 2).

Table 2. Differentially methylated clusters. The top 10 hits for each comparison (MMC1 vs. NMC, MMC2 vs. NMC, and MMC1 vs. MMC2) are shown. The regions are ordered according to their significance (see Supplementary Data for more details). The last column shows the location of overlapping gene transcription start sites and GeneHancer (double elite) promoter or enhancer elements. Methylation status is depicted as + for hypermethylated and – for hypomethylated.

Location	Range	Length	Meth. Status	DNA Elements of Interest
		MMC1 vs. NMC		
chr2	223,163,573–223,172,329	8757	+	CCDC140, PAX3
chr14	10,1505,130–101,515,879	10,750	–	microRNA cluster
chr3	147,122,664–147,131,860	9197	+	ZIC4, ZIC1, GH03J147407
chr14	101,487,756–101,493,252	5497	–	microRNA cluster
chr2	200,328,645–200,336,146	7502	+	ATB2, SAT2B, GH02J199454
chr6	29,520,527–29,521,803	1277	+	OR2I1P, GH06J029552
chr22	22,898,356–22,902,665	4310	–	PRAME
chr3	157,812,018–157,817,678	5661	+	SHOX2, GH03J158097
chr6	31,650,735–31,651,676	942	+	GH06J031682
chr14	60,972,853–60,978,852	6000	+	SIX6

Table 2. Cont.

Location	Range	Length	Meth. Status	DNA Elements of Interest
MMC2 vs. NMC				
chr3	46,446,998–46,449,636	2639	−	CCR5AS, CCRL2, GH03J046404
chr1	160,680,856–160,682,655	1800	−	CD48, GH01J160703
chr1	233,248,709–233,249,314	606	−	-
chr13	102,568,345–102,570,482	2138	−	FGF14
MMC2 vs. NMC (continued)				
chr2	176,963,315–176,965,729	2415	+	HOXD12
chr1	203,320,190–203,321,087	898	−	GH01J203319
chr14	61,108,227–61,110,649	2423	+	SIX1, GH14J060640
chr18	53,068,921–53,070,851	1931	−	TCF4, GH18J055398
chr11	2,846,681–2,848,492	1812	−	GH11J002824
chr1	234,907,722–234,908,514	793	−	GH01J234766
MMC1 vs. MMC2				
chr14	101,487,756–101,493,252	5497	−	microRNA cluster
chr2	166,649,910–166,651,571	1662	+	GALTN3, GH02J165791
chr14	101,518,766–101,522,431	3666	−	microRNA cluster
chr7	157,527,573–157,534,758	7186	−	-
chr1	203,320,190–203,321,854	1665	+	FMOD, GH01J203349
chr10	106,027,915–106,029,358	1444	+	MIR4428, STO2, GSTO2, GH10J104267
chr12	120,241,287–120,242,513	1227	+	GH12J119803
chr2	54,784,402–54,786,148	1747	+	SPTBN1, GH02J05455
chr1	234,667,087–234,668,366	1280	+	LINC01354, GH01J234527
chr1	91,300,215–91,302,117	1903	+	LINC02609

4. Discussion

Our study investigated the genetic and epigenetic landscape of CM and MN. During cohort selection, we specifically aimed to include as many CM cases with a TWT genotype as possible to compare their genetic and epigenetic landscape to the more common MAPK-mutated cases. As a result, the cohort does not reflect the typical distribution of CM subtypes and locations but is enriched for acrally localized tumors, particularly ALM. The main limitation of the cohort is the relatively small sample size, with 19 CM and 11 MN cases. Although a larger number of samples (56 per entity) were initially collected, many had to be excluded due to failing the strict quality and biological requirements for DNA samples used for methylome analysis.

The majority of excluded samples had insufficient DNA yield or showed severe degradation. This is largely due to the retrospective nature of the study, as many of the archived FFPE tissue blocks were up to or over a decade old. Supplementary Figure S1 clearly illustrates that the excluded samples were significantly older than the samples included in the final cohort. The bias toward larger, more advanced tumors also stems from this issue, as these lesions usually provide higher DNA yields. Since fresh tissue generally allows for better DNA quality, future studies should prioritize a multicenter approach focusing on recently diagnosed patients rather than relying on retrospective recruitment limited to only a few local centers.

Another major reason for sample exclusion was the general requirement for high tumor cell content for methylome analysis [35]. To retain as many samples as possible without compromising data integrity, we combined a bioinformatic estimation of tumor purity with an assessment of whether samples clustered distinctly or not. Despite this effort, our approach using the described methods was not able to fully resolve the inherent bias towards samples with high tumor cell contents. CM subtypes with a less dense growth pattern remained underrepresented in the final cohort. Future advances in technology may help address this issue. Methods such as long-read sequencing [36] and artificial intelligence-driven models (e.g., similar to the concept described by Yasumizu et al., 2024 [37]) could enable the analysis of mixed tissues and samples with low tumor cell content in the future, allowing for a more comprehensive view of CM heterogeneity.

The genetic findings in CM—both at molecular and cytogenomic levels—match the described patterns in the literature. The distribution of driver mutations in our study is admittedly slightly skewed compared to the frequencies reported in the literature [2,38]. However, this can be accounted for by the selection bias during the generation of the cohort and the subsequent overrepresentation of cases with a TWT status. CM with one of the three MAPK-activating driver mutations presented with a high mutational burden combined with a heavily distorted genome structure with several or many extensive CNVs. TWT-CMs, on the other hand, had lower mutational burden and a CNV profile shifting towards more focal abnormalities. *TERT* promoter mutations are common alterations in CM, found in approximately 70% of cases [29,39]. In our study, *TERT* promoter mutations were highly common in MAPK-altered CM but much rarer in TWT cases. This is in accordance with previous reports, which found that *TERT* promoter mutations are rare events in acral CMs [40–42], which represent the majority of TWT cases in our study. The differences between the two groups may be even more pronounced if one re-classifies these cases into an MAPK-altered group with (rare) alterations in other MAPK-associated genes such as *MAP2K1* mutations [43], *KIT* alterations [44], *BRAF* gene fusions [45], or other. However, as only a part of those alterations can be reliably detected with the utilized methods, we decided to use the traditional definition established by The Cancer Genome Atlas in 2015 [16]. MN showed—as expected—only a few mutations in addition to the recognized driver mutations (mostly *BRAF* p.V600) and lacked both CNVs and *TERT* promoter mutations.

Dimensional reduction of DMA resulted in a clear separation of CM and MN cases into two methylation clusters. Within the CM cohort, no differences between CM with MAPK-affecting driver mutations and cases with TWT status were found. This is similar to the findings of Jurmeister et al., 2021 [46], who did not detect major differences in the methylome structure when comparing mucosal melanoma (with a high frequency of cases without MAPK driver mutation) and CM. The exception was one single sample, which localized separately from all other CM specimens. This sample additionally showed a unique genetic pattern, with a low mutational burden and only a few but focal CNV abnormalities. Inclusion of an external dataset published by Pradhan et al., 2019 [4] confirmed the existence of a second methylation cluster including this sample. In the external cohort, a higher number of samples belonged to the MMC2 cluster compared to our internal cohort. The majority of them were classified as ALM by the authors. However, no further information about the single sample was provided; therefore, we were not able to assess whether there is a distinct histological or molecular marker that connects these cases.

An in-depth analysis of the three identified methylation clusters revealed extensive differences between the three groups. The top DMRs of MMC1, in comparison to the other two groups, were quite similar and mostly encompassed regulatory elements such as miRNA clusters and gene promoters. When compared to NMC, one of the top hypomethylated DMRs overlapped with the *PRAME* gene. As the full name "Preferentially Expressed in Melanoma" indicates, this tumor marker is expressed in CM but only rarely in MN [47].This is in accordance with the distinct hypomethylation of the gene region detected in our study. Markers in other regions, such as the *CCDC140/PAX3* region on chromosome 2, are in accordance with a previously published study by Conway et al., 2022 [11]. Both comparisons involving MMC2 identified a high proportion of CpGs with intermediate methylation levels.

Despite the relatively small cohort due to the high sample dropout rate, our study demonstrates that DMA combined with dimensional reduction methods such as UMAP can robustly distinguish CM from MN. However, all investigated lesions can be classified as benign or malignant using standard histology. The more intriguing question is how borderline lesions, such as dysplastic, Spitz, or Reed nevi, behave in this approach and whether their DNA methylation patterns contain information about malignant potential. Furthermore, our study identified a possible new molecular CM subtype with a distinct DNA methylation profile. Since most of these samples originated from an external cohort without additional metadata, the commonality underlying this subtype remains unclear. Larger studies focusing on uncommon melanocytic lesions are needed to address this question.

In the future, DNA methylome analysis may be a promising tool for enhancing diagnostic and prognostic accuracy in the clinical workup of melanocytic lesions. While the results of this study should be interpreted with caution, they provide a solid basis for further large, prospective, and independent studies to validate the clinical utility of the potential epigenetic biomarkers identified here.

Supplementary Materials: The following supporting information can be downloaded at: https://www.mdpi.com/article/10.3390/diagnostics15050531/s1, Figure S1: Comparison of FFPE block age of included and excluded samples. (a) Box-and-Whiskers plot depicting the distribution of block age (in years) of excluded/not included (blue) and included (green) BN samples. (b) Simultaneous plot depicting the distribution of block age (in years) of excluded (violet) and included (mustard) CM specimens. For both comparisons, the block age of excluded samples is significantly higher as determined by the Wilcoxon test (p-value: <0.001 for BN and p-value: 0.005 for CM); Figure S2: Biological parameters of excluded and included samples. (a–c) Box-and-Whiskers plot showing tumor size, Breslow's depth, and cell vitality of excluded (violet) and included (mustard) CM samples. (d) Bar plot of ulceration status of excluded (violet) and included (mustard) CM specimens. (e) Distribution of excluded/not included (violet) and included (mustard) CM samples according to their tumor stage depicted as bar plots; Figure S3: Methylation clusters determined by UMAP reduction analysis of the internal cohort. Two-dimensional UMAP reduction plot of all samples. Each dot represents the overall methylome structure of one sample. UMAP reduction was performed on the EpiDip server together with approximately 25,000 other cancer and normal samples. The coordinates of the specimens in this study were subsequently extracted. The individual methylation clusters are called melanoma methylation cluster 1 (MMC1; green), melanoma methylation cluster 2 (MMC2; magenta), nevus methylation cluster (NMC; orange), and skin methylation cluster (SMC; blue). Figures S4–S6: Visualization of the top 20 differentially methylated CpGs in pairwise cluster comparisons. The individual dots in each plot represent the β-value (0 = unmethylated; 1 = methylated) of each sample in the respective groups; Table S1: Overview of the covered regions of the used custom sequencing panel; Supplementary Data.

Author Contributions: Conceptualization, S.S., J.Z., V.A.N., M.S. and E.J.; data curation, S.S., W.J., M.S. and E.J.; formal analysis, S.S. and T.W.; investigation, S.S., T.W. and V.V.; methodology, S.S., T.W. and J.H.; project administration, M.S. and E.J.; resources, J.H., S.F., P.H. and S.H.; software, S.S., T.W. and J.H.; supervision, M.S. and E.J.; visualization, S.S.; writing—original draft preparation, S.S.; writing—review and editing, T.W., W.J., J.Z., V.A.N., M.S. and E.J. All authors have read and agreed to the published version of the manuscript.

Funding: This study was supported by the project MEMS under the Grant agreement ITAT1018 as part of the EU program Interreg V-A Italia-Austria 2014−2020.

Institutional Review Board Statement: The study was conducted in accordance with the Declaration of Helsinki and approved by the Institutional Ethics Committee of the Medical University of Innsbruck (1182/2018, 13 December 2018 and 1170/2019, 24 October 2019).

Informed Consent Statement: Informed consent was obtained from all subjects involved in the study.

Data Availability Statement: The microarray datasets generated during the current study are available in the ArrayExpress repository, E-MTAB-14045. All other relevant datasets can be found in the Supplementary Data File.

Acknowledgments: The results shown here are in whole or part based on data generated by TCGA Research Network (https://www.cancer.gov/tcga, accessed on 7 May 2023). We further want to thank our colleagues at the Italian groups of the Interreg project MEMS-ITAT 1018 from Bolzano, Trieste, and Aviano for their support.

Conflicts of Interest: The authors declare no conflicts of interest.

References

1. Bastian, B.C.; de la Fouchardière, A.; Elder, D.E.; Gerami, P.; Lazar, A.J.; Massi, D.; Nagore, E.; Scolyer, R.A.; Yun, S.J. Genomic landscape of melanoma. In *WHO Classification of Skin Tumours*, 4th ed.; Elder, D.E., Massi, D., Scolyer, R., Willemze, R., Eds.; IARC: Lyon, France, 2018; pp. 72–75.
2. The Cancer Genome Atlas Network. Genomic classification of cutaneous melanoma. *Cell* **2015**, *161*, 1681–1696. [CrossRef] [PubMed]
3. Yun, S.J.; Bastian, B.C.; Duncan, L.M.; Haneke, E.; Uhara, H. Acral melanoma. In *WHO Classification of Skin Tumours*, 4th ed.; Elder, D.E., Massi, D., Scolyer, R., Willemze, R., Eds.; IARC: Lyon, France, 2018; pp. 116–118.
4. Pradhan, D.; Jour, G.; Milton, D.; Vasudevaraja, V.; Tetzlaff, M.T.; Nagarajan, P.; Curry, J.L.; Ivan, D.; Long, L.; Ding, Y.; et al. Aberrant DNA methylation predicts melanoma-specific survival in patients with acral melanoma. *Cancers* **2019**, *11*, 2031. [CrossRef] [PubMed]
5. Moran, B.; Silva, R.; Perry, A.S.; Gallagher, W.M. Epigenetics of malignant melanoma. *Semin. Cancer Biol.* **2018**, *51*, 80–88. [CrossRef] [PubMed]
6. Sharma, S.; Kelly, T.K.; Jones, P.A. Epigenetics in cancer. *Carcinogenesis* **2010**, *31*, 27–36. [CrossRef] [PubMed]
7. Micevic, G.; Theodosakis, N.; Bosenberg, M. Aberrant DNA methylation in melanoma: Biomarker and therapeutic opportunities. *Clin. Epigenetics* **2017**, *9*, 34. [CrossRef]
8. Koroknai, V.; Szász, I.; Hernandez-Vargas, H.; Fernandez-Jimenez, N.; Cuenin, C.; Herceg, Z.; Vízkeleti, L.; Ádány, R.; Ecsedi, S.; Balázs, M. DNA hypermethylation is associated with invasive phenotype of malignant melanoma. *Exp. Dermatol.* **2020**, *29*, 39–50. [CrossRef]
9. Tanemura, A.; Terando, A.M.; Sim, M.-S.; van Hoesel, A.Q.; de Maat, M.F.G.; Morton, D.L.; Hoon, D.S.B. CpG Island Methylator Phenotype predicts progression of malignant melanoma. *Clin. Cancer Res.* **2009**, *15*, 1801–1807. [CrossRef]
10. Yamamoto, Y.; Matsusaka, K.; Fukuyo, M.; Rahmutulla, B.; Matsue, H.; Kaneda, A. Higher methylation subtype of malignant melanoma and its correlation with thicker progression and worse prognosis. *Cancer Med.* **2020**, *9*, 7194–7204. [CrossRef]
11. Conway, K.; Tsai, Y.S.; Edmiston, S.N.; Parker, J.S.; Parrish, E.A.; Hao, H.; Kuan, P.F.; Scott, G.A.; Frank, J.S.; Googe, P.; et al. Characterization of the CpG island hypermethylated phenotype subclass in primary melanomas. *J. Investig. Dermatol.* **2022**, *142*, 1869–1881. [CrossRef]
12. Barrett, T.; Wilhite, S.E.; Ledoux, P.; Evangelista, C.; Kim, I.F.; Tomashevsky, M.; Marshall, K.A.; Phillippy, K.H.; Sherman, P.M.; Holko, M.; et al. NCBI GEO: Archive for functional genomics data sets—Update. *Nucleic Acids Res.* **2013**, *41*, D991–D995. [CrossRef]
13. Aryee, M.J.; Jaffe, A.E.; Corrada-Bravo, H.; Ladd-Acosta, C.; Feinberg, A.P.; Hansen, K.D.; Irizarry, R.A. Minfi: A flexible and comprehensive Bioconductor package for the analysis of Infinium DNA methylation microarrays. *Bioinformatics* **2014**, *30*, 1363–1369. [CrossRef] [PubMed]
14. Maksimovic, J.; Phipson, B.; Oshlack, A. A cross-package Bioconductor workflow for analysing methylation array data. *F1000Res* **2016**, *5*, 1281. [CrossRef] [PubMed]
15. Johann, P.D.; Jäger, N.; Pfister, S.M.; Sill, M. RF_Purify: A novel tool for comprehensive analysis of tumor-purity in methylation array data based on random forest regression. *BMC Bioinform.* **2019**, *20*, 428. [CrossRef] [PubMed]
16. Chang, K.; Creighton, C.J.; Davis, C.A.; Donehower, L.; Drummond, J.; Wheeler, D.; Ally, A.; Balasundaram, M.; Birol, I.; Butterfield, Y.S.N.; et al. The Cancer Genome Atlas Pan-Cancer analysis project. *Nat. Genet.* **2013**, *45*, 1113–1120. [CrossRef]

17. Ritchie, M.E.; Phipson, B.; Wu, D.; Hu, Y.; Law, C.W.; Shi, W.; Smyth, G.K. limma powers differential expression analyses for RNA-sequencing and microarray studies. *Nucleic Acids Res.* **2015**, *43*, e47. [CrossRef]
18. Peters, T.J.; Buckley, M.J.; Statham, A.L.; Pidsley, R.; Samaras, K.; Lord, R.V.; Clark, S.J.; Molloy, P.L. De novo identification of differentially methylated regions in the human genome. *Epigenetics Chromatin* **2015**, *8*, 6. [CrossRef]
19. Kent, W.J.; Sugnet, C.W.; Furey, T.S.; Roskin, K.M.; Pringle, T.H.; Zahler, A.M.; Haussler, D. The human genome browser at UCSC. *Genome Res.* **2002**, *12*, 996–1006. [CrossRef]
20. Fishilevich, S.; Nudel, R.; Rappaport, N.; Hadar, R.; Plaschkes, I.; Iny Stein, T.; Rosen, N.; Kohn, A.; Twik, M.; Safran, M.; et al. GeneHancer: Genome-wide integration of enhancers and target genes in GeneCards. *Database* **2017**, *2017*, bax028. [CrossRef]
21. Karczewski, K.J.; Francioli, L.C.; Tiao, G.; Cummings, B.B.; Alföldi, J.; Wang, Q.; Collins, R.L.; Laricchia, K.M.; Ganna, A.; Birnbaum, D.P.; et al. The mutational constraint spectrum quantified from variation in 141,456 humans. *Nature* **2020**, *581*, 434–443. [CrossRef]
22. Thorvaldsdóttir, H.; Robinson, J.T.; Mesirov, J.P. Integrative Genomics Viewer (IGV): High-performance genomics data visualization and exploration. *Brief. Bioinform.* **2013**, *14*, 178–192. [CrossRef]
23. Tate, J.G.; Bamford, S.; Jubb, H.C.; Sondka, Z.; Beare, D.M.; Bindal, N.; Boutselakis, H.; Cole, C.G.; Creatore, C.; Dawson, E.; et al. COSMIC: The Catalogue of Somatic Mutations in Cancer. *Nucleic Acids Res.* **2019**, *47*, D941–D947. [CrossRef] [PubMed]
24. Landrum, M.J.; Chitipiralla, S.; Brown, G.R.; Chen, C.; Gu, B.; Hart, J.; Hoffman, D.; Jang, W.; Kaur, K.; Liu, C.; et al. ClinVar: Improvements to accessing data. *Nucleic Acids Res.* **2020**, *48*, D835–D844. [CrossRef] [PubMed]
25. Holt, M.E.; Mittendorf, K.F.; LeNoue-Newton, M.; Jain, N.M.; Anderson, I.; Lovly, C.M.; Osterman, T.; Micheel, C.; Levy, M. My Cancer Genome: Coevolution of precision oncology and a molecular oncology knowledgebase. *JCO Clin. Cancer Inform.* **2021**, *5*, 995–1004. [CrossRef] [PubMed]
26. Ng, P.C.; Henikoff, S. SIFT: Predicting amino acid changes that affect protein function. *Nucleic Acids Res.* **2003**, *31*, 3812–3814. [CrossRef] [PubMed]
27. Adzhubei, I.; Jordan, D.M.; Sunyaev, S.R. Predicting functional effect of human missense mutations using PolyPhen-2. *Curr. Protoc. Hum. Genet.* **2013**, *76*, 7–20. [CrossRef] [PubMed]
28. Nagore, E.; Rachakonda, S.; Kumar, R. TERT promoter mutations in melanoma survival. *Oncotarget* **2019**, *10*, 1546–1548. [CrossRef]
29. Hugdahl, E.; Kalvenes, M.B.; Mannelqvist, M.; Ladstein, R.G.; Akslen, L.A. Prognostic impact and concordance of *TERT* promoter mutation and protein expression in matched primary and metastatic cutaneous melanoma. *Br. J. Cancer* **2018**, *118*, 98–105. [CrossRef]
30. Benjamini, Y.; Hochberg, Y. Controlling the false discovery rate: A practical and powerful approach to multiple testing. *J. R. Stat. Soc. Series B Stat. Methodol.* **1995**, *57*, 289–300. [CrossRef]
31. De Martino, E.; Brunetti, D.; Canzonieri, V.; Conforti, C.; Eisendle, K.; Mazzoleni, G.; Nobile, C.; Rao, F.; Zschocke, J.; Jukic, E.; et al. The association of residential altitude on the molecular profile and survival of melanoma: Results of an Interreg study. *Cancers* **2020**, *12*, 2796. [CrossRef]
32. Curtin, J.A.; Fridlyand, J.; Kageshita, T.; Patel, H.N.; Busam, K.J.; Kutzner, H.; Cho, K.-H.; Aiba, S.; Bröcker, E.-B.; LeBoit, P.E.; et al. Distinct sets of genetic alterations in melanoma. *NEJM* **2005**, *353*, 2135–2147. [CrossRef]
33. McInnes, L.; Healy, J.; Saul, N.; Großberger, L. UMAP: Uniform Manifold Approximation and Projection. *J. Open Source Softw.* **2018**, *3*, 861. [CrossRef]
34. Hench, J.; Vlajnic, T.; Soysal, S.D.; Obermann, E.C.; Frank, S.; Muenst, S. An integrated epigenomic and genomic view on Phyllodes and Phyllodes-like breast tumors. *Cancers* **2022**, *14*, 667. [CrossRef] [PubMed]
35. Hench, J.; Tolnay, M.; Frank, S. Die DNA-Methylomanalyse. *Swiss Med. Forum* **2020**, *20*, 150–154. [CrossRef]
36. Marx, V. Method of the year: Long-read sequencing. *Nat. Methods* **2023**, *20*, 6–11. [CrossRef]
37. Yasumizu, Y.; Hagiwara, M.; Umezu, Y.; Fuji, H.; Iwaisako, K.; Asagiri, M.; Uemoto, S.; Nakamura, Y.; Thul, S.; Ueyama, A.; et al. Neural-net-based cell deconvolution from DNA methylation reveals tumor microenvironment associated with cancer prognosis. *NAR Cancer* **2024**, *6*, zcae022. [CrossRef]
38. Hayward, N.K.; Wilmott, J.S.; Waddell, N.; Johansson, P.A.; Field, M.A.; Nones, K.; Patch, A.-M.; Kakavand, H.; Alexandrov, L.B.; Burke, H.; et al. Whole-genome landscapes of major melanoma subtypes. *Nature* **2017**, *545*, 175–180. [CrossRef]
39. Huang, F.W.; Hodis, E.; Xu, M.J.; Kryukov, G.V.; Chin, L.; Garraway, L.A. Highly recurrent *TERT* promoter mutations in human melanoma. *Science* **2013**, *339*, 957–959. [CrossRef]
40. Bai, X.; Kong, Y.; Chi, Z.; Sheng, X.; Cui, C.; Wang, X.; Mao, L.; Tang, B.; Li, S.; Lian, B.; et al. MAPK Pathway and *TERT* promoter gene mutation pattern and its prognostic value in melanoma patients: A retrospective study of 2,793 cases. *Clin. Cancer Res.* **2017**, *23*, 6120–6127. [CrossRef]
41. Liau, J.Y.; Tsai, J.H.; Jeng, Y.M.; Chu, C.Y.; Kuo, K.T.; Liang, C.W. *TERT* promoter mutation is uncommon in acral lentiginous melanoma. *J. Cutan. Pathol.* **2014**, *41*, 504–508. [CrossRef]

42. de Lima Vazquez, V.; Vicente, A.L.; Carloni, A.; Berardinelli, G.; Soares, P.; Scapulatempo, C.; Martinho, O.; Reis, R.M. Molecular profiling, including *TERT* promoter mutations, of acral lentiginous melanomas. *Melanoma Res.* 2016, 26, 93–99. [CrossRef]
43. Williams, E.A.; Montesion, M.; Shah, N.; Sharaf, R.; Pavlick, D.C.; Sokol, E.S.; Alexander, B.; Venstrom, J.; Elvin, J.A.; Ross, J.S.; et al. Melanoma with in-frame deletion of *MAP2K1*: A distinct molecular subtype of cutaneous melanoma mutually exclusive from *BRAF*, *NRAS*, and *NF1* mutations. *Mod. Pathol.* 2020, 33, 2397–2406. [CrossRef] [PubMed]
44. Pham, D.D.M.; Guhan, S.; Tsao, H. *KIT* and melanoma: Biological insights and clinical implications. *Yonsei Med. J.* 2020, 61, 562–571. [CrossRef] [PubMed]
45. Ross, J.S.; Wang, K.; Chmielecki, J.; Gay, L.; Johnson, A.; Chudnovsky, J.; Yelensky, R.; Lipson, D.; Ali, S.M.; Elvin, J.A.; et al. The distribution of *BRAF* gene fusions in solid tumors and response to targeted therapy. *Int. J. Cancer* 2016, 138, 881–890. [CrossRef] [PubMed]
46. Jurmeister, P.; Wrede, N.; Hoffmann, I.; Vollbrecht, C.; Heim, D.; Hummel, M.; Wolkenstein, P.; Koch, I.; Heynol, V.; Schmitt, W.D.; et al. Mucosal melanomas of different anatomic sites share a common global DNA methylation profile with cutaneous melanoma but show location-dependent patterns of genetic and epigenetic alterations. *J. Pathol.* 2022, 256, 61–70. [CrossRef]
47. Lezcano, C.; Jungbluth, A.A.; Nehal, K.S.; Hollmann, T.J.; Busam, K.J. PRAME Expression in Melanocytic Tumors. *Am J Surg Pathol.* 2018, 42, 1456–1465. [CrossRef]

Disclaimer/Publisher's Note: The statements, opinions and data contained in all publications are solely those of the individual author(s) and contributor(s) and not of MDPI and/or the editor(s). MDPI and/or the editor(s) disclaim responsibility for any injury to people or property resulting from any ideas, methods, instructions or products referred to in the content.

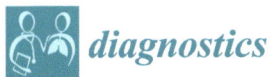

Article

Zoom-in Dermoscopy for Facial Tumors

Martina D'Onghia [1,*], Francesca Falcinelli [1], Lorenzo Barbarossa [1], Alberto Pinto [1], Alessandra Cartocci [1], Linda Tognetti [1], Giovanni Rubegni [2], Anastasia Batsikosta [3], Pietro Rubegni [1] and Elisa Cinotti [1]

[1] Dermatology Unit, Department of Medical, Surgical and Neurological Sciences, University of Siena, 51300 Siena, Italy; f.falcinelli@student.unisi.it (F.F.); lorenzobarbarossa1993@gmail.com (L.B.); alberto.pinto@student.unisi.it (A.P.); alessandra.cartocci@dbm.unisi.it (A.C.); linda.tognetti@dbm.unisi.it (L.T.); pietro.rubegni@unisi.com (P.R.); elisa.cinotti@unisi.it (E.C.)
[2] Department of Clinical Medicine and Immunological Sciences, Section of Ophthalmology, University of Siena, 51300 Siena, Italy; giovannirubegni@gmail.com
[3] Pathological Anatomy Section, University of Siena, 51300 Siena, Italy; natasha.batsikosta@gmail.com
* Correspondence: martina.donghia@gmail.com

Abstract: Background/Objectives: Facial lesions, including lentigo maligna and lentigo maligna melanoma (LM/LMM), both malignant, present significant diagnostic challenges due to their clinical similarity to benign conditions. Although standard dermoscopy is a well-established tool for diagnosis, its inability to reveal cellular-level details highlights the necessity of new magnified techniques. This study aimed to assess the role of standard dermoscopy, high-magnification dermoscopy, and fluorescence-advanced videodermatoscopy (FAV) in diagnosing LM/LMM and differentiating them from benign facial lesions. **Methods**: This retrospective, observational, multicenter study evaluated 85 patients with facial skin lesions (including LM, LMM, basal-cell carcinoma, solar lentigo, seborrheic keratosis, actinic keratosis, and nevi) who underwent dermatological examination for skin tumor screening. Standard dermoscopy at 30× magnification (D30), high-magnification dermoscopy at 150× magnification (D150), and FAV examination were performed. Dermoscopic images were retrospectively evaluated for the presence of fifteen 30× and twenty-one 150× dermoscopic features, and their frequency was calculated. To compare D30 with D150 and D150 with FAV, the Gwet AC1 concordance index and the correct classification rate (CCR) were estimated. **Results**: Among 85 facial lesions analyzed, LM/LMM exhibited distinctive dermoscopic features at D30, including a blue–white veil (38.9% vs. 1.7%, $p < 0.001$), regression structures (55.6% vs. 21.7%, $p = 0.013$), irregular dots or globules (50.0% vs. 10%, $p = 0.001$), angulated lines (72.2% vs. 6.7%, $p < 0.001$), an annular granular pattern (61.1% vs. 20%, $p = 0.002$), asymmetrical pigmented follicular openings (100.0% vs. 21.7%; $p < 0.001$), and follicular obliteration (27.8% vs. 3.3%). At D150, roundish melanocytes (87.5% vs. 18.2%, $p < 0.001$) and melanophages (43.8% vs. 14.5%, $p = 0.019$) were predominant. FAV examination identified large dendritic cells, isolated melanocytes, and free melanin in LM/LMM (all $p < 0.001$) with high concordance to D150. **Conclusions**: Integrating D30, D150, and FAV into clinical practice may enhance diagnostic precision for facial lesions by combining macroscopic and cellular insights, thereby reducing unnecessary biopsies. However, future studies are essential to confirm these results.

Keywords: dermoscopy; high magnification; FAV; melanocyte; lentigo maligna; melanoma

1. Introduction

Diagnosing pigmented skin lesions on the face is challenging for dermatologists, mainly because of the clinical overlap between benign and malignant conditions [1]. In fact, typical lesions of photo-aged skin, such as solar lentigo (SL), seborrheic keratosis (SK), and actinic keratosis (AK), especially in pigmented forms, frequently mimic melanocytic lesions, complicating diagnosis [2]. Lentigo maligna (LM) and lentigo maligna melanoma (LMM) are slow-growing tumors that primarily affect white elderly individuals, typically developing on chronically sun-exposed areas of the head and neck. LM refers to in situ lesions, while invasive forms are classified as LMM [3]. These tumors usually present as irregularly pigmented macules and can often grow to a significant size before being detected [3].

Standard dermoscopy with magnifications up to 30× (D30) is a widely recognized tool that enhances diagnostic accuracy for skin tumors. Indeed, the use of criteria based on distinct patterns and structures in both melanocytic and non-melanocytic lesions significantly improves diagnostic precision [4]. This technique is especially valuable for reducing unnecessary biopsies, especially in the facial areas.

The unique characteristics of facial skin, such as thin epidermis and high exposure to sunlight, contribute to the diverse dermoscopic patterns observed. Benign lesions, including SK or SL, often display features such as milia-like cysts or comedo-like openings, whereas AK commonly presents with a pseudonetwork pattern and a strawberry-like appearance [5]. In contrast, dermoscopic criteria to identify LM and LMM include dots, gray globules, asymmetric follicular openings, rhomboidal structures, and pigmentation surrounding hair follicles up to follicular obliteration [3,6]. Despite these diagnostic clues, differentiating between benign and malignant lesions on the face is still challenging due to overlapping features and subtle presentations. This highlights the need for further advancements in dermoscopic techniques, such as magnified dermoscopy, to improve the diagnostic accuracy of those lesions.

The advent of high-magnification videodermoscopy with magnification up to 150× (D150) has significantly enhanced diagnostic capabilities by providing unprecedented detail, enabling the visualization and differentiation of individual pigmented cells, such as keratinocytes and melanocytes, particularly in cases where standard magnification is insufficient to identify critical diagnostic features, thereby offering a more precise evaluation of complex lesions [7,8].

Fluorescence-advanced videodermoscopy (FAV) has also emerged as a new technique for the non-invasive, rapid, and dynamic examination of superficial skin structures at cellular-level resolution [9]. By using the fluorescence emitted by endogenous molecules upon absorption at specific wavelengths, FAV enables in vivo imaging through direct application to the skin. This method facilitates real-time scanning across various skin depths, presenting grayscale images in which the fluorescence intensity ranges from black to white [9]. Although previous studies have highlighted the potential of FAV for improving the diagnostic accuracy of flat pigmented facial lesions, research on this emerging technique remains limited, with only a few studies conducted to date [10]. Moreover, comparative studies between FAV and high-magnification dermoscopy are scarce, underscoring the need for more comprehensive research to clarify their respective roles in dermatological diagnostics.

Against this background, we evaluated the diagnostic value of high-magnification dermoscopy for pigmented facial lesions by comparing its findings with those of traditional dermoscopy. In addition, we investigated whether higher magnification could uncover previously undetectable structures, thereby aiding in the differentiation of LM, LMM, and benign facial lesions. Finally, FAV was used to analyze facial lesions, and its findings were compared with those of high-magnification dermoscopy to further explore its diagnostic utility.

2. Materials and Methods

We conducted an observational and retrospective study between November 2023 and June 2024 on non-consecutive patients who underwent dermatological examination for skin tumor screening at the Dermatology Department of the University Hospital of Siena, Italy.

This study enrolled patients presenting with facial lesions that, based on the evaluation of an expert dermatologist (E.C.), required either removal or 12-month follow-up due to atypical clinical or dermoscopic features. The following lesions were included: LM, LMM, basal-cell carcinoma (BCC), SL, SK, AK, pigmented AK (PAK), lichenoid keratosis (LK), and nevi.

Double-magnification, polarized light videodermatoscopy images were captured at $30\times$ and $150\times$ magnification using Horus System HS600® (Adamo Srl., Trapani, Italy). Specialists in skin imaging (E.C. and F.F.), acquired at least 5 images for each lesion. In addition, in some cases, advanced fluorescence videodermatoscopy (Horus® handled probe, Adamo Srl.) at $500\times$ magnification was performed.

Images at $150\times$ magnification were captured from the most characteristic areas identified at $30\times$ magnification by rotating the ring on the videodermoscope probe, allowing for real-time zooming into the details of the $30\times$ images. FAV images were obtained using a separate probe connected to the same computer system as the $30\times/150\times$ probe. The field of view has a diameter of 8 mm, 1.7 mm, and 0.34 mm for $30\times$, $150\times$, and FAV, respectively.

According to the current literature, the following dermoscopic patterns were assessed for $30\times$ evaluation: blue–white veil, atypical vascular pattern, regression structures, irregular blotches, irregular dots or globules, white and wide follicular opening, reticular or parallel brown lines, sharply demarcated borders, milia-like cysts or comedo-like openings, erythematous pseudonetwork pattern, pseudonetwork pattern, angulated lines (which include polygons or rhomboids or a zig-zag pattern), annular granular pattern or gray circles, asymmetrical pigmented follicular openings, and follicular obliteration [11,12].

For high magnification, we considered the following variables identified in our previous studies: the presence of pigmented cells (keratinocytes, roundish or dendritic melanocytes, melanophages) and their features (distribution, size, or shape regularity); dots (round pigmented areas smaller than a cell); nests of cells (roundish pigmented areas formed by >1 cell); structureless areas that do not follow the DEJ architecture; vessels and their shape (linear, glomerular, arborizing, dilated inside the dermal papilla, or irregular); hyperkeratotic, roundish, concentric structures; pigmented network delimiting well-defined dermal papillae (edged papillae) or undefined dermal papillae (nonedged papillae, not delimited by single cells); and keratin plug inside hair follicle, multiple shades of brown, out-of-focus purple-bluish structureless area, and folliculotrophism [13].

Finally, we identified the following terms to describe the parameters observed with FAV: small, pigmented cells, large isolated cells with clearly visible sharp borders, large isolated dendritic cells, and free melanin [10].

For all selected cases, a correlation between $30\times$ and $150\times$ and between $150\times$ and FAV features was performed. The images were evaluated by a group of three expert dermatologists (L.B., M.D., and F.F.), who were blinded to the histological diagnoses.

Descriptive statistics included the mean and standard deviation (SD) for quantitative variables, whereas frequency and percentage were reported for categorical variables. To compare D30 with D150 and D150 with FAV, the Gwet AC1 concordance index and the correct classification rate (CCR) were estimated. $p < 0.05$ was considered statistically significant. All analyses were performed using R software version 4.1.0 (R Foundation for Statistical 100 Computing, Vienna, Austria).

3. Results

A total of 85 patients were included in this study, with a mean age (SD) at diagnosis of 64.24 (13.04) years (Table 1). Most of the patients were female (55.3%). All pigmented lesions were located on the face, with the cheeks being the most affected site (35.3%), followed by the nose (23.6%), forehead (16.5%), and scalp (13%). Less frequent locations included the eyelids, which were involved in five cases, the neck in three cases, and the ears and chin, with each contributing one case. Overall, histological examination was performed in 47 patients (55.3%). Among benign lesions, LS was the most frequently identified subtype, observed in 24 cases (28.2%), followed by SK (10.6%), PAK (9.4%), nevi (9.4%), and AK (8.2%). LM and LMM were identified in 14 and 4 patients, respectively.

Table 1. Clinical and histological characteristics of facial lesions in our study population.

	Overall n = 85 n (%)
Female	47 (55.3)
Age at diagnosis, mean (SD)	64.24 (13.04)
Specific areas involved	
Cheeks	30 (35.3)
Nose	20 (23.6)
Forehead	14 (16.5)
Scalp	11 (13)
Eyelids	5 (5.9)
Neck	3 (3.5)
Ears	1 (1.2)
Chin	1 (1.2)
Histological examination	47 (55.3)
Lesion subtypes	
SL	24 (28.2)
LM	14 (16.5)
SK	9 (10.6)
Naevus	8 (9.4)
PAK	8 (9.4)
AK	7 (8.2)
BCC	7 (8.2)
KL	4 (4.7)
LMM	4 (4.7)

Legend: AK, actinic keratosis; BCC, basal-cell carcinoma; KL, lichenoid keratosis; LM, lentigo maligna; LMM, lentigo maligna melanoma; SL, solar lentigo; PAK, pigmented actinic keratosis; SK, seborrheic keratosis.

3.1. Dermoscopy at 30× Magnification

The D30 features are listed in Table 2.

Concerning malignant benchmarks, the blue–white veil (38.9% vs. 1.7%, $p < 0.001$), regression structures (55.6% vs. 21.7%, $p = 0.013$), irregular dots or globules (50.0% vs. 10%, $p = 0.001$), angulated lines (72.2% vs. 6.7%, $p < 0.001$), annular granular pattern (61.1% vs. 20%, $p = 0.002$), asymmetrical pigmented follicular openings (100.0% vs. 21.7%; $p < 0.001$), and follicular obliteration (27.8% vs. 3.3%) were more commonly observed in LM or LMM lesions compared to other skin lesions. As for white and wide follicular openings (76.7% vs. 27.8%, <0.001), reticular or parallel brown lines (38.3% vs. 0%, $p = 0.005$), and pseudonetwork pattern (56.7% vs. 0%, $p < 0.001$), these patterns were primarily observed in non-LM/LMM lesions.

Table 2. Dermoscopy features of facial lesions at 30× magnification.

	Other * N = 60 n (%)	LM or LMM N = 18 n (%)	p
White and wide follicular opening	46 (76.7)	5 (27.8)	<0.001
Reticular or parallel brown lines	23 (38.3)	0 (0.0)	0.005
Sharply demarcated borders	30 (50.0)	5 (27.8)	0.164
Milia-like cysts or comedo-like openings	4 (6.7)	0 (0.0)	0.606
Blue–white veil	1 (1.7)	7 (38.9)	<0.001
Atypical vascular pattern	1 (1.7)	1 (5.6)	0.948
Regression structures	13 (21.7)	10 (55.6)	0.013
Blotches irregularly distributed	2 (3.3)	1 (5.6)	1.000
Irregular dots or globules	6 (10.0)	9 (50.0)	0.001
Erythematous pseudonetwork pattern	8 (13.3)	4 (22.2)	0.586
Pseudonetwork pattern	34 (56.7)	0 (0.0)	<0.001
Angulated lines	4 (6.7)	13 (72.2)	<0.001
Annular granular pattern or gray circles	12 (20.0)	11 (61.1)	0.002
Asymmetrical pigmented follicular openings	13 (21.7)	18 (100.0)	<0.001
Follicular obliteration	2 (3.3)	5 (27.8)	0.007

Legend: * this group included actinic keratosis; lichenoid keratosis; solar lentigo; pigmented actinic keratosis, and seborrheic keratosis. LM, lentigo maligna; LMM, lentigo maligna melanoma.

3.2. Dermoscopy at 150× Magnification

The D150 features are presented in Table 3.

Keratinocytes (100% vs. 71.4%, $p = 0.005$) and regular cell distribution (65.5% vs. 14.3%, $p = 0.038$) were significantly more common in other facial lesions than BCC. Roundish melanocytes were more indicative of LM/LMM, compared to non-LM/LMM lesions ($p < 0.001$). Similarly, dendritic melanocytes (43.8% vs. 14.5%, $p = 0.019$), melanophages (43.8% vs. 14.5%, $p = 0.019$), pigmentation without edged papillae (93.8% vs. 40%, $p < 0.001$), multiple shades of brown (81.2% vs. 23.6%, $p < 0.001$), and out-of-focus purple-bluish structureless areas (37.5% vs. 5.5%, $p = 0.001$) were present in LM/LMM lesions compared to other facial lesions (Figure 1).

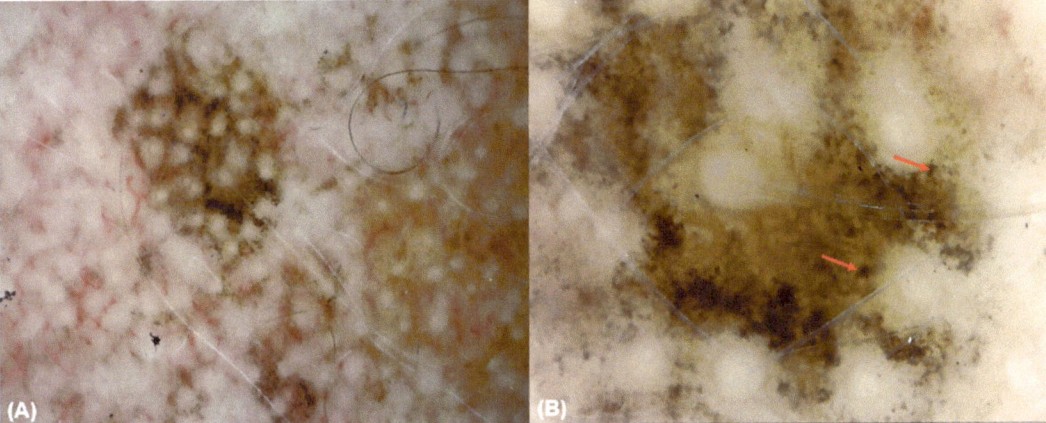

Figure 1. A lentigo maligna at 30× (**A**) and 150× (**B**) magnification. The 30× magnification dermoscopy (**A**) reveals asymmetrical pigmented follicular openings and annular granular pattern. The 150× magnification dermoscopy (**B**) shows a network without well-defined dermal papillae and the presence of large, irregular (in size and shape) roundish (red arrow) cells, corresponding to melanocytes.

Conversely, pigmentation with edged papillae was more indicative of non-LM/LMM than LM/LMM lesions (50.9% vs. 18.8%, $p = 0.005$) (Figure 2). Finally, vessel shape showed significant differences, being predominant in BCC lesions (71.4%), compared to other lesions (27.3% and 25%, non-LM/LMM and LM/LMM, respectively).

Table 3. Dermoscopy features of facial lesions at 150× magnification.

	BCC N = 7 n (%)	Other * N = 55 n (%)	LM or LMM N = 16 n (%)	p
Cell presence	6 (85.7)	55 (100.0)	16 (100.0)	0.090
Cell type				
Keratinocytes	5 (71.4)	55 (100.0)	15 (93.8)	0.005 a
Roundish melanocytes	1 (14.3)	10 (18.2)	14 (87.5)	<0.001 b,c
Dendritic melanocytes	-	8 (14.5)	7 (43.8)	0.019
Melanophages	-	8 (14.5)	7 (43.8)	0.019
Cell irregularity in shape and size	3 (42.9)	12 (21.8)	13 (81.2)	<0.001 c
Cell distribution				
Regular cell distribution	1 (14.3)	36 (65.5)	9 (56.2)	0.038 a
Roundish nests	1 (14.3)	5 (9.1)	0 (0.0)	0.362
Dots	3 (42.9)	12 (21.8)	7 (43.8)	0.132
Structureless area that do not follow DEJ architecture	1 (14.3)	7 (12.7)	4 (25.0)	0.458
Vessels	5 (71.4)	15 (27.3)	4 (25.0)	0.065
Vessel shape				<0.001
No vessels	1 (14.3)	41 (74.5)	12 (75.0)	
Linear	-	9 (16.4)	4 (25.0)	
Arborizing	6 (85.7)	3 (5.5)	-	
Polymorphous	-	2 (3.6)	-	
Out of focus purple-bluish, structureless areas	3 (42.9)	3 (5.5)	6 (37.5)	0.001 a,c
Multiple shades of brown	2 (28.6)	13 (23.6)	13 (81.2)	<0.001 b,c
Hyperkeratotic roundish concentric areas	-	8 (14.5)	1 (6.2)	0.608
Pigmentation with edged papillae	-	28 (50.9)	3 (18.8)	0.005 c
Pigmentation without edged papillae	5 (71.4)	22 (40.0)	15 (93.8)	<0.001 c
Keratin plugs inside hair follicles	1 (14.3)	10 (18.2)	-	0.172

Legend: * this group included actinic keratosis, lichenoid keratosis, solar lentigo, pigmented actinic keratosis, and seborrheic keratosis (SK). LM, lentigo maligna; LMM, lentigo maligna melanoma. (a) BCC significantly different from others, (b) BCC significantly different from LM/LMM, (c) others significantly different from LM/LMM.

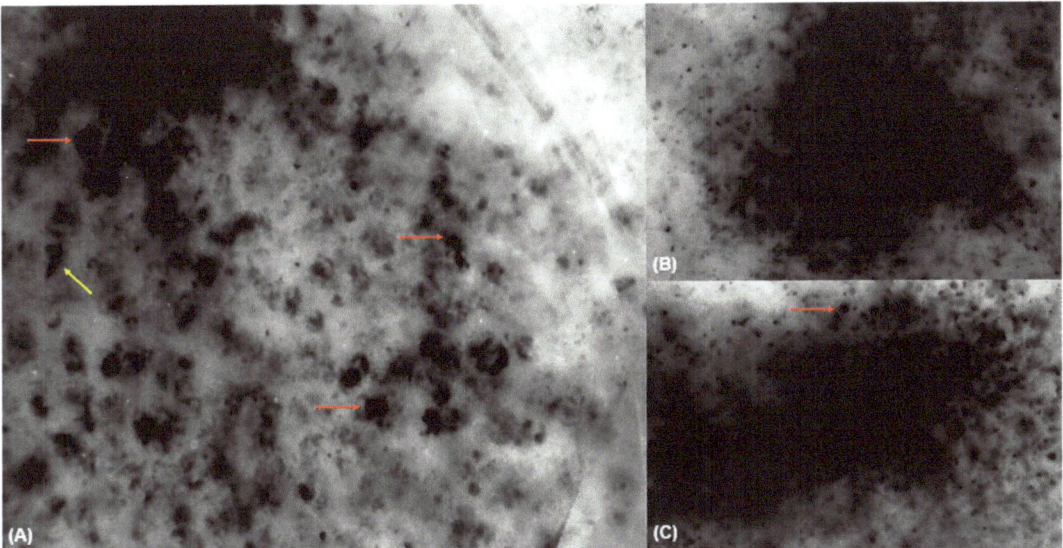

Figure 2. Fluorescence-advanced videodermoscopy of a lentigo maligna (**A–C**). FAV (**A,C**) shows large isolated cells with clearly visible sharp borders (red arrow) and (**C**) isolated dendritic cells (yellow arrow) corresponding to malignant melanocytes.

3.3. Dermoscopy at 30× Compared with 150× Magnification

The agreement between D30× and D150× magnifications was generally moderate to good across all parameters evaluated (all $p < 0.001$) (Table 4). However, significant differences in the prevalence of features were observed between D150× and D30×. These included roundish or dendritic melanocytes and angulated lines (41% vs. 20%, $p = 0.006$), roundish or dendritic melanocytes and follicular obliteration (41% vs. 8.2%, $p < 0.001$), melanophages and follicular obliteration (19.2% vs. 8.2%, $p = 0.010$), cell irregularity in morphology and follicular obliteration (35.9% vs. 8.2%, $p < 0.001$), and folliculotropism with asymmetrical pigmented follicular openings (15.4% vs. 8.2%, $p = 0.001$).

3.4. Fluorescence-Advanced Videodermatoscopy Imaging

Large isolated cells with clearly visible sharp borders (93.8% vs. 2.4%, $p < 0.001$), large isolated dendritic cells (68.8% vs. 9.5%, $p < 0.001$), and free melanin (93.8% vs. 8.1%, $p < 0.01$) were mainly observed in skin lesions diagnosed as LM/LMM lesions compared to other lesions (Table 5) (Figures 2 and 3).

Overall, the prevalence of D150 and FAV features assumed was consistent across the two techniques (all $p > 0.05$), with a strong concordance between the two methods ($p < 0.001$), although a slightly lower agreement was noted for dendritic melanocytes and large isolated cells (Gwet AC1: 0.50) (Table 6).

Table 4. Relative frequencies and agreement between D150 and D30 features.

150×	30×	Agreement Gwet AC1	p	Accuracy	Prevalence 150×	Prevalence 30×	p
Roundish or dendritic melanocytes	Angulated lines	0.579	<0.001	75.6	41.0%	20.0	0.006
	Annular granular pattern or gray circles	0.531	<0.001	74.4%	41.0	27.1	0.085
	Asymmetrical pigmented follicular openings	0.481	<0.001	73.1	41.0	38.8	0.899
	Follicular obliteration	0.432	<0.001	64.1	41.0	8.2	<0.001
Melanophages	Angulated lines	0.591	<0.001	71.8	19.2	20.0	1.000
	Annular granular pattern or gray circles	0.658	<0.001	78.2	19.2	27.1	0.319
	Asymmetrical pigmented follicular openings	0.385	<0.001	64.1	19.2	38.8	0.010
	Follicular obliteration	0.749	<0.001	80.7	19.2	8.2	0.068
Cell irregularity in shape and size	Angulated lines	0.552	<0.001	73.1	35.9	20.0	0.036
	Annular granular pattern/gray circles	0.591	<0.001	76.9	35.9	27.1	0.295
	Asymmetrical pigmented follicular openings	0.492	<0.001	73.0	35.9	38.8	0.823
	Follicular obliteration	0.533	<0.001	69.2	35.9	8.2	<0.001
Pigmentation with edged papillae	Pseudonetwork pattern	0.603	<0.001	79.5	39.7	40.0	1.00
Polymorphus vessels	Atypical vascular pattern	0.854	<0.001	87.2	2.6	9.4	0.135
Folliculotropism	Angulated lines	0.802	<0.001	85.9	15.4	20.0	0.572
	Annular granular pattern or gray circles	0.650	<0.001	76.9	15.4	27.1	0.104
	Asymmetrical pigmented follicular openings	0.552	<0.001	73.1	15.4	38.8	0.001
	Follicular obliteration	0.871	<0.001	89.7	15.4	8.2	0.239

Table 5. Fluorescence-advanced videodermatoscopy features of facial lesions.

	Other * N = 42 n (%)	LM/LMM N = 16 n (%)	p
Small pigmented cells with sharp borders	38 (90.5)	16 (100.0)	0.484
Large isolated cells with clearly visible sharp borders	1 (2.4)	15 (93.8)	<0.001
Large isolated dendritic cells	4 (9.5)	11 (68.8)	<0.001
Free melanin	16 (8.1)	15 (93.8)	<0.001

Legend: * this group included actinic keratosis, basal-cell carcinoma, lichenoid keratosis, solar lentigo, pigmented actinic keratosis, and seborrheic keratosis.

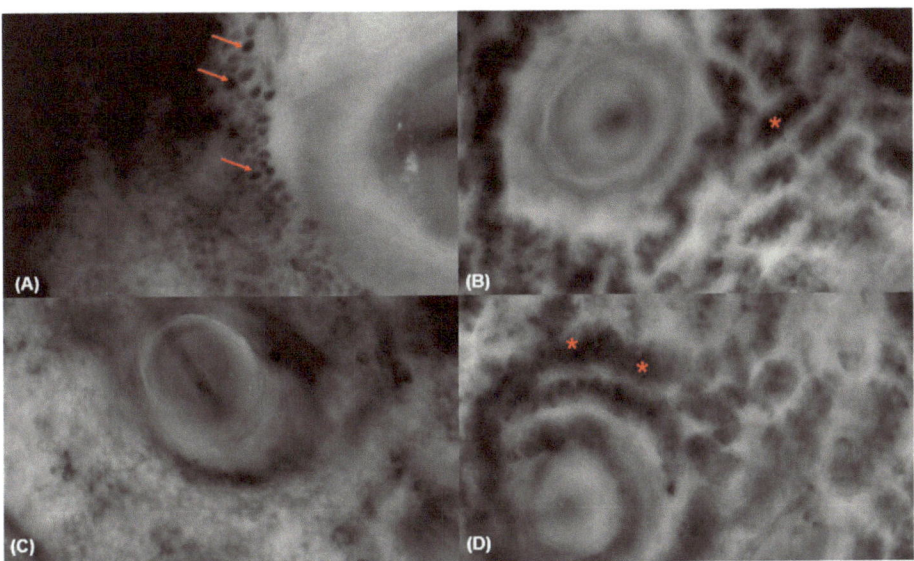

Figure 3. Fluorescence-advanced videodermoscopy of a solar lentigo (A–D). FAV (A) shows interfollicular arrangement of the pigmented cell with follicle sparing corresponding to keratinocytes (red arrow) and (B–D) pseudo-tubular formations (red asterisks).

Table 6. Relative frequencies and agreement between D150 and FAV.

150×	FAV	Agreement Gwet AC1	p	Accuracy p	Prevalence 150×	Prevalence Prevalence FAV	p
Keratinocytes	Small pigmented cells with sharp borders	0.86	<0.001	0.88	96.1%	93.7%	0.772
Roundish melanocytes	Large isolated cells with clearly visible sharp borders	0.70	<0.001	0.82	32.1%	25.4%	0.497
Dendritic melanocytes	Large isolated dendritic cells	0.50	0.001	0.68	19.2%	23.8%	0.650

4. Discussion

This study provides a comprehensive evaluation of standard dermoscopy, high-magnification dermoscopy, and FAV in diagnosing pigmented lesions, emphasizing their complementary contributions to enhancing diagnostic accuracy for LM/LMM and their benign mimics.

As expected, conventional dermoscopy at D30 magnification is a reliable tool for detecting the distinctive features of both malignant and benign lesions, which is consistent with previous findings in the existing literature [14]. According to our results, LM/LMM lesions exhibited the well-documented dermoscopic criteria for malignancy compared to benign lesions, including blue–white veil (38.9% vs. 1.7%, $p < 0.001$), regression structures (55.6% vs. 21.7%, $p = 0.013$), irregular dots or globules (50.0% vs. 10%, $p = 0.001$), angulated lines (72.2% vs. 6.7%, $p < 0.001$), annular granular pattern (61.1% vs. 20%, $p = 0.002$), asymmetrical pigmented follicular openings (100.0% vs. 21.7%; $p < 0.001$) and follicular obliteration (27.8% vs. 3.3%). On the other hand, benign benchmarks, including white and wide follicular openings (76.7% vs. 27.8%, <0.001), reticular or parallel brown lines (38.3% vs. 0%, $p = 0.005$), and pseudonetwork pattern (56.7% vs. 0%, $p < 0.001$), were mainly present in non-LM/LMM lesions.

Although conventional dermoscopy is an essential tool for diagnosing LM/LMM, its ability to reveal cellular and subcellular details remains inherently limited. This limitation highlights the value of complementary magnified techniques, which enable cellular-level visualization and help bridge the gap between traditional imaging and histopathology [15]. These advanced methods offer a promising opportunity to correlate dermoscopic findings with histopathological findings, thereby enhancing diagnostic precision (Figures 4 and 5).

In this context, the Horus videodermoscope allows for real-time zoom into a selected area of a conventional dermoscopy image at 30× magnification, providing highly magnified images with cytological detail. This approach mirrors the histopathological process, where an initial examination is conducted at a lower magnification, followed by a closer inspection of specific areas at higher magnification to observe finer details (Figure 6).

Consistent with previous studies on the use of magnified dermoscopy for evaluating facial lesions [16], our findings demonstrated that features such as roundish melanocytes (87.5% vs. 18.2%, $p < 0.001$), dendritic melanocytes (43.8% vs. 14.5%, $p = 0.019$), melanophages (43.8% vs. 14.5%, $p = 0.019$), pigmentation without edged papillae (93.8% vs. 40%, $p < 0.001$), multiple shades of brown (81.2% vs. 23.6%, $p < 0.001$), and out-of-focus purple-bluish structureless areas (37.5% vs. 5.5%, $p = 0.001$) observed at D150× were significantly more common in LM/LMM compared with other lesions (Figure 7).

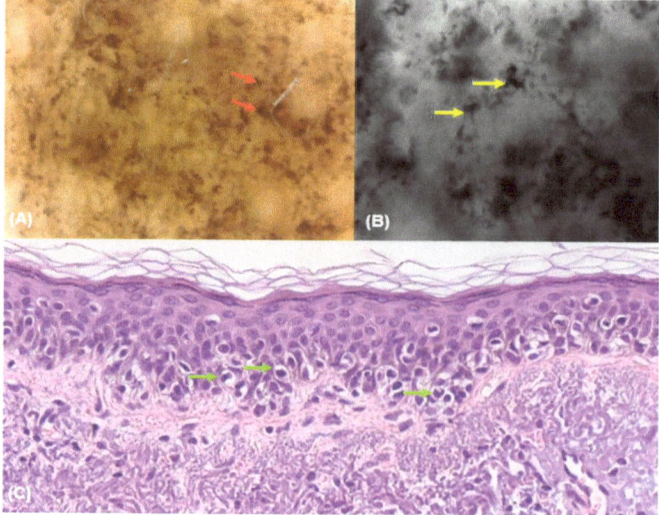

Figure 4. Dermoscopy at 150× magnification (**A**), fluorescence-advanced videodermoscopy, (**B**) and histological image (**C**) of a lentigo maligna melanoma. Dermoscopy at 150× magnification (**A**) reveals

melanocytes and melanocytic invasion of a hair follicle (red arrow). FAV (**B**) reveals pigmented cells that are irregular in shape and size and correspond to malignant melanocytes (yellow arrow). Histological image (**C**) shows a proliferation of intraepidermal melanocytes overlying solar elastosis (green arrow). Hematoxylin and eosin; original magnification 20×.

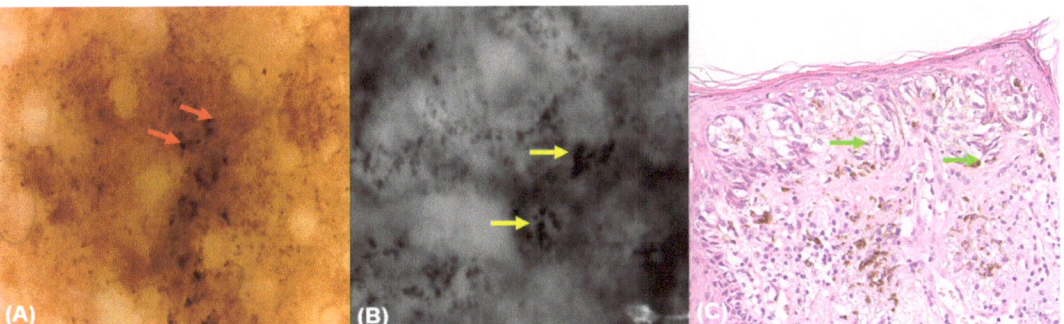

Figure 5. Dermoscopy at 150× magnification (**A**), fluorescence-advanced videodermoscopy, (**B**) and histological image (**C**) of a lentigo maligna melanoma. Dermoscopy at 150× magnification (**A**) reveals melanocytes and melanocytic invasion of a hair follicle (red arrow). FAV (**B**) reveals pigmented cells that are irregular in shape and size and correspond to malignant melanocytes (yellow arrow). Histological image (**C**) shows a proliferation of intraepidermal melanocytes with irregular distribution of nests (green arrow). Hematoxylin and eosin; original magnification 20×.

Notably, a pilot study by Cinotti et al. [17] demonstrated that images acquired with a videodermoscope offering similar magnification (D400 or super-high magnification dermoscopy, Fotofinder Medicam 1000, Bad Birnbach, Germany) can assist in the non-invasive diagnosis of MM by visualizing individual pigmented cells [17]. However, unlike the Fotofinder system, the Horus device offers a significant advantage because operators can acquire magnified dermoscopy images simply by rotating a ring on the probe to zoom in on the area of interest without changing the final lens.

Regarding vascular structures, our analysis revealed significant differences at D150, with vessels being more prevalent in BCC lesions (71.4%) compared with AK/LS (27.3%) and LM/LMM (25%). Notably, BCC lesions predominantly exhibited arborizing vessels (85.7%). The dermoscopic diagnosis of BCC largely depends on the absence of a pigment network and the identification of one or more of six key dermoscopic criteria, including arborizing telangiectasia [18]. In this context, magnified dermoscopy has the potential to visualize vascular structures with unprecedented clarity, and it is particularly valuable when characteristic pigmented features are absent in standard dermoscopy.

As shown in Table 4, our comparative analysis of conventional and magnified dermoscopy parameters revealed moderate to good agreement for most of the evaluated features, with concordance levels ranging from 0.432 to 0.871. These findings suggest that the two techniques are not entirely concordant. A distinctive, albeit not entirely specific, feature of LM/LMM is the invasion of follicular structures, which can be indirectly observed as pigmentation surrounding hair follicles [19]. At the cellular level, this phenomenon is likely explained by the migration of melanocytes and melanophages into follicular structures as the lesion progresses [19]. These cellular elements, as previously mentioned, can be directly visualized using D150 dermoscopy.

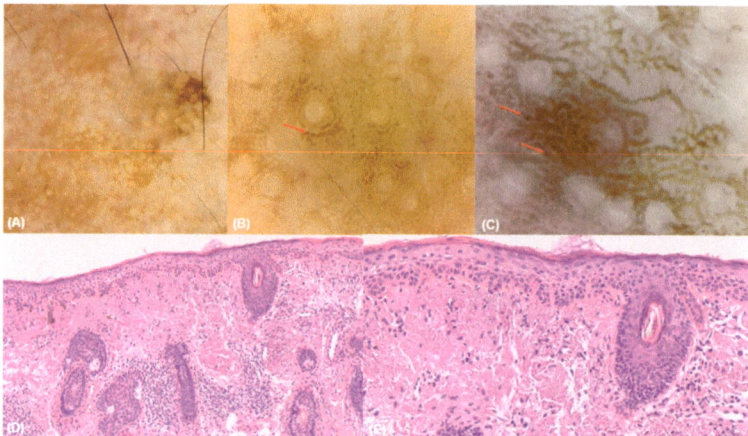

Figure 6. Dermoscopy at 30× (**A**) and 150× (**B**,**C**) magnification and histological images (**D**,**E**) of a solar lentigo. Dermoscopy at 30× magnification (**A**) reveals white and wide follicular openings. Dermoscopy at 150× magnification (**B**,**C**) shows round keratinocytes with a pseudo-tubular distribution (red arrows) around the follicular openings. Histological images (**D**,**E**) reveal atypia of basal keratinocytes with loss of polarization and intense solar elastosis. Hematoxylin and eosin; original magnification 10× (**D**), and 20× (**E**).

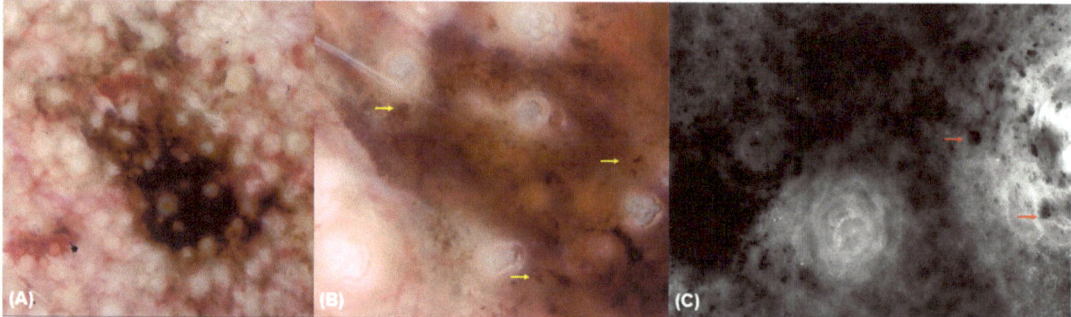

Figure 7. Dermoscopy at 30× (**A**) and 150× (**B**) magnification and fluorescence-advanced videodermoscopy of a lentigo maligna. Dermoscopy at 30× magnification (**A**) reveals asymmetrical pigmented follicular openings and follicular obliteration. Dermoscopy at 150× magnification (**B**) shows melanocytes and melanocytic invasion of a hair follicle (yellow arrow). FAV (**C**) shows pigmented cells that are irregular in shape and size and correspond to malignant melanocytes (red arrow).

In our analysis, the differences in the prevalence of analyzed parameters, such as melanophages at D150 (19.2%) and follicular obliteration at D30 (8.2%), confirm that the two techniques, due to their differing levels of magnification, provide different details of the lesion. However, the high level of concordance (Gwet AC1 0.749, $p < 0.001$) indicates that in cases where follicular obliteration was identified at 30× magnification, melanophages were consistently visible at 150× magnification. This synergistic relationship enhances diagnostic specificity for facial lesions, highlighting the added value of integrating both approaches and emphasizing the importance of employing both methods for comprehensive evaluation. Furthermore, these findings underscore the utility of high-magnification imaging for identifying diagnostic features that remain undetectable in conventional dermoscopy alone.

Similarly to D150, FAV is an innovative non-invasive imaging technique that combines videodermoscopy with information derived from the autofluorescence of skin molecules such as hemoglobin and melanin, enabling the visualization of pigmented keratinocytes and melanocytes [9]. Recently, Scrafi et al. [10] analyzed 21 consecutive suspected facial lesions, including LM, LMM, SL, SK, and PAK, and concluded that FAV features offer an enhanced diagnostic approach for differentiating flat pigmented facial lesions.

Our results further confirmed the diagnostic potential of FAV for identifying malignant features. Specifically, we observed that large, isolated cells with sharp, well-defined borders, large dendritic cells, and free melanin were significantly more prevalent in LM/LMM than in other lesions (all $p < 0.001$). Notably, the high concordance between FAV and D150 in our study suggested that FAV could serve as a reliable alternative to D150 in clinical practice (Table 6).

The current study highlights the importance of integrating traditional and magnified dermoscopy techniques to achieve a more comprehensive understanding of facial lesions.

The ability of D150 and FAV to reveal cellular details that are not detectable with D30 may offer valuable insights into the histopathological correlates of dermoscopic features, ultimately enhancing diagnostic accuracy and informing clinical decision making. Notably, the features observed at 30× magnification often differ from those seen at 150×, with each level offering unique advantages. While 150× magnification enables the visualization of fine cytological details, 30× magnification provides a broader perspective, allowing for a clearer assessment of pigmentation patterns of the skin. Moreover, the observed concordance between the modalities underscores the potential of these techniques to complement each other, providing unique diagnostic information.

However, our study has some limitations. First, the acquisition of D150 and FAV images was operator-dependent, potentially introducing variability in the selection of areas for examination. Second, the image interpretation was retrospective. Finally, this study did not assess correlations between histopathological images.

5. Conclusions

Integrating D30, D150, and FAV into routine clinical practice may improve the diagnosis of facial lesions and minimize unnecessary biopsies. Moreover, a deeper understanding of these techniques could bridge the gap between dermoscopy and histology, advancing the field of dermoscopic imaging. Nevertheless, further research is required in this field.

Author Contributions: Conceptualization, E.C. and M.D.; methodology, E.C.; formal analysis, A.C.; investigation, E.C., M.D., F.F. and L.B.; resources, A.P., A.B., G.R. and L.B.; data curation, A.C.; writing—original draft preparation, M.D.; writing—review and editing, E.C. and M.D.; visualization, P.R.; supervision, L.T. All authors have read and agreed to the published version of the manuscript.

Funding: This research received no external funding.

Institutional Review Board Statement: Ethical review and approval were waived for this study because it was an observational and retrospective study that did not change our clinical practice.

Informed Consent Statement: Informed consent was obtained from all of the subjects involved in this study.

Data Availability Statement: The data presented in this study are available on request from the corresponding author.

Conflicts of Interest: The authors declare no conflict of interest.

References

1. Akay, B.N.; Kocyigit, P.; Heper, A.O.; Erdem, C. Dermatoscopy of flat pigmented facial lesions: Diagnostic challenge between pigmented actinic keratosis and lentigo maligna. *Br. J. Dermatol.* **2010**, *163*, 1212–1217. [CrossRef] [PubMed]

2. Star, P.; Guitera, P. Lentigo Maligna, Macules of the Face, and Lesions on Sun-Damaged Skin: Confocal Makes the Difference. *Dermatol. Clin.* **2016**, *34*, 421–429. [CrossRef]
3. DeWane, M.E.; Kelsey, A.; Oliviero, M.; Rabinovitz, H.; Grant-Kels, J.M. Melanoma on chronically sun-damaged skin: Lentigo maligna and desmoplastic melanoma. *J. Am. Acad. Dermatol.* **2019**, *81*, 823–833. [CrossRef]
4. Tschandl, P.; Rosendahl, C.; Kittler, H. Dermatoscopy of flat pigmented facial lesions. *J. Eur. Acad. Dermatol. Venereol.* **2015**, *29*, 120–127. [CrossRef]
5. Ozbagcivan, O.; Akarsu, S.; Ikiz, N.; Semiz, F.; Fetil, E. Dermoscopic Differentiation of Facial Lentigo Maligna from Pigmented Actinic Keratosis and Solar Lentigines. *Acta Dermatovenerol. Croat.* **2019**, *27*, 146–152.
6. Lallas, A.; Paschou, E.; Manoli, S.M.; Papageorgiou, C.; Spyridis, I.; Liopyris, K.; Bobos, M.; Moutsoudis, A.; Lazaridou, E.; Apalla, Z. Dermatoscopy of melanoma according to type, anatomic site and stage. *Ital. J. Dermatol. Venerol.* **2021**, *156*, 274–288. [CrossRef] [PubMed]
7. Pogorzelska-Dyrbus, J.; Szepietowski, J.C. Melanoma cells in optical super-high magnification dermoscopy. *Br. J. Dermatol.* **2023**, *189*, e55. [CrossRef] [PubMed]
8. Daviti, M.; Papadimitriou, I.; Cinotti, E.; Lallas, A. Atypical melanocytes of an atypical Spitz tumour observed with optical super-high magnification dermoscopy. *Br. J. Dermatol.* **2024**, *191*, 853. [CrossRef] [PubMed]
9. Sanlorenzo, M.; Vujic, I.; De Giorgi, V.; Tomasini, C.; Deboli, T.; Quaglino, P.; Fierro, M.T.; Broganelli, P. Fluorescence-advanced videodermatoscopy: A new method for in vivo skin evaluation. *Br. J. Dermatol.* **2017**, *177*, e209–e210. [CrossRef] [PubMed]
10. Scarfi, F.; Trane, L.; Maio, V.; Silvestri, F.; Venturi, F.; Zuccaro, B.; Massi, D.; De Giorgi, V. Fluorescence-advanced videodermatoscopy (FAV) for the differential diagnosis of suspicious facial lesions: A single-centre experience with pattern analysis and histopathological correlation. *Photodermatol. Photoimmunol. Photomed.* **2022**, *38*, 266–276. [CrossRef] [PubMed]
11. Argenziano, G.; Catricala, C.; Ardigo, M.; Buccini, P.; De Simone, P.; Eibenschutz, L.; Ferrari, A.; Mariani, G.; Silipo, V.; Sperduti, I.; et al. Seven-point checklist of dermoscopy revisited. *Br. J. Dermatol.* **2011**, *164*, 785–790. [CrossRef] [PubMed]
12. Tognetti, L.; Cartocci, A.; Cinotti, E.; D'Onghia, M.; Zychowska, M.; Moscarella, E.; Dika, E.; Farnetani, F.; Guida, S.; Paoli, J.; et al. Dermoscopy of atypical pigmented lesions of the face: Variation according to facial areas. *Exp. Dermatol.* **2023**, *32*, 2166–2172. [CrossRef]
13. Cinotti, E.; Cioppa, V.; Tognetti, L.; Perrot, J.L.; Rossi, R.; Gnone, M.; Cartocci, A.; Rubegni, P.; Cortonesi, G. Super-High Magnification Dermoscopy in 190 Clinically Atypical Pigmented Lesions. *Diagnostics* **2023**, *13*, 2238. [CrossRef] [PubMed]
14. Kaminska-Winciorek, G.; Spiewak, R. Tips and tricks in the dermoscopy of pigmented lesions. *BMC Dermatol.* **2012**, *12*, 14. [CrossRef] [PubMed]
15. Radi, G.; Rossi, R.; Diotallevi, F.; Giannoni, M.; Molinelli, E.; Paolinelli, M.; Ferrara, G.; Offidani, A. The role of the optical super high magnification dermoscopy (O.S.H.M.D) in the management of melanocytic lesions. *J. Eur. Acad. Dermatol. Venereol.* **2023**, *37*, e122–e124. [CrossRef]
16. Cinotti, E.; Cartocci, A.; Liso, F.G.; Cioppa, V.; Falcinelli, F.; Tognetti, L.; Rubegni, P.; Perrot, J.L. Super-High Magnification Dermoscopy Can Help for the Diagnosis of Lentigo Maligna: A Pilot Study on 61 Cases. *Dermatol. Pract. Concept.* **2023**, *13*, e2023101. [CrossRef] [PubMed]
17. Cinotti, E.; Tognetti, L.; Campoli, M.; Liso, F.; Cicigoi, A.; Cartocci, A.; Rossi, R.; Rubegni, P.; Perrot, J.L. Super-high magnification dermoscopy can aid the differential diagnosis between melanoma and atypical naevi. *Clin. Exp. Dermatol.* **2021**, *46*, 1216–1222. [CrossRef] [PubMed]
18. Altamura, D.; Menzies, S.W.; Argenziano, G.; Zalaudek, I.; Soyer, H.P.; Sera, F.; Avramidis, M.; DeAmbrosis, K.; Fargnoli, M.C.; Peris, K. Dermatoscopy of basal cell carcinoma: Morphologic variability of global and local features and accuracy of diagnosis. *J. Am. Acad. Dermatol.* **2010**, *62*, 67–75. [CrossRef] [PubMed]
19. Dika, E.; Lambertini, M.; Patrizi, A.; Misciali, C.; Scarfi, F.; Pellacani, G.; Mandel, V.D.; Di Tullio, F.; Stanganelli, I.; Chester, J.; et al. Folliculotropism in head and neck lentigo maligna and lentigo maligna melanoma. *J. Dtsch. Dermatol. Ges.* **2021**, *19*, 223–229. [CrossRef] [PubMed]

Disclaimer/Publisher's Note: The statements, opinions and data contained in all publications are solely those of the individual author(s) and contributor(s) and not of MDPI and/or the editor(s). MDPI and/or the editor(s) disclaim responsibility for any injury to people or property resulting from any ideas, methods, instructions or products referred to in the content.

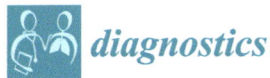

Article

High Incidence of Isolated Tumor Cells in Sentinel Node Biopsies of Thin Melanomas: A Potential Factor in the Paradoxical Prognosis of Stage IIIA Cutaneous Melanoma?

Andrea Ronchi [1], Giuseppe D'Abbronzo [1], Emma Carraturo [1], Giuseppe Argenziano [2], Gabriella Brancaccio [2], Camila Scharf [2], Elvira Moscarella [2], Teresa Troiani [3], Francesco Iovino [4], Salvatore Tolone [5], Mario Faenza [6], Gerardo Cazzato [7] and Renato Franco [1,*]

[1] Pathology Unit, Department of Mental and Physical Health and Preventive Medicine, University of Campania Luigi Vanvitelli, 81100 Naples, Italy; andrea.ronchi@unicampania.it (A.R.); dabbronzogiuseppe@gmail.com (G.D.); em.carraturo@gmail.com (E.C.)
[2] Dermatology Unit, Department of Mental and Physical Health and Preventive Medicine, University of Campania Luigi Vanvitelli, 81100 Naples, Italy; giuseppe.argenziano@unicampania.it (G.A.); gabriella.brancaccio@unicampania.it (G.B.); camila.araujoscharfpinto@unicampania.it (C.S.); elvira.moscarella@unicampania.it (E.M.)
[3] Medical Oncology Unit, Department of Precision Medicine, University of Campania Luigi Vanvitelli, 81100 Naples, Italy; teresa.troiani@unicampania.it
[4] Department of Translational Medicine Science, School of Medicine, University of Campania Luigi Vanvitelli, 81100 Naples, Italy; francesco.iovino@unicampania.it
[5] Department of Advanced Medical and Surgical Sciences, University of Campania Luigi Vanvitelli, 81100 Naples, Italy; salvatore.tolone@unicampania.it
[6] Plastic Surgery Unit, Multidisciplinary Department of Medical-Surgical and Dental Specialties, University of Campania Luigi Vanvitelli, 81100 Naples, Italy; mario.faenza@unicampania.it
[7] Section of Molecular Pathology, Department of Precision and Regenerative Medicine and Ionian Area (DiMePRe-J), University of Bari "Aldo Moro", 70121 Bari, Italy; gerycazzato@hotmail.com
* Correspondence: renato.franco@unicampania.it; Tel.: +39-0815664000

Abstract: Background/Objectives: This study aims to evaluate whether the presence of isolated tumor cells (ITCs) correlates with specific stages of cutaneous melanoma, potentially shedding light on their prognostic significance and the paradoxical survival outcomes in stage IIIA. **Methods**: This study analyzed cases of sentinel lymph node biopsies for cutaneous melanoma between 2021 and 2023. It included patients with CM diagnoses, available histological slides, and clinical information about the neoplasia stage. The correlation between the primary tumor stage and the presence of isolated tumor cells was statistically analyzed. **Results**: This study analyzed 462 sentinel lymph node biopsies, revealing 77.1% negative cases and 22.9% positive cases. Isolated tumor cells were observed in 24 cases (5.2%), most commonly in the early stages (e.g., pT1b and pT2a). Statistical analysis confirmed a significant correlation between ITC presence and early-stage neoplasms ($p = 0.014$). **Conclusions**: Although ITCs prompt upstaging, their prognostic impact appears limited, especially in thin melanomas, where survival aligns more closely with stage IB than stage IIIA. This aligns with findings from breast cancer studies where ITCs are not equated to metastases in staging due to their minimal impact on prognosis. Current melanoma staging practices could benefit from differentiating ITCs from larger metastatic deposits to better reflect the actual metastatic burden and guide treatment decisions.

Keywords: sentinel node biopsy; cutaneous melanoma; isolated tumor cells; staging; prognosis

1. Introduction

Cutaneous melanoma (CM) is currently the fifth most prevalent malignancy and one of the cancers with the greatest incidence increase over the past 50 years [1]. According to the latest SEER data, there were an estimated 100,640 new cases of CM in 2024 in the United States, accounting for 5.0% of all new cancer cases [2]. CM staging is the primary prognostic factor for this cancer, encompassing Breslow thickness, ulceration, and the presence of lymph node metastases and distant metastases. The management of the patient, therefore, primarily depends on the stage of the cancer. According to the AJJC 8th edition, 11 stage classes are defined, including 0, IA, IB, IIA, IIB, IIC, IIIA, IIIB, IIIC, IIID, and IV. Mortality strictly depends on stage, and the 5-year relative survival rates for localized (stages 0, I, and II), regional (stage III), and metastatic (stage IV) CMs are >99%, 74%, and 35%, respectively [3]. Although staging is the most important tool for predicting patient prognosis and consequently making appropriate clinical decisions, there seems to be a discrepancy in the current staging system when assessing prognosis: The survival rate for patients in stage IIIA is paradoxically higher than that for patients in a lower stage, specifically stage IIC [4,5]. Thus, patients with a high Breslow thickness and no lymph node metastases (stage IIC) have a worse prognosis compared to those with a lower Breslow thickness but with lymph node metastases (stage IIIA). Indeed, the 5-year disease-specific survival (DSS) rates for stages IIIA and IIC are 93% and 82%, respectively [6].

Sentinel node biopsy (SNB) is indicated for all cases ranging from pT1b to pT4b and currently serves a primarily prognostic and staging role [7]. The histological examination of the sentinel lymph node is widely based on the protocol by Cook et al., based on the examination of multiple sections at various depths, stained with hematoxylin and eosin and complemented by immunohistochemistry [8]. This extensive examination of the lymph node parenchyma is highly sensitive and can even detect isolated tumor cells (ITCs) [8]. Notably, when evaluating a sentinel lymph node biopsy (SNB), the lymph node should be considered positive for metastasis even if only a few ITCs are present [9]. This assessment applies specifically to CM, whereas for other neoplasms, such as breast carcinoma, ITCs are not considered prognostically significant; therefore, their presence is not an indication that the lymph node is metastatic. Recent evidence suggests that ITCs also do not have a significant prognostic impact in thin melanomas [10]. So, it can be hypothesized that the paradoxically favorable outcome of stage IIIA may be due to the presence of cases of thin melanoma where only isolated cells are found in the sentinel lymph node.

The aim of this study is to examine a series of sentinel lymph nodes analyzed between 2021 and 2023 in order to investigate the frequency of ITCs in SNBs and whether they correlate with a specific stage of the neoplasm.

2. Materials and Methods

All cases of SNBs for CM managed at the University "Luigi Vanvitelli" Hospital (Naples, Italy) from 1 January 2021 to 31 December 2023 were obtained from the archives of the Pathology Unit. The inclusion criteria were as follows: (1) SNB performed for the diagnosis of CM; (2) availability of corresponding histological slides; and (3) availability of clinical information regarding the stage of the neoplasm. Written informed consent, including permission to utilize the diagnostic data for scientific purposes, was obtained from each patient. This study was conducted according to the guidelines of the Declaration of Helsinki and approved by the ethics committee of "Vanvitelli" University (protocol code 282; approval date 6 October 2020).

All cases of sentinel lymph nodes included in this study were processed according to the protocol defined by Cook et al. [8]. For the immunohistochemical staining, we substituted SOX10 for S100, as previously proposed by several authors, because of its higher specificity and equal sensitivity [11–14]. Immunohistochemistry was performed on 4 µm thick formalin-fixed and paraffin-embedded (FFPE) slices using a fully automated assay on the Ventana® Benchmark XT platform (Ventana-Roche Diagnostics, Meylan, France). The procedure was performed according to the manufacturer's instructions.

All histological slides were retrieved from the archives, including both hematoxylin and eosin-stained slides and immunostained slides. Expert pathologists reviewed all the slides, assessing the presence or absence of metastases and the quantity of tumor present in the lymph node (single cells vs. metastatic aggregates).

Data on SNBs performed at our institution during the period 2019–2020, prior to the implementation of the protocol established by Cook et al., were retrieved from institutional archives. This retrospective analysis aimed to compare the frequency of ITCs between these cases and the samples under investigation.

The statistical correlation between the stage of the primary neoplasm and the presence of ITCs in the SNB was assessed using Spearman's correlation, employing "IBM SPSS Statistics version 27" software. Values of $p < 0.05$ were considered statistically significant.

3. Results

3.1. Clinicopathological Features

The series included 462 patients affected by CM and submitted for SNBs. The clinicopathological features of the series are detailed in Table 1.

Table 1. Clinicopathological features.

Stage	N	%
pT1b	112	24.2
pT2a	131	28.4
pT2b	34	7.4
pT3a	52	11.3
pT3b	54	11.7
pT4a	24	5.2
pT4b	55	11.8
Histological type	**N**	**%**
SSM	342	74.0
NM	105	22.7
Other	15	3.3
Location	**N**	**%**
H/N	98	21.2
Trunk	174	37.7
Upper limb	78	16.9
Lower limb	112	24.2

Abbreviations: N: number; SSM: superficial spreading melanoma; NM: nodular melanoma; H/N: head and neck.

Overall, 356 (77.1%) cases were negative and 106 (22.9%) cases were positive, indicating the presence of neoplasia.

Regarding the stage of the neoplasm, 112 cases were classified as pT1b; of these, in 6 cases, the SNBs (5.4%) were positive for neoplasia, while in the remaining 106 (94.6%) cases, the SNBs were negative. A total of 131 cases were classified as stage pT2a; of these, in 21 (16.0%) cases, SNBs were positive, and in the remaining 110 (84.0%) cases, the SNBs were negative. A total of 34 cases were classified as stage pT2b. In 9 (26.5%) cases, the SNBs were positive, and in 25 (73.5%) cases, the SNBs were negative. The pT3a stage included 52 cases, with 12 (23.1%) cases showing positive SNBs and 40 (76.9%) cases showing negative SNBs. A total of 54 cases were classified as pT3b; of these, in 20 (37.0%) cases, the SNBs were positive, and in 34 (63.0%) cases, the SNBs were negative. A total of 24 cases were classified as pT4a; in 8 (33.3%) cases, the SNBs were positive, while in 16 (66.7%) cases, the SNBs were negative. Lastly, 55 cases were classified as pT4b; of these, in 30 (54.5%) cases, the SNBs were positive, and in 25 (45.5%) cases, the SNBs were negative. The results are presented in Table 2 and Figure 1.

Table 2. SNB assessment according to the stage.

Stage	Positive SNB (N; %)	Negative SNB (N; %)
pT1b	6; 5.4	106; 94.6
pT2a	21; 16.0	110; 84.0
pT2b	9; 26.5	25; 73.5
pT3a	12; 23.1	40; 76.9
pT3b	20; 37.0	34; 63.0
pT4a	8; 33.3	16; 66.7
pT4b	30; 54.5	25; 45.5

Abbreviation: SNB: sentinel node biopsy; N: number.

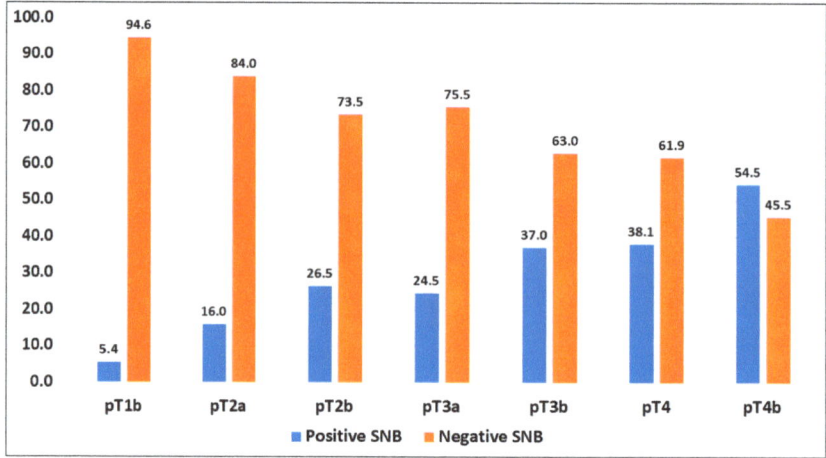

Figure 1. SNB assessment according to the stage.

ITCs were observed in 24 out of 462 (5.2%) cases, including 4 cases in stage pT1b (66.7% of positive SNBs in stage pT1b; 3.8% of all SNBs), 8 cases in stage pT2a (38.1% of positive SNBs in stage pT2a; 7.5% of all SNBs), 3 cases in stage pT2b (33.3% of positive SNBs in stage pT2b; 2.8% of all SNBs), 4 cases in stage pT3a (33.3% of positive SNBs in stage pT3a; 3.8% of all SNBs), 1 case in stage pT3b (5.0% of positive SNBs in stage pT3b; 0.9% of all SNBs), 1 case in stage pT4a (12.5% of positive SNBs in stage pT1b; 0.9% of all SNBs), and 4 cases in stage pT4b (13.3% of positive SNBs in stage pT1b; 3.8% of all SNBs), as shown in Figure 2.

An example of ITCs in an SNB sample is shown in Figure 3.

A total of 90 SNBs were performed at our institution in 2019 and 2020. Retrospective analysis of these cases revealed the presence of ITCs in only three cases, accounting for 3.3% of the total.

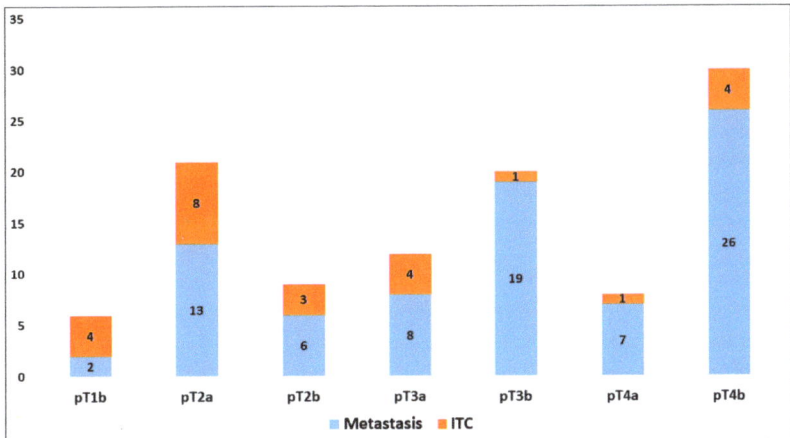

Figure 2. Assessment of metastases and isolated neoplastic cells (ITCs) in positive sentinel node biopsies according to the stage.

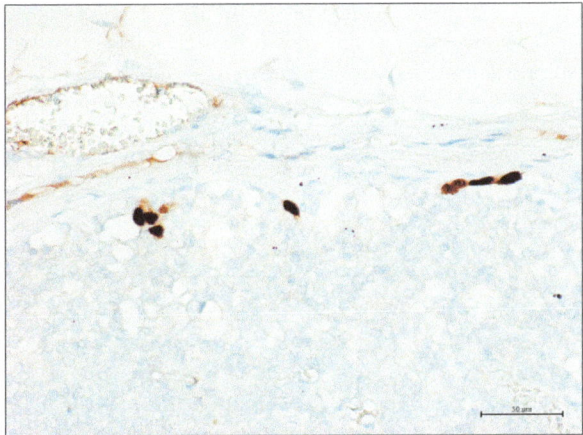

Figure 3. SOX10-positive isolated tumor cells in a sentinel node biopsy (SOX10 immunohistochemical stain, original magnification 200×).

3.2. Statistical Analysis

Spearman's correlation demonstrated a statistically significant correlation between the presence of ITCs in the sentinel lymph node and early stages of primary neoplasm (pT1b or pT2a), with an rs (Spearman's Rank Correlation Coefficient) of 0.265 (p-value: 0.014).

4. Discussion

Sentinel node biopsy (SNB) is a cornerstone in the staging of cutaneous melanoma (CM). This procedure is carried out on the basis of the Breslow thickness of primary tumors, specifically for cases classified from pT1b to pT4b. Examination of SNB samples is worldwide based on the protocol proposed by Cook et al., including multiple histological sections stained by hematoxylin and eosin, complemented by immunohistochemistry, to ensure precise staging and assessment. SNB plays a critical role in determining the neoplasm stage, and its results significantly impact CM outcomes. Thin cutaneous melanomas (classified as pT1a, pT1b, and pT2a) with a positive SNB are assigned to stage IIIA, while thicker melanomas (pT3 and pT4) with a negative SNB result are classified as stages IIB and IIC (see Table 1). Importantly, in the evaluation of an SNB, the lymph node should be classified as positive for metastasis even if only a small number of ITCs are detected [9]. However, stage IIC patients typically have a worse prognosis than stage IIIA patients, with 5-year disease-specific survival (DSS) rates of 82% and 93%, respectively, suggesting that thickness rather than the SNB result impacts the prognosis more [6]. The paradoxical survival outcomes between stages IIC and IIIA may be explained by the interpretation that is currently given to ITCs detected in SNBs.

This study evaluated the presence of ITCs in SNBs from patients with cutaneous melanoma (CM) at various stages. ITCs were detected in 24 out of 462 (5.2%) cases, including 4 cases in stage pT1b, 8 cases in stage pT2a, 3 cases in stage pT2b, 4 cases in stage pT3a, 1 case in stage pT3b, 1 case in stage pT4a, and 4 cases in stage pT4b. A notable finding was the higher prevalence of ITCs in early-stage melanomas (pT1b and pT2a), as indicated by the statistically significant Spearman correlation ($p = 0.014$). The histological evaluation of sentinel lymph nodes typically adheres to the protocol outlined by Cook et al., which entails examining multiple tissue sections at varying depths. These sections are stained using hematoxylin and eosin and further analyzed through immunohistochemical methods. This meticulous approach to lymph node analysis proves highly effective in detecting metastases, and it also has a high sensitivity in detecting ITCs. In our institution, Cook's protocol has been adopted since 2021, while previously SNBs were examined by hematoxylin and eosin staining and a single immunohistochemical staining for each block. Interestingly, 90 SNBs were examined in our institution in 2019 and 2020, and ITCs were detected only in 3 cases (3.3% of cases), while ITCs were detected in 5.2% (24 out of 462) of cases in the 2021–2023 period, when Cook's protocol was applied, with an increase in positivity of 63.5%. Notably, two out of the three cases of ITCs detected in 2019–2020 were thin melanomas staged pT2a, confirming the data showing that ITCs are more frequently observed in cases of thin melanoma. These data support the hypothesis that ITCs have become particularly frequent in recent years, applying a very sensitive protocol. However, the real prognostic impact of ITCs in thin melanomas is not yet well defined. Although ITC-positive thin melanomas are classified as stage IIIA, the presence of ITCs in the sentinel lymph node may not have a significant prognostic impact, potentially undermining the rationale for assigning a higher stage. The case series analyzed in this study is relatively recent, as it is associated with the implementation of a relatively new protocol. Consequently, the prognostic evaluation is significantly limited by the overly short follow-up period, which limits the ability to perform a comprehensive multivariate statistical analysis. However, it is noteworthy that in our series, disease progression occurred in only one case of melanoma with ITCs. This case involved a patient with pT4b melanoma who declined adjuvant therapy and experienced lymph node progression and brain metastases within 8 months of diagnosis. On the other hand, disease progression was observed in six cases of thick melanomas (one case of pT3a, one case of pT4a, and four cases of pT4b) which presented a metastasis in the SNB. The progression occurred between 2 and 23 months after the diagnoses and involved lymph node metastases in all cases. In one instance, a cutaneous metastasis was also identified in addition to the lymph node metastasis. Regarding thin melanomas with ITCs (stage IIIA melanomas), no cases showed disease progression in a follow-up ranging from 1 to 3 years. Therefore, in our series, thin melanomas with ITCs, staged as IIIA, exhibited the same biological behavior as thin melanomas without ITCs. These data align with studies suggesting that ITCs in thin melanomas correlate with a prognosis similar to that of stage IB [10]. Thus, while the presence of ITCs traditionally leads to categorizing the lymph node as metastatic, it may not necessarily indicate a worse prognosis in the early stages. This supports the hypothesis that ITCs might represent a minimal metastatic burden with limited prognostic impact, especially in the context of thin CMs, where clinical outcomes remain favorable despite SNB positivity, implying that their detection should be considered cautiously in the staging process.

An important issue in CM staging involves understanding the biological and clinical implications of ITCs in SNBs compared to more extensive metastatic deposits. In other cancers, such as breast carcinoma, ITCs are not considered equivalent to metastatic disease and do not typically affect the staging classification. The presence of ITCs in breast cancer lymph nodes does not lead to upstaging, since studies have demonstrated that ITCs alone generally do not confer an increased risk of recurrence or poor outcomes. In contrast, lymph nodes with ITCs are currently classified as metastatic in melanoma staging, leading to upstaging and potentially overtreatment for patients whose prognosis might otherwise be favorable, as seen with patients in stage IIIA. In breast cancer, isolated tumor cells (ITCs) detected in lymph nodes have been a subject of extensive study, particularly regarding their impact on prognosis and implications for staging and treatment. ITCs are defined as single cells or small clusters not exceeding 0.2 mm and are commonly identified through immunohistochemical staining. Unlike more extensive lymph node metastases, ITCs are considered to represent a minimal tumor burden, and research has demonstrated that their presence does not significantly affect overall survival or recurrence rates in breast cancer. Several large studies have investigated the prognostic impact of ITCs in breast cancer lymph nodes, suggesting that these cells do not confer a worse prognosis when present in isolation. For example, the MIRROR study, including over 2700 patients with early-stage breast cancer, demonstrated that ITCs alone did not significantly impact disease-free survival when compared to patients with node-negative disease [15]. Thus, the presence of ITCs alone is not an indication of the same aggressive treatment strategies used in patients with larger metastatic deposits, since the risk of recurrence is minimal. Similarly, findings from the ACOSOG Z0010 trial, a large multicenter study of sentinel lymph node biopsies in breast cancer, demonstrated that patients with ITCs had no significant difference in survival outcomes compared to patients without nodal involvement [16]. This reinforces the notion that ITCs do not carry the same prognostic weight as larger nodal metastases, and that their presence does not address upstaging or intensified systemic therapy. The NSABP B-32 trial, another major study that included over 5000 breast cancer patients, also explored the clinical significance of ITCs and micrometastases in sentinel lymph nodes. The researchers found that micrometastases (0.2–2.0 mm) were associated with a slightly higher risk of recurrence than ITCs, but the overall impact on survival was modest [17]. This trial further supported the position that ITCs alone are not strong prognostic markers in breast cancer. As a result of these findings, current guidelines from the American Joint Committee on Cancer (AJCC) and the Union for International Cancer Control (UICC) recommend that ITCs in breast cancer lymph nodes should not lead to upstaging. The AJCC classifies ITCs separately from micrometastases and macrometastases, acknowledging their limited clinical impact. Accordingly, the detection of ITCs in breast cancer is typically recorded but does not alter staging or prompt the same treatment escalation that would be warranted for larger nodal metastases. The distinction between ITCs and larger metastatic deposits may be particularly relevant in melanoma, where staging relies on detecting nodal involvement as a critical prognostic indicator. The absence of a distinction between ITCs and larger metastatic foci in melanoma staging could therefore contribute to some of the paradoxical outcomes observed between stages IIC and IIIA. The clinical significance of this distinction also raises questions about how melanoma staging could evolve to better reflect the actual metastatic burden. If ITCs in SNBs do not contribute to poorer outcomes in patients with thin melanomas, differentiating them from more substantial metastases could refine staging, allowing for more accurate prognosis and treatment planning.

Several studies have examined the prognostic implications of isolated tumor cells (ITCs) in the sentinel lymph nodes (SLNs) of melanoma patients, emphasizing the correlation between lymph node tumor burden and survival outcomes. Research conducted by the Italian Melanoma Intergroup (IMI) indicated that a higher tumor burden in sentinel nodes correlates with poorer survival. Specifically, the study found that an increased metastatic deposit diameter in the sentinel nodes serves as a significant predictor of adverse prognosis. By integrating tumor burden with other variables such as ulceration and Breslow thickness, the multivariate models effectively stratified risk, thereby underscoring the prognostic relevance of tumor burden in SLN-positive melanoma patients [18]. Another investigation explored the prognostic utility of disseminated melanoma cell density within sentinel lymph nodes. Using immunocytology, the researchers quantified disseminated cancer cell (DCC) density and found a strong association between increased DCC density and elevated melanoma-specific mortality risk. This quantitative approach, leveraging metastatic cell counts, significantly enhanced predictive accuracy for patient outcomes beyond traditional histopathological measures [19]. Additionally, European research efforts, notably the EORTC-DeCOG, have developed nomograms to predict recurrence and survival outcomes based on SLN tumor burden, patient age, and other clinical parameters. Validated in extensive cohorts, these models indicate that isolated tumor cells in sentinel nodes hold significant clinical weight in melanoma staging, often predicting recurrence risk when assessed alongside primary tumor characteristics such as Breslow depth [20]. Akkooi et al. analyzed a series of 388 positive SNBs and confirmed that higher tumor burden in the SNB is associated with worse overall survival (OS) and disease-free survival (DFS) [21]. The study showed that patients with micrometastases < 0.1 mm have a significantly better prognosis than patients with metastases > 0.1 mm, and a comparable prognosis to patients with negative lymph nodes [21]. In the study by Madu et al., an SNB metastasis size threshold of 1 mm demonstrated a clear distinction in survival outcomes for stage IIIA melanoma in both the seventh and eighth editions of the staging guidelines. Patients with SN metastases smaller than 1 mm exhibited outstanding distant metastasis-free survival and melanoma-specific survival rates [22]. The study by Verver et al. analyzed the role of SNB micrometastases in patients with CM to better define surgical management and adjuvant therapies. The main results confirm that tumor burden in the sentinel lymph node is a crucial prognostic factor: patients with micrometastases smaller than 1 mm show a significantly better prognosis than those with more extensive metastases [23].

5. Conclusions

In conclusion, our findings contribute to the understanding of staging complexities in CM, specifically the prognostic discrepancies observed between stages IIC and IIIA and the potential significance of isolated cells in SNBs. Future research is warranted to confirm the long-term outcomes associated with ITCs in melanoma and to assess whether alternative staging criteria, which consider the metastatic burden rather than solely the presence of neoplastic cells, might better align with patient prognosis. Until such adjustments are widely accepted, clinicians should exercise caution in interpreting ITCs as equivalent to established metastases, particularly in cases of early-stage melanoma, where ITCs may represent a minimal risk factor rather than an indicator of advanced disease.

Author Contributions: Conceptualization, A.R. and R.F.; methodology, A.R. and G.C.; software, G.D.; formal analysis, A.R., G.B., C.S., G.A. and E.M.; investigation, F.I., M.F., S.T. and T.T.; data curation, E.C.; writing—original draft preparation, A.R. and G.D.; writing—review and editing, R.F. and G.A.; supervision, R.F. All authors have read and agreed to the published version of the manuscript.

Funding: This research received no external funding.

Institutional Review Board Statement: This study was conducted in accordance with the Declaration of Helsinki and approved by the ethics committee of Vanvitelli University (protocol code 282; approval date 6 October 2020).

Informed Consent Statement: Informed consent was obtained from all subjects involved in the study. Written informed consent was obtained from the patients to publish this paper.

Data Availability Statement: The original contributions presented in this study are included in the article. Further inquiries can be directed to the corresponding author.

Conflicts of Interest: The authors declare no conflicts of interest.

References

1. Saginala, K.; Barsouk, A.; Aluru, J.S.; Rawla, P.; Barsouk, A. Epidemiology of Melanoma. *Med. Sci.* **2021**, *9*, 63. [CrossRef] [PubMed]
2. National Cancer Institute Melanoma of the Skin-Cancer Stat Facts. Available online: https://seer.cancer.gov/statfacts/html/melan.html (accessed on 5 August 2024).
3. Survival Rates for Melanoma Skin Cancer. Available online: https://www.cancer.org/cancer/types/melanoma-skin-cancer/detection-diagnosis-staging/survival-rates-for-melanoma-skin-cancer-by-stage.html (accessed on 5 August 2024).
4. Tan, S.Y.; Najita, J.; Li, X.; Strazzulla, L.C.; Dunbar, H.; Lee, M.Y.; Seery, V.J.; Buchbinder, E.I.; Tawa, N.E.; McDermott, D.F.; et al. Clinicopathologic features correlated with paradoxical outcomes in stage IIC versus IIIA melanoma patients. *Melanoma Res.* **2019**, *29*, 70–76. [CrossRef] [PubMed]
5. Miller, R.; Walker, S.; Shui, I.; Brandtmüller, A.; Cadwell, K.; Scherrer, E. Epidemiology and survival outcomes in stages II and III cutaneous melanoma: A systematic review. *Melanoma Manag.* **2020**, *7*, MMT39. [CrossRef]
6. Gershenwald, J.E.; Scolyer, R.A.; Hess, K.R.; Sondak, V.K.; Long, G.V.; Ross, M.I.; Lazar, A.J.; Faries, M.B.; Kirkwood, J.M.; McArthur, G.A.; et al. Melanoma staging: Evidence-based changes in the American Joint Committee on Cancer eighth edition cancer staging manual. *CA Cancer J. Clin.* **2017**, *67*, 472–492. [CrossRef] [PubMed]
7. Brancaccio, G.; Briatico, G.; Scharf, C.; Colella, G.; Docimo, G.; Docimo, L.; Faenza, M.; Iovino, F.; Tolone, S.; Verolino, P.; et al. The role of sentinel node biopsy in the era of adjuvant therapy for melanoma. *Dermatol. Pract. Concept.* **2024**, *14*, e2024038. [CrossRef] [PubMed]
8. Cook, M.G.; Massi, D.; Szumera-Ciećkiewicz, A.; Van den Oord, J.; Blokx, W.; van Kempen, L.C.; Balamurugan, T.; Bosisio, F.; Koljenović, S.; Portelli, F.; et al. An updated European Organisation for Research and Treatment of Cancer (EORTC) protocol for pathological evaluation of sentinel lymph nodes for melanoma. *Eur. J. Cancer* **2019**, *114*, 1–7. [CrossRef]
9. Trinidad, C.M.; Torres-Cabala, C.A.; Curry, J.L.; Prieto, V.G.; Aung, P.P. Update on eighth edition American Joint Committee on Cancer classification for cutaneous melanoma and overview of potential pitfalls in histological examination of staging parameters. *J. Clin. Pathol.* **2019**, *72*, 265–270. [CrossRef]
10. Amaral, T.; Nanz, L.; Stadler, R.; Berking, C.; Ulmer, A.; Forschner, A.; Meiwes, A.; Wolfsperger, F.; Meraz-Torres, F.; Chatziioannou, E.; et al. Isolated melanoma cells in sentinel lymph node in stage IIIA melanoma correlate with a favorable prognosis similar to stage IB. *Eur. J. Cancer* **2024**, *201*, 113912. [CrossRef] [PubMed]
11. Willis, B.C.; Johnson, G.; Wang, J.; Cohen, C. SOX10: A useful marker for identifying metastatic melanoma in sentinel lymph nodes. *Appl. Immunohistochem. Mol. Morphol.* **2015**, *23*, 109–112. [CrossRef] [PubMed]
12. Szumera-Ciećkiewicz, A.; Bosisio, F.; Teterycz, P.; Antoranz, A.; Delogu, F.; Koljenović, S.; van de Wiel, B.A.; Blokx, W.; van Kempen, L.C.; Rutkowski, P.; et al. SOX10 is as specific as S100 protein in detecting metastases of melanoma in lymph nodes and is recommended for sentinel lymph node assessment. *Eur. J. Cancer* **2020**, *37*, 175–182. [CrossRef] [PubMed]
13. Jennings, C.; Kim, J. Identification of nodal metastases in melanoma using SOX-10. *Am. J. Dermatopathol.* **2011**, *33*, 474–482. [CrossRef] [PubMed]
14. Ronchi, A.; Zito Marino, F.; Toni, G.; Pagliuca, F.; Russo, D.; Signoriello, G.; Moscarella, E.; Brancaccio, G.; Argenziano, G.; Franco, R.; et al. Diagnostic performance of melanocytic markers for immunocytochemical evaluation of lymph-node melanoma metastases on cytological samples. *J. Clin. Pathol.* **2022**, *75*, 45–49. [CrossRef]
15. de Boer, M.; van Deurzen, C.H.; van Dijck, J.A.; Borm, G.F.; van Diest, P.J.; Adang, E.M.; Nortier, J.W.; Rutgers, E.J.; Seynaeve, C.; Menke-Pluymers, M.B.; et al. Micrometastases or isolated tumor cells and the outcome of breast cancer. *N. Engl. J. Med.* **2009**, *361*, 653–663. [CrossRef]
16. Hunt, K.K.; Ballman, K.V.; McCall, L.M.; Boughey, J.C.; Mittendorf, E.A.; Cox, C.E.; Whitworth, P.W.; Beitsch, P.D.; Leitch, A.M.; Buchholz, T.A.; et al. Factors associated with local-regional recurrence after a negative sentinel node dissection: Results of the ACOSOG Z0010 trial. *Ann. Surg.* **2012**, *256*, 428–436. [CrossRef] [PubMed]

17. Krag, D.N.; Anderson, S.J.; Julian, T.B.; Brown, A.M.; Harlow, S.P.; Costantino, J.P.; Ashikaga, T.; Weaver, D.L.; Mamounas, E.P.; Jalovec, L.M.; et al. Sentinel-lymph-node resection compared with conventional axillary-lymph-node dissection in clinically node-negative patients with breast cancer: Overall survival findings from the NSABP B-32 randomised phase 3 trial. *Lancet Oncol.* **2010**, *11*, 927–933. [CrossRef] [PubMed]
18. Tropea, S.; Del Fiore, P.; Maurichi, A.; Patuzzo, R.; Santinami, M.; Ribero, S.; Quaglino, P.; Caliendo, V.; Borgognoni, L.; Sestini, S.; et al. The role of sentinel node tumor burden in modeling the prognosis of melanoma patients with positive sentinel node biopsy: An Italian melanoma intergroup study (N = 2086). *BMC Cancer* **2022**, *22*, 610. [CrossRef]
19. Ulmer, A.; Dietz, K.; Hodak, I.; Polzer, B.; Scheitler, S.; Yildiz, M.; Czyz, Z.; Lehnert, P.; Fehm, T.; Hafner, C.; et al. Quantitative measurement of melanoma spread in sentinel lymph nodes and survival. *PLoS Med.* **2014**, *11*, e1001604. [CrossRef]
20. Verver, D.; Rekkas, A.; Garbe, C.; van Klaveren, D.; van Akkooi, A.C.J.; Rutkowski, P.; Powell, B.W.E.M.; Robert, C.; Testori, A.; van Leeuwen, B.L.; et al. The EORTC-DeCOG nomogram adequately predicts outcomes of patients with sentinel node-positive melanoma without the need for completion lymph node dissection. *Eur. J. Cancer* **2020**, *134*, 9–18. [CrossRef]
21. van Akkooi, A.C.; Nowecki, Z.I.; Voit, C.; Schäfer-Hesterberg, G.; Michej, W.; de Wilt, J.H.; Rutkowski, P.; Verhoef, C.; Eggermont, A.M. Sentinel node tumor burden according to the Rotterdam criteria is the most important prognostic factor for survival in melanoma patients: A multicenter study in 388 patients with positive sentinel nodes. *Ann. Surg.* **2008**, *248*, 949–955. [CrossRef]
22. Madu, M.F.; Franke, V.; Van de Wiel, B.A.; Klop, W.M.C.; Jóźwiak, K.; van Houdt, W.J.; Wouters, M.W.J.M.; van Akkooi, A.C.J. External validation of the American Joint Committee on Cancer 8th edition melanoma staging system: Who needs adjuvant treatment? *Melanoma Res.* **2020**, *30*, 185–192. [CrossRef] [PubMed]
23. Verver, D.; van Klaveren, D.; van Akkooi, A.C.J.; Rutkowski, P.; Powell, B.W.E.M.; Robert, C.; Testori, A.; van Leeuwen, B.L.; van der Veldt, A.A.M.; Keilholz, U.; et al. Risk stratification of sentinel node-positive melanoma patients defines surgical management and adjuvant therapy treatment considerations. *Eur. J. Cancer* **2018**, *96*, 25–33. [CrossRef]

Disclaimer/Publisher's Note: The statements, opinions and data contained in all publications are solely those of the individual author(s) and contributor(s) and not of MDPI and/or the editor(s). MDPI and/or the editor(s) disclaim responsibility for any injury to people or property resulting from any ideas, methods, instructions or products referred to in the content.

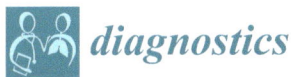

Article

PRAME Immunohistochemistry in Thin Melanomas Compared to Melanocytic Nevi

Iulia Zboraș [1], Loredana Ungureanu [1,*], Simona Șenilă [1], Bobe Petrushev [2], Paula Zamfir [2], Doinița Crișan [3], Flaviu Andrei Zaharie [4], Ștefan Cristian Vesa [5] and Rodica Cosgarea [1]

[1] Department of Dermatology, "Iuliu Hațieganu" University of Medicine and Pharmacy, 400006 Cluj-Napoca, Romania; iuliazboras@yahoo.com (I.Z.); simonasenila@yahoo.com (S.Ș.); cosgearr@yahoo.com (R.C.)
[2] Department of Pathology, Regional Institute of Gastroenterology and Hepatology, 400162 Cluj-Napoca, Romania; bobe.petrushev@gmail.com (B.P.); paulacristinela@yahoo.com (P.Z.)
[3] Department of Pathology, "Iuliu Hațieganu" University of Medicine and Pharmacy, 400006 Cluj-Napoca, Romania; doinitacrisan@gmail.com
[4] Faculty of Medicine, "Iuliu Hațieganu" University of Medicine and Pharmacy, 400012 Cluj-Napoca, Romania; zandrei75@yahoo.com
[5] Department of Pharmacology, Toxicology and Clinical Pharmacology, "Iuliu Hațieganu" University of Medicine and Pharmacy, 400337 Cluj-Napoca, Romania; stefanvesa@gmail.com
* Correspondence: loredanaungureanu08@gmail.com; Tel.: +40-740961845

Abstract: PRAME (PReferentially expressed Antigen in Melanoma) immunohistochemistry has proven helpful in distinguishing malignant from benign melanocytic tumors. We studied PRAME IHC expression in 46 thin melanomas and 39 melanocytic nevi, mostly dysplastic nevi. Twenty-six percent (26.09%) of the melanomas showed diffuse PRAME staining in over 76% of the tumor cells (4+), and 34.78% of the melanomas showed PRAME expression in over 51% of the tumor cells (3+ or 4+), while 8% were entirely negative for PRAME. No melanocytic nevi were PRAME 4+ or 3+. More than half of the nevi (64%) were entirely negative for PRAME staining, and 36% of the nevi showed staining expression in 1–25% (1+) or 26–50% of the cells (2+). No nevi were stained with a color intensity of 3, while 16.67% of the melanomas were stained with this color intensity. Most nevi (78.57%) were stained with an intensity of 1. With a lower positivity threshold, sensitivity increases with still reasonable specificity. The best accuracy was obtained for the 2+ positivity threshold. In conclusion, PRAME staining helps distinguish thin melanomas from dysplastic nevi. However, the threshold of positivity should be lowered in order not to miss thin melanomas.

Keywords: PRAME; immunohistochemistry; melanoma; nevus

1. Introduction

PRAME (PReferentially expressed Antigen in Melanoma) immunohistochemistry (IHC) has proven its diagnostic utility in differentiating between benign melanocytic tumors and malignant melanocytic tumors [1]. Melanocytic neoplasms are classified according to the latest WHO classification of melanocytic skin tumors, 5th edition and are shown in Table 1 [2]. PRAME was mostly positive in superficial spreading melanomas (SSMs), acral melanomas (AMs), nodular melanomas (NMs) or lentigo maligna melanomas (LMMs) and only in a few desmoplastic melanomas (DMs) [3,4]. It was also observed to be positive in most melanoma in situ cases [4]. PRAME immunohistochemistry can be positive in some cases of Spitz nevi (SN) or atypical Spitz tumors (ASTs) but in a lower proportion of cases compared to spitzoid melanomas (SMs), and the proportion is lower in SMs compared to SSMs and LMMs [5–7].

PRAME immunohistochemistry was sometimes interpreted as positive in dysplastic nevi (DN) but in a lower proportion compared to melanomas [8]. In challenging melanocytic tumors, a higher positivity of PRAME staining was observed when compared to nevi, but a lower positivity compared to melanomas, thus supporting the histopathological result [9]. There was good concordance between PRAME IHC results in challenging melanocytic tumors and other cytogenetic test results like fluorescence in situ hybridization (FISH) and single-nucleotide polymorphism (SNP) array and between PRAME IHC results and the final diagnostic interpretation [10]. Compared to FISH testing, PRAME staining had lower sensitivity in spitzoid neoplasms and other atypical melanocytic neoplasms [11]. McAfee et al. found no statistically significant correlation between PRAME staining and FISH testing in spitzoid tumors [12].

Table 1. Classification of melanocytic neoplasms according to WHO classification of melanocytic skin tumors, 5th edition.

Melanocytic Neoplasms	Subtypes	
Melanocytic Neoplasms in Intermittently Sun-Exposed Skin	Nevi	Junctional, compound and dermal nevi
		Simple lentigo and lentiginous melanocytic nevus
		Dysplastic nevus
		Nevus spilus
		Special-site nevus (of the breast, axilla, scalp and ear)
		Halo nevus
		Meyerson nevus
		Recurrent nevus
		Combined nevus
	Melanocytomas	WNT-activated deep-penetrating/plexiform melanocytoma (nevus)
		Pigmented epithelioid melanocytoma
		BAP1-inactivated melanocytoma
		MITF pathway-activated melanocytic tumor
	Melanomas in intermittently sun-exposed skin	Melanoma on skin with low cumulative sun damage (low CSD); includes superficial spreading melanoma
Melanocytic Neoplasms in Chronically Sun-Exposed Skin	Lentigo maligna melanomas	
	Desmoplastic melanomas	
Spitz Tumors	Spitz nevi	Pigmented spindle cell nevus (Reed nevus)
		Spitz nevus
	Spitz melanocytomas	Spitz melanocytoma (atypical Spitz tumor)
	Spitz melanomas	
Melanocytic Tumors in Acral Skin	Acral nevi	
	Acral melanomas	
Genital and Mucosal Melanocytic Tumors	Mucosal and genital nevi	Melanosis
		Genital nevus
	Mucosal melanomas	
Blue Nevi and Related Tumors	Blue nevi and melanocytoses	Nevus of Ito and nevus of Ota
		Congenital dermal melanocytosis
		Blue nevus
	Melanomas arising in blue nevi	
Congenital Melanocytic Tumors	Congenital nevi	Congenital melanocytic nevus
		Proliferative nodules in congenital melanocytic nevus
	Melanomas arising in congenital nevi	Melanoma arising in giant congenital nevus

Table 1. Cont.

Melanocytic Neoplasms	Subtypes	
Ocular and Central Nervous System (CNS) Melanocytic Tumors	Conjunctival melanocytic tumors	Conjunctival nevus
		Conjunctival melanocytic intraepithelial lesion
		Conjunctival melanoma
	Uveal melanocytic tumors	Uveal melanocytoma
		Uveal melanoma
	CNS melanocytic tumors	Diffuse meningeal melanocytic neoplasms: melanocytosis and melanomatosis
		Circumscribed meningeal melanocytic neoplasms: melanocytoma and melanoma
Nodular, Nevoid and MetaStatic Melanomas	Nodular and other melanomas	Nodular melanoma
		Nevoid melanoma
		Dermal melanoma
	Metastatic melanomas	Melanoma metastatic to the skin
		Melanoma metastatic to other organs

PRAME immunohistochemistry can be used for a better margin assessment of lentigo maligna (LM) and lentigo maligna melanomas [1,13,14]. Slow Mohs micrographic surgery is the best procedure to assess the margins in LM and LMM cases [15]. Adding special immunohistochemistry like PRAME or combined immunohistochemistry PRAME/Melan A to slow Mohs micrographic surgery could help assess the margins in lentigo maligna and lentigo maligna melanoma cases [16].

Combining nuclear staining PRAME with membranous staining like Melan A and HMB-45 could be of potential use in the diagnosis of melanoma, especially in complex cases [16–18]. The double staining with the two melanocytic markers Melan A and HMB-45 helps to assess PRAME immunohistochemistry on melanocytes better [19]. PRAME immunohistochemistry can differentiate nodal nevi from metastatic melanomas, but it is recommended to use prior H&E and other melanocytic markers (SOX 10 or Melan A) to confirm the presence of melanocytes in the sentinel lymph node biopsy or to use double staining PRAME/Melan A [20]. PRAME staining is superior to HMB-45 in differentiating benign from malignant melanocytic tumors, but combining nuclear PRAME staining with membranous HMB-45 staining can increase specificity [21]. Combining PRAME with p16 staining has proven helpful in distinguishing between benign and malignant melanocytic lesions, with PRAME being mostly positive in malignant lesions and p16 being mostly positive in benign lesions [22].

Regarding the prognostic value of PRAME immunohistochemistry, it seems to have no impact on disease-specific survival [23]. Lo Bello et al. observed no statistically significant correlation between PRAME positivity and relapse or survival rate [24].

Our study aimed to evaluate whether PRAME immunohistochemistry can effectively differentiate thin melanomas, defined as melanomas with a Breslow index of ≤ 1 mm, from nevi, primarily dysplastic nevi, which are the main histopathological differential diagnoses for melanomas. There are only a few published studies that focus specifically on thin melanomas or melanomas in situ with regard to PRAME immunohistochemistry. However, some studies have included these groups alongside more advanced melanoma cases. Our research focused on a Romanian patient population, and to the best of our knowledge, no previous studies on PRAME immunohistochemistry in a Romanian population have been published.

2. Materials and Methods

2.1. Study Design and Patients

This retrospective study included 46 thin melanomas and 39 melanocytic nevi (Figure 1) diagnosed in the Department of Dermatology and Venereology of Cluj-Napoca Emergency County Hospital between 2014 and 2019. The study was approved by the Ethics Committee of Iuliu Hatieganu University of Medicine and Pharmacy Cluj-Napoca, Romania. All participants gave their informed consent. All melanocytic lesions were reviewed by a pathologist (D.C.).

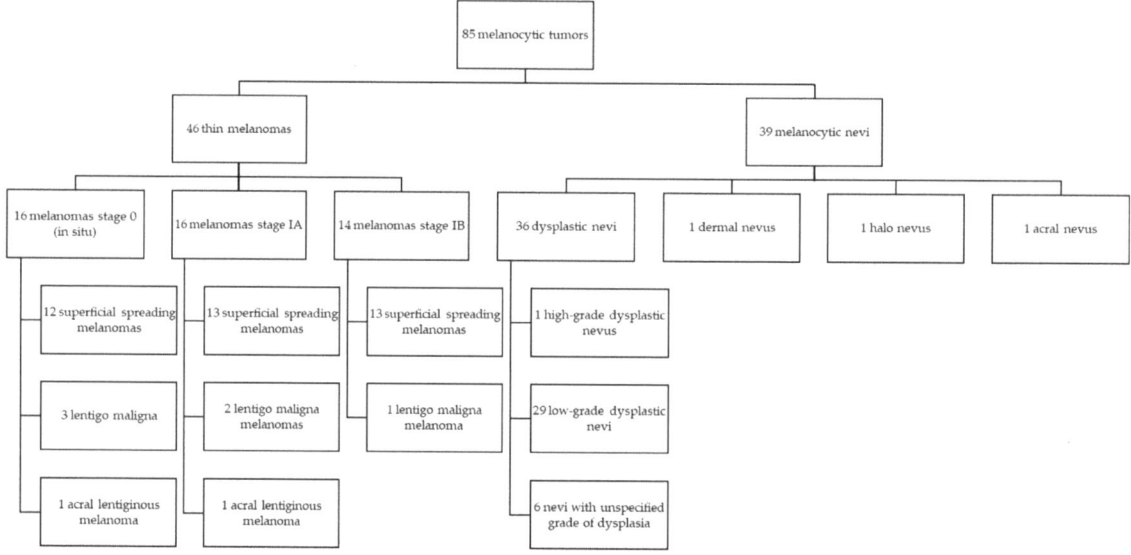

Figure 1. Study design (Melanocytic tumor distribution).

2.2. Immunohistochemistry

The paraffin-embedded blocks were retrieved from the Department of Pathology of Cluj-Napoca Emergency County Hospital and were cut into 5 mm thick tissue sections for immunohistochemical analysis. We performed depigmentation with hydrogen peroxide 3% to remove the excessive melanin. The immunohistochemistry staining was performed with the recombinant anti-PRAME antibody [ERP20330] (ab219650) from Abcam (Cambridge, UK) on an automated Leica Bond-Max stainer platform from Leica Biosystems (Melbourne, Australia) at a 1:100 dilution using a DAB brown chromogen. We used sebaceous glands as positive internal controls, while non-melanocytic and non-sebaceous cells were used as negative internal controls.

The staining results were recorded as the percentage and intensity of immunoreactive tumor cells with nuclear labeling. No staining at all indicated 0%; staining of 1% to 25% of tumor cells was scored as 1+; staining of 26% to 50% of tumor cells was scored as 2+; staining of 51% to 75% of tumor cells was scored 3+; and staining of more than 76% of tumor cells was scored as 4+. Staining intensity was recorded as negative (0), weak (1), moderate (2) and strong (3).

2.3. Statistical Analysis

Statistical analysis was performed in R version 4.4.0–"Puppy Cup". Descriptive statistics were reported for all variables. Continuous variables were presented as mean and standard, while categorical variables were reported as frequency and percentage. The Student's t-test was used for the comparison of continuous variables between two groups, while the chi-square test was used to test for differences in frequency between groups. Sensitivity, specificity, negative predictive value (NPV), positive predictive value (PPV) and accuracy parameters were computed for different thresholds of PRAME staining to assess the discriminatory capacity between nevi and melanomas. A *p*-value of less than 0.05 was considered statistically significant.

3. Results

We examined 46 melanomas for PRAME immunohistochemistry in this study: 16 stage 0 melanomas, 16 stage IA melanomas and 14 stage IB melanomas. The group of melanomas included 38 superficial spreading melanomas, two acral lentiginous melanomas (ALMs), three lentigo maligna and three lentigo maligna melanomas. Eighteen patients were female, and twenty-eight patients were male. Patient age ranged between 26 and 85 years, with a mean age of 57.56 and a median age of 60. The Breslow thickness ranged between 0 and 1 mm, with a mean Breslow thickness of 0.45 mm and a median Breslow thickness of 0.5 mm. Regarding localization, 24 melanomas were located on the trunk, eight on the head and neck regions, eight on the lower limbs and six on the upper limbs. Of all melanomas, 31 were in a horizontal growth phase, while 15 were in a vertical growth phase. The mitotic rate ranged from 0 to 12 mitosis/mm^2, with a mean of 1.41 mitosis/mm^2 and a median of 0 mitosis/mm^2.

Twenty-six (26.09%) of the melanomas showed diffuse PRAME staining in over 76% of the tumor cells (4+) (Figures 2–4), and 8.7% showed PRAME staining in 51 to 75% of the cells (3+), while 8% were entirely negative for PRAME. In total, 34.78% of the melanomas showed PRAME staining in over 51% of the tumor cells. Considering only melanoma in situ cases, from 16 melanoma in situ cases, only 2 stained in over 76% (4+) of the tumor cells, meaning only 12.5% of the cases and 1 case stained 3+, accounting for 6.25% of the cases. However, all melanomas showed slight staining, with the majority in the 2+ group (11/16), accounting for 68.75% of the cases.

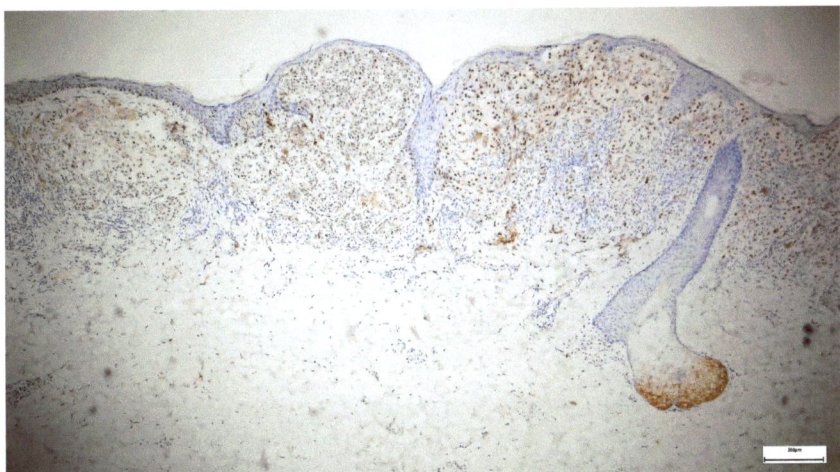

Figure 2. PRAME immunohistochemistry in melanoma (staining in over 76% of the cells 4+, staining intensity 3)—sebaceous gland as positive internal control 50×.

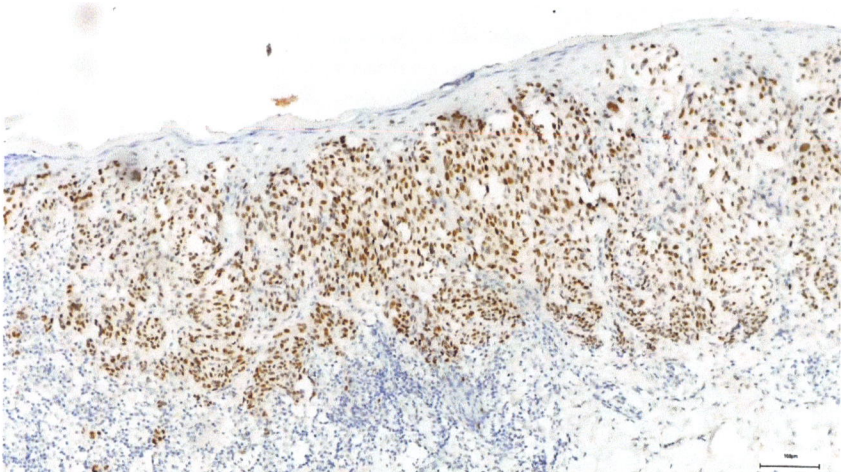

Figure 3. PRAME immunohistochemistry in melanoma (staining in over 76% of the cells 4+, staining intensity 3) 100×.

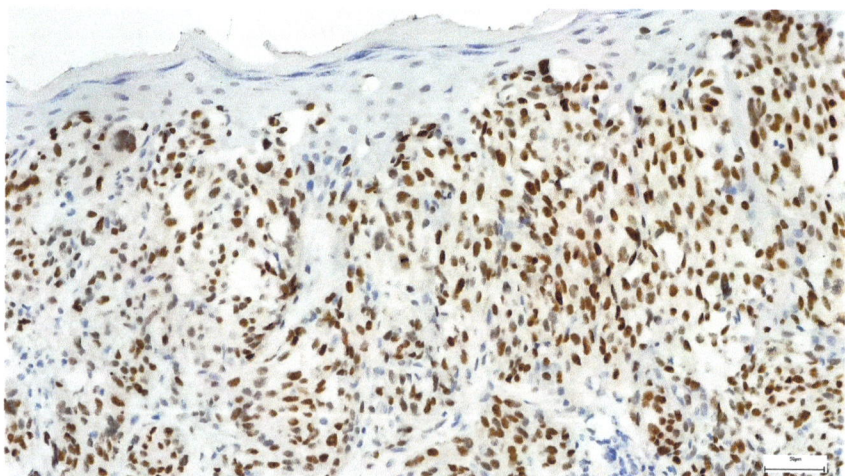

Figure 4. PRAME immunohistochemistry in melanoma (staining in over 76% of the cells 4+, staining intensity 3) 200×.

In comparison to melanomas, we examined 39 melanocytic nevi: 36 dysplastic nevi, one dermal nevus, one halo nevus and one acral nevus. One nevus was a high-grade dysplastic nevus; 29 nevi were low-grade dysplastic nevi, and six nevi had unspecified grades of dysplasia. From the dysplastic nevi, two were in acral location. No nevi showed positive PRAME staining in over 76% (4+) or 51 to 75% of the cells (3+). A total of 64% of the nevi were entirely negative for PRAME staining, and 36% of the nevi stained in 1–25% of the cells (1+) or 26–50% (Table 2). There was no statistically significant difference in color intensity of PRAME staining between the nevi and the melanoma group. No nevi stained with a color intensity of 3, while 16.67% of the melanomas stained with a color intensity of 3. Most nevi (78.57%) stained with an intensity of 1. The high-grade dysplastic nevus stained 1+ with a color intensity of 1. The dermal and the halo nevus did not show PRAME staining in any cells (0). The acral nevus stained in 1–25% (1+) of the cells.

Table 2. Comparison between PRAME immunohistochemistry in melanomas vs. nevi.

		Nevi	Melanomas	p-Value
Staining percentage N (%)	0% (0)	25 (64.1)	4 (8.7)	<0.001
	1–25% (1+)	8 (20.51)	7 (15.22)	
	26–50% (2+)	6 (15.38)	19 (41.3)	
	51–75% (3+)	0 (0)	4 (8.7)	
	>76% (4+)	0 (0)	12 (26.09)	
Staining percentage N (%)	0, 1+, 2+	39 (100)	30 (65.22)	<0.001
	3+, 4+	0 (0)	16 (34.78)	
Staining percentage N (%)	0, 1+, 2+, 3+	39 (100)	34 (73.91)	0.001
	4+	0 (0)	12 (26.09)	
Color intensity N (%)	1	11 (78.57)	24 (57.14)	0.202
	2	3 (21.43)	11 (26.19)	
	3	0 (0)	7 (16.67)	

In the melanoma patient group, melanomas with vertical growth were positive for PRAME immunohistochemistry in over 76% of the tumor cells (4+), more frequently than other groups in terms of staining percentage ($p < 0.05$) (Table 3). Different variables like sex, age, localization, histopathological subtype, stage, ulceration, regression, Breslow index, mitotic rate, personal or family history of melanoma or development on pre-existent nevus showed no statistically significant association with PRAME staining.

Table 3. Comparison between PRAME staining in melanomas in over 76% of the tumor cells (4+) and under 75% of the tumor cells (0, 1+, 2+ and 3+) according to clinical and histopathological variables.

Variable		Melanoma PRAME Staining Groups 0, 1+, 2+ and 3+ N = 34	Melanoma PRAME Staining Group 4+ N = 12	p-Value
Sex N (%)	F	14 (41.18)	4 (33.33)	0.632 $
	M	20 (58.82)	8 (66.67)	
Age [years] Median ± sd		58.68 ± 13.82	54.42 ± 15	0.374 #
Localization N (%)	Head and neck	8 (23.53)	0	0.111 $
	Trunk	16 (47.06)	8 (66.67)	
	Upper limb	3 (8.82)	3 (25)	
	Lower limb	7 (20.59)	1 (8.33)	
Histopathological subtype N (%)	SSM	26 (76.47)	12 (100)	0.332 $
	LMM	3 (8.82)	0	
	LM	3 (8.82)	0	
	ALM	2 (5.88)	0	
Vertical growth N (%)	No	26 (76.47)	5 (41.67)	0.027 $
	Yes	8 (23.53)	7 (58.33)	
Stage N (%)	In situ	14 (41.18)	2 (16.67)	0.167 $
	IA	12 (35.29)	4 (33.33)	
	IB	8 (23.53)	6 (50)	

Table 3. Cont.

Variable		Melanoma PRAME Staining Groups 0, 1+, 2+ and 3+ N = 34	Melanoma PRAME Staining Group 4+ N = 12	p-Value
Ulceration N (%)	No	34 (100)	11 (91.67)	0.089 $
	Yes	0	1 (8.33)	
Regression N (%)	No	27 (79.41)	10 (83.33)	0.768 $
	Yes	7 (20.59)	2 (16.67)	
Breslow index Median ± sd		0.4 ± 0.36	0.61 ± 0.35	0.080 #
Mitotic rate Median ± sd		1.38 ± 2.63	1.5 ± 1.57	0.885 #
Family history of melanoma	No	32 (94.12)	12 (100)	0.390
	Yes	2 (5.88)	0 (0)	
Personal history of melanoma	No	28 (82.35)	12 (100)	0.119
	Yes	6 (17.65)	0 (0)	
Nevus-associated melanoma	No	26 (76.47)	7 (58.33)	0.230
	Yes	8 (23.53)	5 (41.67)	

$ Chi-Square test; # t-test.

In the LM group, all three cases stained 26–50% (2+) of the tumor cells, while in the LMM group, one case stained 51–75% (3+), one case stained 1–25% (1+) of the tumor cells, and one case was completely negative.

In our study, sensitivity for a cutoff value of >76% (4+) or >51% (3+ and 4+) was low, 26% and 35%, respectively, but specificity was 100% for both (Table 4). The cutoff value of >26% (2+) provided the best accuracy and Youden's index.

Table 4. Diagnostic values by different cutoff values for PRAME.

Cutoff	Sensitivity (%)	Specificity (%)	Positive Predictive Value (%)	Negative Predictive Value (%)	Accuracy (%)	Youden's Index
>76% (4+)	26%	100%	100%	53%	60%	0.26
>51% (3+, 4+)	35%	100%	100%	56%	64%	0.35
>26% (2+, 3+, 4+)	76%	85%	85%	75%	80%	0.61
>1% (1+, 2+, 3+, 4+)	91%	64%	75%	86%	79%	0.55

Considering a lower positivity threshold and interpreting 0 and 1+ as PRAME-negative and 2+, 3+ and 4+ as PRAME-positive, 76.09% of the melanomas were PRAME-positive, while 84.61% of the nevi were negative.

Regarding survival, 45 patients out of 46 were alive by July 2024, while one patient died of another cause.

4. Discussion

4.1. PRAME Staining in Melanoma

In the study conducted by Lezcano et al., 83.2% of the melanomas were diffusely PRAME-positive (4+) [1], while in the Gassenmeier et al. study conducted on thin melanomas (Breslow index ≤ 1 mm), the melanomas were PRAME-positive (4+) in 58.6% of them [25]. Our study included only thin melanomas with a Breslow index ≤ 1 mm, similarly to the study conducted by Gassenmeier et al., and our percentage of PRAME-positive melanoma cases was 26.09%, almost half compared to the previously mentioned study [25]. The mean

Breslow thickness in their study was 0.7 mm (range 0.3–1.0) [25], higher than our mean Breslow thickness of only 0.45 mm (range 0–1.0), which is probably the reason for our lower proportion of positive cases, or probably because Gassenmeier et al. used a different dilution (1:50) of the antibody compared to our dilution (1:100), and they used another clone (clone QR005, DCS, Hamburg, Germany). In addition, they included stage III and stage IV metastasizing and non-metastasizing melanomas, while our study included only non-metastasizing stage 0 (in situ) and stage I melanomas. In our study, 16/46 melanomas were in situ. In Lezcano et al.'s study [1], the melanoma in situ cases showed positive PRAME staining (4+) in 93.8% of the cases compared to our study group of melanoma in situ cases in which only 12.5% of the cases stained 4+. However, although they used the same antibody as ours, they did not mention the dilution. Moreover, the entirely negative melanoma cases were similar to those of other studies, 8.7%, compared to the Lezcano et al. [1] study in which 8% of the melanoma cases were entirely negative for PRAME IHC. The difference is that we observed many cases in the intermediate staining groups (3+ and 2+).

Parra et al. observed no impact on disease-specific survival regarding PRAME immunohistochemistry, but they observed a positive correlation between PRAME-positive staining in melanomas and a higher mitotic rate ($p = 0.047$) [23]. We observed a positive correlation between PRAME positivity and vertical growth in melanomas ($p = 0.027$) but no statistically significant correlation with the mitotic rate. Out of 46 melanoma patients, 45 are alive and one patient died of another cause.

In other studies, lentigo maligna and lentigo maligna melanomas have similar PRAME expressions compared to superficial spreading melanomas [1]. Tio et al. observed a higher expression of PRAME in lentigo maligna melanomas than in lentigo maligna [26]. In our study, no lentigo maligna or lentigo maligna melanoma case stained in over 76% of the tumor cells (4+), but all three lentigo maligna cases and 2/3 lentigo maligna melanoma cases stained for PRAME, but in a lower proportion of the cells. However, the included cases were too few.

In acral melanocytic tumors, PRAME staining proved to help distinguish benign from malignant lesions. Still, the proportion of PRAME-positive cases was higher for invasive melanomas than for melanomas in situ [27]. It proved its diagnostic utility in both subungual and non-subungual acral melanomas [28]. PRAME staining proved superior in distinguishing acral melanomas from acral nevi compared to p16 staining [29]. In our study, both acral lentiginous melanoma cases were stained in 26–50% (2+) of the tumor cells with a 2 and 1 intensity score, respectively. If considering a 4+ or 3+ positivity threshold, both cases would be negative, suggesting that PRAME staining is not always helpful in distinguishing benign from malignant lesions. If a positivity threshold of 2+ was considered, both cases would be positive.

4.2. PRAME Staining in Melanocytic Nevi

No nevi in our study were positive for PRAME staining in over 50% of the cells. Although 36% of melanocytic nevi were focally positive 1+ or 2+ for PRAME staining, a higher percentage compared to the study conducted by Lezcano et al., where only 13.6% were described [1], this can also be due to the fact that our study mainly included DN. In the study conducted by Cazzato et al., 96.4% of the nevi were PRAME-negative or had a score of 1+ [30]. The results in our study are similar, with 84.61% PRAME-negative nevi or with a score of 1+. DN can sometimes be diffusely positive for PRAME immunohistochemistry in over 76% of the tumor cells (4+). Turner et al. found a 10% positivity of DN in over 75% of the cells (4+) [8], but in our study, no nevi showed diffuse positive staining. Rasic et al. observed a higher diffuse positivity of PRAME staining in high-grade dysplastic nevi compared to low-grade dysplastic nevi and common nevi [21]. In the study carried out by Innocenti et al., PRAME staining could differentiate between high-grade dysplastic nevi and cutaneous melanomas or between low-grade dysplastic nevi and cutaneous melanomas, but not between high-grade dysplastic nevi and low-grade dysplastic nevi [31]. Lezcano et al. found a single melanocytic nevus to be diffusely positive for PRAME (4+), which was described as a Spitz nevus, and more nevi showed focal positive PRAME staining (1+ or 2+) [1]. Raghavan et al. also found one Spitz nevus to be diffusely positive (4+) for PRAME staining, but no dysplastic nevi, recurrent nevi, mitotically active nevi or traumatized nevi showed diffuse positive PRAME staining (4+) [7].

4.3. Interpretation of PRAME Staining

Although the first studies considered PRAME staining positive if it was diffusely present in over 76% of the tumor cells (4+) [1], more recently, Kunc et al. suggested in their meta-analysis that PRAME positivity should be interpreted as both 4+ (>75% of the cells) and 3+ (51–75% of the cells) cases in clinical practice due to better sensitivity with reasonable specificity [32]. In the study conducted by Rawson et al., 35% of the melanomas showed 4+ staining, an outcome closer to our study. If 3+ and 4+ represented positive staining, the percentage of PRAME-positive melanomas was 64%. No nevi showed 4+ staining, similarly to our study, while only 4% showed 3+ staining, with both cases being dysplastic nevi. Thus, the author suggested considering PRAME as positive for 3+ staining (present in 50–76% of the tumor cells) or 4+ staining (present in over 76% of the tumor cells [3]. As in our study no nevi showed 3+ or 4+ staining, we can say that the previous statement is also suitable for our research, although we found more melanomas with 4+ staining than 3+. Raghavan et al. considered PRAME as positive if staining was present in over 60% of the tumor cells in order to improve sensitivity. Their study included atypical melanocytic proliferations of indeterminate behavior and atypical Spitz tumors. In both groups, the expression of PRAME was low; only one atypical melanocytic proliferation was positive for PRAME staining in 10% of the cells, and one atypical Spitz tumor was positive for PRAME staining in over 60% of the cells [7]. O'Connor et al. suggested that the results should be interpreted as favoring nevus if PRAME staining is present in <25% of the cells, noncontributory if PRAME staining is present in 26–75% of the cells and favoring melanoma if PRAME staining is present in >76% of the cells. In their study, most melanomas were in situ and pT1a, like in our research. They found 64% of the melanomas positive for PRAME staining in >76% of the cells compared to 26% of the melanomas in our study. However, staining was performed on another automated platform (BenchMark ULTRA IHC/ISH System, Roche Diagnostics, Indianapolis, IN, USA) using PRAME EPR20330 antibody from Biocare Medical [33]. Alomari et al. described positive staining cases with 'hotspot' staining, defined as cases with diffuse staining (over 75% of the tumor cells) in at least two adjacent high-power fields [9]. Warbasse et al. considered cases 2+, 3+ and 4+ positive for PRAME staining with low sensitivity (29.6%) on a series of spitzoid and challenging melanocytic neoplasms [11]. Umano et al. recorded the percentage of positive cells, staining intensity (1+: slight positivity, 2+: moderate positivity and 3+: intense positivity) and the location of positive cells (junctional or intradermal) [34]. Forchhamer et al. observed a lower proportion of PRAME-positive melanoma cases in the pediatric population than in the adult population, suggesting that age might be considered when interpreting PRAME staining in melanomas [35]. In our study, no nevi stained 3+ or 4+, while the majority of melanomas stained 2+, 3+ or 4+ with the best accuracy and Youden's index for the 2+, 3+ and 4+ groups; therefore, we suggest considering at least 3+ as a threshold for positivity, but further studies are needed with a higher number of cases included. The results should be interpreted according to the dilution of the antibody, the technique used, the stainer vendor and the previous results of the given histopathological laboratory so as not to miss any thin melanomas.

5. Conclusions

PRAME immunohistochemistry is a powerful diagnostic tool for distinguishing melanocytic nevi from thin melanomas, but the interpretation should be performed carefully. Combining more immunohistochemistry antibodies would probably give more specific results with better sensitivity and specificity, but further studies are needed. We suggest a lower positivity threshold for PRAME staining to avoid missing any thin melanomas, but differences could appear between different histopathological laboratories.

Author Contributions: Conceptualization, I.Z., L.U., S.Ș. and R.C.; Methodology, L.U., S.Ș., B.P., P.Z. and D.C.; Formal analysis, Ș.C.V.; Investigation, I.Z. and P.Z.; Resources, I.Z., P.Z., D.C. and F.A.Z.; Data curation, I.Z.; Writing—original draft preparation, I.Z. and R.C.; Writing—review and editing, L.U., S.Ș., B.P., P.Z., D.C., F.A.Z. and Ș.C.V.; Visualization, B.P.; Supervision, R.C.; Project administration, I.Z. All authors have read and agreed to the published version of the manuscript.

Funding: This research received no external funding.

Institutional Review Board Statement: The study was conducted in accordance with the Declaration of Helsinki and approved by The Ethics Committee of Iuliu Hatieganu University of Medicine and Pharmacy Cluj-Napoca, Romania (protocol code 39 from 31 March 2023) for studies involving humans.

Informed Consent Statement: Informed consent was obtained from all subjects involved in the study.

Data Availability Statement: The datasets used and/or analyzed during the current study are available from the corresponding author on reasonable request.

Conflicts of Interest: The authors declare no conflicts of interest.

References

1. Lezcano, C.; Jungbluth, A.A.; Nehal, K.S.; Hollmann, T.J.; Busam, K.J. PRAME Expression in Melanocytic Tumors. *Am. J. Surg. Pathol.* **2018**, *42*, 1456–1465. [CrossRef]
2. WHO Classification. Available online: https://www.pathologyoutlines.com/topic/skintumormelanocyticWHO.html (accessed on 4 September 2024).
3. Rawson, R.V.; Shteinman, E.R.; Ansar, S.; Vergara, I.A.; Thompson, J.F.; Long, G.V.; Scolyer, R.A.; Wilmott, J.S. Diagnostic Utility of PRAME, P53 and 5-hmC Immunostaining for Distinguishing Melanomas from Naevi, Neurofibromas, Scars and Other Histological Mimics. *R. North. Shore Mater. Hosp.* **2022**, *4*, 863–873. [CrossRef]
4. Lezcano, C.; Jungbluth, A.A.; Busam, K.J. PRAME Immunohistochemistry as an Ancillary Test for the Assessment of Melanocytic Lesions. *Surg. Pathol. Clin.* **2021**, *14*, 165–175. [CrossRef]
5. Koh, S.S.; Lau, S.K.; Scapa, J.V.; Cassarino, D.S. PRAME Immunohistochemistry of Spitzoid Neoplasms. *J. Cutan. Pathol.* **2022**, *49*, 709–716. [CrossRef]
6. Gerami, P.; Benton, S.; Zhao, J.; Zhang, B.; Lampley, N.; Roth, A.; Boutko, A.; Olivares, S.; Busam, K.J. PRAME Expression Correlates with Genomic Aberration and Malignant Diagnosis of Spitzoid Melanocytic Neoplasms. *Am. J. Dermatopathol.* **2022**, *44*, 575. [CrossRef]
7. Raghavan, S.S.; Wang, J.Y.; Kwok, S.; Rieger, K.E.; Novoa, R.A.; Brown, R.A. PRAME Expression in Melanocytic Proliferations with Intermediate Histopathologic or Spitzoid Features. *J. Cutan. Pathol.* **2020**, *47*, 1123–1131. [CrossRef]
8. Turner, N.; Ko, C.J.; McNiff, J.M.; Galan, A. Pitfalls of PRAME Immunohistochemistry in a Large Series of Melanocytic and Nonmelanocytic Lesions With Literature Review. *Am. J. Dermatopathol.* **2024**, *46*, 21–30. [CrossRef]
9. Alomari, A.K.; Tharp, A.W.; Umphress, B.; Kowal, R.P. The Utility of PRAME Immunohistochemistry in the Evaluation of Challenging Melanocytic Tumors. *J. Cutan. Pathol.* **2021**, *48*, 1115–1123. [CrossRef]
10. Lezcano, C.; Jungbluth, A.A.; Busam, K.J. Comparison of Immunohistochemistry for PRAME with Cytogenetic Test Results in the Evaluation of Challenging Melanocytic Tumors. *Am. J. Surg. Pathol.* **2020**, *44*, 893. [CrossRef]
11. Warbasse, E.; Mehregan, D.; Utz, S.; Stansfield, R.B.; Abrams, J. PRAME Immunohistochemistry Compared to Traditional FISH Testing in Spitzoid Neoplasms and Other Difficult to Diagnose Melanocytic Neoplasms. *Front. Med.* **2023**, *10*, 1265827. [CrossRef]
12. McAfee, J.L.; Scarborough, R.; Jia, X.S.; Azzato, E.M.; Astbury, C.; Ronen, S.; Andea, A.A.; Billings, S.D.; Ko, J.S. Combined Utility of P16 and BRAF V600E in the Evaluation of Spitzoid Tumors: Superiority to PRAME and Correlation with FISH. *J. Cutan. Pathol.* **2023**, *50*, 155–168. [CrossRef]
13. Gradecki, S.E.; Valdes-Rodriguez, R.; Wick, M.R.; Gru, A.A. PRAME Immunohistochemistry as an Adjunct for Diagnosis and Histological Margin Assessment in Lentigo Maligna. *Histopathology* **2021**, *78*, 1000–1008. [CrossRef]
14. De Wet, J.; Plessis, P.J.D.; Schneider, J.W. Staged Excision of Lentigo Maligna of the Head and Neck: Assessing Surgical Excision Margins With Melan A, SOX10, and PRAME Immunohistochemistry. *Am. J. Dermatopathol.* **2023**, *45*, 107–112. [CrossRef]
15. Bittar, P.G.; Bittar, J.M.; Etzkorn, J.R.; Brewer, J.D.; Aizman, L.; Shin, T.M.; Sobanko, J.F.; Higgins, H.W.; Giordano, C.N.; Cohen, J.V.; et al. Systematic Review and Meta-Analysis of Local Recurrence Rates of Head and Neck Cutaneous Melanomas after Wide Local Excision, Mohs Micrographic Surgery, or Staged Excision. *J. Am. Acad. Dermatol.* **2021**, *85*, 681–692. [CrossRef]
16. Salih, R.; Ismail, F.; Orchard, G.E. Double Immunohistochemical Labelling of PRAME and Melan A in Slow Mohs Biopsy Margin Assessment of Lentigo Maligna and Lentigo Maligna Melanoma. *Br. J. Biomed. Sci.* **2024**, *81*, 12319. [CrossRef]

17. Grillini, M.; Ricci, C.; Pino, V.; Pedrini, S.; Fiorentino, M.; Corti, B. HMB45/PRAME, a Novel Double Staining for the Diagnosis of Melanocytic Neoplasms: Technical Aspects, Results, and Comparison With Other Commercially Available Staining (PRAME and Melan A/PRAME). *Appl. Immunohistochem. Mol. Morphol.* **2022**, *30*, 14–18. [CrossRef]
18. Carvajal, P.; Zoroquiain, P. PRAME/MELAN-A Double Immunostaining as a Diagnostic Tool for Conjunctival Melanocytic Lesions: A South American Experience. *Pathol. Res. Pract.* **2023**, *250*, 154776. [CrossRef]
19. Ricci, C.; Dika, E.; Ambrosi, F.; Lambertini, M.; Veronesi, G.; Barbara, C. Cutaneous Melanomas: A Single Center Experience on the Usage of Immunohistochemistry Applied for the Diagnosis. *Int. J. Mol. Sci.* **2022**, *23*, 5911. [CrossRef]
20. Lezcano, C.; Pulitzer, M.; Moy, A.P.; Hollmann, T.J.; Jungbluth, A.A.; Busam, K.J. Immunohistochemistry for PRAME in the Distinction of Nodal Nevi From Metastatic Melanoma. *Am. J. Surg. Pathol.* **2020**, *44*, 503–508. [CrossRef]
21. Rasic, D.; Korsgaard, N.; Marcussen, N.; Precht Jensen, E.M. Diagnostic Utility of Combining PRAME and HMB-45 Stains in Primary Melanocytic Tumors. *Ann. Diagn. Pathol.* **2023**, *67*, 152211. [CrossRef]
22. Bahmad, H.F.; Oh, K.S.; Alexis, J. Potential Diagnostic Utility of PRAME and P16 Immunohistochemistry in Melanocytic Nevi and Malignant Melanoma. *J. Cutan. Pathol.* **2023**, *50*, 763–772. [CrossRef]
23. Parra, O.; Ma, W.; Li, Z.; Coffing, B.N.; Linos, K.; LeBlanc, R.E.; Momtahen, S.; Sriharan, A.; Cloutier, J.M.; Wells, W.A.; et al. PRAME Expression in Cutaneous Melanoma Does Not Correlate with Disease-Specific Survival. *J. Cutan. Pathol.* **2023**, *50*, 903–912. [CrossRef]
24. Lo Bello, G.; Pini, G.M.; Giagnacovo, M.; Patriarca, C. PRAME Expression in 137 Primary Cutaneous Melanomas and Comparison with 38 Related Metastases. *Pathol. Res. Pract.* **2023**, *251*, 154915. [CrossRef]
25. Gassenmaier, M.; Hahn, M.; Metzler, G.; Bauer, J.; Yazdi, A.S.; Keim, U.; Garbe, C.; Wagner, N.B.; Forchhammer, S. Diffuse Prame Expression Is Highly Specific for Thin Melanomas in the Distinction from Severely Dysplastic Nevi but Does Not Distinguish Metastasizing from Non-Metastasizing Thin Melanomas. *Cancers* **2021**, *13*, 3864. [CrossRef]
26. Tio, D.; Willemsen, M.; Krebbers, G.; Kasiem, F.R.; Hoekzema, R.; Van Doorn, R.; Bekkenk, M.W.; Luiten, R.M. Differential Expression of Cancer Testis Antigens on Lentigo Maligna and Lentigo Maligna Melanoma. *Am. J. Dermatopathol.* **2020**, *42*, 625–627. [CrossRef]
27. Parra, O.; Linos, K.; Li, Z.; Yan, S. PRAME Expression in Melanocytic Lesions of the Nail. *J. Cutan. Pathol.* **2022**, *49*, 610–617. [CrossRef]
28. Rothrock, A.T.; Torres-Cabala, C.A.; Milton, D.R.; Cho, W.C.; Nagarajan, P.; Vanderbeck, K.; Curry, J.L.; Ivan, D.; Prieto, V.G.; Aung, P.P. Diagnostic Utility of PRAME Expression by Immunohistochemistry in Subungual and Non-Subungual Acral Melanocytic Lesions. *J. Cutan. Pathol.* **2022**, *49*, 859–867. [CrossRef]
29. McBride, J.D.; McAfee, J.L.; Piliang, M.; Bergfeld, W.F.; Fernandez, A.P.; Ronen, S.; Billings, S.D.; Ko, J.S. Preferentially Expressed Antigen in Melanoma and P16 Expression in Acral Melanocytic Neoplasms. *J. Cutan. Pathol.* **2022**, *49*, 220–230. [CrossRef]
30. Cazzato, G.; Cascardi, E.; Colagrande, A.; Belsito, V.; Lospalluti, L.; Foti, C.; Arezzo, F.; Dellino, M.; Casatta, N.; Lupo, C.; et al. PRAME Immunoexpression in 275 Cutaneous Melanocytic Lesions: A Double Institutional Experience. *Diagnostics* **2022**, *12*, 2197. [CrossRef]
31. Innocenti, L.; Scarpitta, R.; Corraro, S.; Ortenzi, V.; Bonadio, A.G.; Loggini, B.; De Ieso, K.; Naccarato, A.G.; Fanelli, G.N.; Scatena, C. Shedding Light on PRAME Expression in Dysplastic Nevi: A Cohort Study. *Virchows Arch.* **2023**, *485*, 97–104. [CrossRef]
32. Kunc, M.; Żemierowska, N.; Skowronek, F.; Biernat, W. Diagnostic Test Accuracy Meta-Analysis of PRAME in Distinguishing Primary Cutaneous Melanomas from Benign Melanocytic Lesions. *Histopathology* **2023**, *83*, 3–14. [CrossRef]
33. O'Connor, M.K.; Dai, H.; Fraga, G.R. PRAME Immunohistochemistry for Melanoma Diagnosis: A STARD-Compliant Diagnostic Accuracy Study. *J. Cutan. Pathol.* **2022**, *49*, 780–786. [CrossRef]
34. Umano, G.R.; Errico, M.E.; D'Onofrio, V.; Delehaye, G.; Trotta, L.; Spinelli, C.; Strambi, S.; Franco, R.; D'Abbronzo, G.; Ronchi, A.; et al. The Challenge of Melanocytic Lesions in Pediatric Patients: Clinical-Pathological Findings and the Diagnostic Value of PRAME. *Front. Oncol.* **2021**, *11*, 688410. [CrossRef]
35. Forchhammer, S.; Aebischer, V.; Lenders, D.; Seitz, C.M.; Schroeder, C.; Liebmann, A.; Abele, M.; Wild, H.; Bien, E.; Krawczyk, M.; et al. Characterization of PRAME Immunohistochemistry Reveals Lower Expression in Pediatric Melanoma Compared to Adult Melanoma. *Pigment. Cell Melanoma Res.* **2024**, *37*, 453–461. [CrossRef]

Disclaimer/Publisher's Note: The statements, opinions and data contained in all publications are solely those of the individual author(s) and contributor(s) and not of MDPI and/or the editor(s). MDPI and/or the editor(s) disclaim responsibility for any injury to people or property resulting from any ideas, methods, instructions or products referred to in the content.

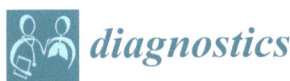 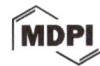

Article

Cutaneous Adverse Reactions and Survival Outcomes of Advanced Melanoma Treated with Immune Checkpoint Inhibitors in an Academic Medical Centre in Singapore

Agnes Yeok-Loo Lim [1], Jason Yongsheng Chan [2,3,*] and Choon Chiat Oh [1,2,*]

[1] Department of Dermatology, Singapore General Hospital, Singapore 169608, Singapore; agnes.lim@mohh.com.sg
[2] Duke-NUS Medical School, Singapore 169857, Singapore
[3] Division of Medical Oncology, National Cancer Centre Singapore, Singapore 168583, Singapore
* Correspondence: jason.chan.y.s@nccs.com.sg (J.Y.C.); oh.choon.chiat@singhealth.com.sg (C.C.O.)

Abstract: Programmed cell death-1 (PD1) inhibitors, a form of immune checkpoint inhibitor, are efficacious for metastatic melanoma but are associated with cutaneous adverse reactions (CARs). Studies in Europe and North America showed that CARs are associated with an increased overall survival. However, studies from Asia showed mixed results. There is a paucity of data regarding the efficacy of PD1 inhibitors and the effect of CARs on overall survival from Southeast Asia. A retrospective study of patients in the National Cancer Centre Singapore who were diagnosed with melanoma between 2015 and 2020 was conducted. Patients were included in the study if they had stage IV melanoma (advanced melanoma). Sixty-two patients were included in the study. The median age was 62.5 years and acral melanoma was the commonest subtype. Forty-three patients received PD1 inhibitors. Comparing patients who did not receive PD1 inhibitors to patients who received PD1 inhibitors, the former had a median overall survival of 6 months (95% CI: 5.07, 6.93), whereas the latter had a median overall survival of 21 months (95% CI: 13.33, 28.67; $p < 0.001$) (Hazard ratio 0.32; 95% CI: 0.16, 0.63; $p = 0.001$). Amongst patients who received PD1 inhibitors, patients who developed CARs had a greater median overall survival of 33 months (95% CI: 17.27, 48.73) compared to 15 months (95% CI: 9.20, 20.80; $p = 0.013$) for patients who did not (HR 0.29; 95% CI: 0.098, 0.834; $p = 0.022$). This study provides insight into the outcomes of metastatic melanoma in Singapore, and adds to the body of evidence supporting the use of PD1 inhibitors in Asians.

Keywords: melanoma; PD1 inhibitor; immunotherapy; cutaneous adverse reaction

1. Introduction

Metastatic melanoma is associated with poor prognosis and high mortality [1]. The development of immune checkpoint inhibitors (ICIs) targeting programmed cell death-1 (PD1) pathways has changed the landscape of melanoma therapy [2]. By blocking the inhibitory pathway between T lymphocytes and antigen-presenting cells or tumour cells, ICIs restore the immune response of effector T cells to tumour cells [2]. Nivolumab and pembrolizumab are examples of ICIs that bind PD1 on T cells, inhibiting the binding of PD1 to its ligand on tumour cells [2].

Multiple large-scale phase III trials studying the impact of PD1 inhibitors on metastatic melanoma outcomes have shown favourable results, but were conducted primarily in white populations [3–5]. As the spectrum of melanoma differs between Asian and white populations, it is important to investigate if these findings can be extended to Asian populations. However, there are limited data on the efficacy of PD1 inhibitors in Asian melanoma populations, with few studies on advanced melanoma conducted in Japan and China [6–10]. At present, there are no studies on PD1 inhibitor outcomes for metastatic melanoma in Singapore or Southeast Asia, where Singapore is located.

The use of immune checkpoint inhibitors can result in the development of immune-related adverse events. The development of cutaneous adverse reactions (CARs) was associated with increased overall survival in many studies of predominantly white patients in Europe [11–14], Canada [15] and America [16]. On the other hand, the impact of CARs on overall survival in Asian populations is less clear, with reports of CARs being associated with increased [6,17–19] or decreased [20] overall survival, with multiple reports showing inconclusive data [21,22]. Of note, there is a paucity of data from Southeast Asia.

The aims of this study are two-fold: to investigate the impact of anti-PD1 inhibitors on overall survival in metastatic melanoma, and to describe the cutaneous adverse reactions to anti-PD1 inhibitors in Singapore melanoma patients and their effect on overall survival.

2. Materials and Methods

A total of 195 patients with melanoma diagnosed between 2015 and 2021 at the National Cancer Centre Singapore (NCCS) were retrospectively analysed. Consent was obtained from the Institutional Review Board of the NCCS (CIRB: 2018/3065). The details of the patients' baseline demographics, clinical presentation, treatment and survival data were collected.

Staging was carried out according to the American Joint Committee on Cancer (AJCC) staging system (8th Edition) [23]. *BRAF* and *cKIT* mutations were analysed using next generation sequencing. Overall survival (OS) was computed from the date of diagnosis of stage IV melanoma to the date of demise or last follow-up (for surviving patients). Alive or lost to follow-up patients were censored at the last follow-up date. The median survival time was analysed using the Kaplan–Meier method and differences in survival curves between groups of patients were compared using the log-rank test. A univariate analysis of the association between prognostic factors and survival was performed using the Cox proportional hazard model. For continuous variables, the Mann–Whitney U test was used to compare the medians between the two groups. Counts and percentages were reported for categorical variables, and the chi-squared test or Fisher's exact test (when more than 20% of the cells had expected frequencies < 5) were used to test for differences between groups. A 2-sided *p*-value < 0.05 was considered statistically significant. Statistical analyses were performed using the IBM SPSS Statistics software version 28.

3. Results

3.1. Patient Demographics

A total of 62 patients with stage IV melanoma diagnosed between 2015 and 2021 at the National Cancer Centre Singapore (NCCS) were identified (Table 1). Patients who were diagnosed at stage IV or who subsequently progressed to stage IV disease were included in the study. The median age was 62.5 years. There was a predominance of Chinese (74.2%) followed by Malay patients (9.7%), reflecting the ethnic composition of Singapore. Acral melanoma was the commonest subtype seen (38.7%), followed by cutaneous (33.9%) and mucosal melanoma (27.4%). Further details of each subtype can be found in Supplementary Tables S1 and S2. Most patients had metastases in non-central nervous system (CNS) visceral organs (74.2%). A subset of patients opted to undergo testing for *BRAF* and/or *cKIT* mutations. Amongst the patients who were tested for *BRAF* or *cKIT* mutations, 28% had *BRAF* mutations and 19.5% had *cKIT* mutations.

Forty-three patients received treatment with PD1 inhibitors, either pembrolizumab (22.6%), nivolumab (24.2%) or both (22.6%). Nineteen patients did not receive PD1 inhibitors; these patients were given the best supportive care (seven patients), dabrafenib with trametinib (four patients), imatinib (three patients), other systemic therapies (three patients) or radiotherapy (three patients) alone or in combination with other previously mentioned therapies. For the entire cohort of 62 patients, the median overall survival was 10 months, and the median follow-up time was 9.5 months (Table 1).

Table 1. Stage IV melanoma population characteristics ($n = 62$).

Characteristics	Number (%)
Median age (range), years	62.5 (30–86)
Gender	
Female	39 (62.9)
Male	23 (37.1)
Ethnicity	
Chinese	46 (74.2)
Malay	6 (9.7)
Indian	2 (3.2)
White	3 (4.8)
Others	5 (8.1)
Subtype	
Acral	24 (38.7)
Cutaneous	21 (33.9)
Mucosal	17 (27.4)
M category	
1a	11 (17.7)
1b	16 (25.8)
1c	30 (48.4)
1d	5 (8.1)
BRAF status [a]	
Wild type	36 (72)
Mutation	14 (28)
cKIT status [b]	
Wild type	33 (80.5)
Mutation	8 (19.5)
PD1 inhibitor	
Pembrolizumab	14 (22.6)
Nivolumab	15 (24.2)
Both	14 (22.6)
None	19 (30.6)
Any administration of systemic non-PD1 therapy	
No	34 (54.8)
Yes	28 (45.2)
Dabrafenib/Trametinib	8
Imatinib	6
Clinical Trial drug	5
Paclitaxel/Carboplatin	4
Temozolamide	2
Decarbazine	1
Vemurafenib	1
Encorafenib/Binimetinib	1
Overall survival (range), months	10 (1–76)
Follow-up time (range), months	9.5 (1–75)

[a] A total of 12 patients were not tested for *BRAF* mutations. [b] A total of 21 patients were not tested for *cKIT* mutations.

3.2. Survival Analysis

The prognostic impact of age, gender, ethnicity, melanoma subtype, M category (extent of distant metastasis), *BRAF* mutational status, *cKIT* mutational status, PD1 inhibitor therapy and the use of non-PD1 inhibitor systemic therapies on overall survival was analysed. In univariable analysis, only the use of the PD1 inhibitor was associated with increased overall survival (Table 2). Comparing patients who did not receive PD1 inhibitors to patients who received PD1 inhibitors, the former had a median overall survival of 6 months, whereas the latter had a median overall survival of 21 months ($p < 0.001$, Figure 1a, Table 3). Amongst those who received PD1 inhibitors, 25 patients received PD1 inhibitors alone, and 18 also received non-PD1 therapy. The median overall survival for patients receiving PD1 inhibitors alone was 25 months compared to 17 months for patients who also received other therapies ($p = 0.197$). Although patients who received PD1 inhibitors had a lower median age (60 years) than patients who did not receive PD1 inhibitors (69 years, $p = 0.008$), age was not a significant prognostic factor in the univariate analysis for overall survival (Table 2). In addition, the multivariable analysis of overall survival in patients receiving PD1 inhibitors showed that age was not a significant factor in affecting overall survival, whereas the development of cutaneous adverse reactions was significant (Supplementary Table S3).

Table 2. Univariate analysis for overall survival in stage IV melanoma.

Characteristics	E/N	Hazard Ratio (95% CI)	p-Value
Age at diagnosis			
<60 years old	12/22	1	ref
≥60 years old	28/40	1.74 (0.87, 3.47)	0.119
Gender			
Female	24/39	1	ref
Male	16/23	0.86 (0.64, 1.22)	0.450
Ethnicity			
Chinese	31/46	1	ref
Malay	4/6	1.10 (0.36, 3.13)	0.862
Indian	2/2	1.02 (0.24, 4.34)	0.983
White	2/3	0.72 (0.17, 3.03)	0.649
Others	1/5	1.73 (0.22, 13.69)	0.605
Subtype			
Acral	14/24	1	ref
Cutaneous	16/21	1.61 (0.78, 3.32)	0.195
Mucosal	10/17	1.13 (0.50, 2.56)	0.762
M category			
1a	6/11	1	ref
1b	9/16	0.82 (0.29, 2.33)	0.704
1c	22/30	2.10 (0.85, 5.23)	0.110
1d	3/5	1.48 (0.36, 6.05)	0.586
BRAF status			
Wild type	24/36	1	ref
Mutation	9/14	1.72 (0.78, 3.78)	0.176
cKIT status			
Wild type	21/33	1	ref
Mutation	6/8	1.45 (0.57, 3.71)	0.436
PD1 inhibitor			
No	14/19	1	ref
Yes	26/43	0.32 (0.16, 0.63)	0.001
Any administration of systemic non-PD1 therapy			
No	18/34	1	ref
Yes	22/28	1.55 (0.82, 2.95)	0.182

CI: Confidence interval. p value calculated using the Cox proportional hazards model. E/N: Events/Number of cases. Ref: reference.

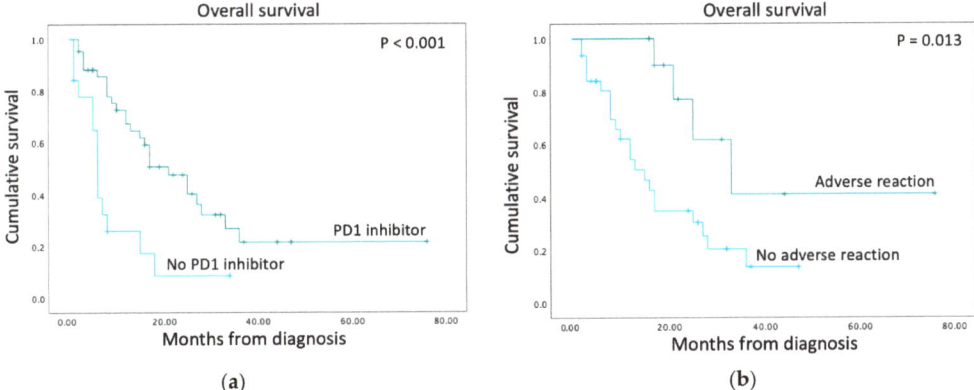

Figure 1. Kaplan–Meier curves for overall survival. (**a**) Patients who received PD1 inhibitors (n = 43) had increased overall survival compared to patients who did not (n = 19). (**b**) For patients who received PD1 inhibitors, the development of cutaneous adverse reactions (n = 11) was associated with increased overall survival compared to no adverse reactions (n = 32). p values were calculated using the log-rank test.

Table 3. Comparing patients who received PD1 vs. no PD1 inhibitor.

Characteristics	No PD1 (n = 19)	PD1 (n = 43)	p-Value
Median age (range), years	69 (30–86)	60 (31–76)	0.008 [a]
Gender			
Female	10 (52.6)	29 (67.4)	0.266 [b]
Male	9 (47.4)	14 (32.6)	
Ethnicity			
Chinese	14 (73.7)	32 (74.4)	0.186 [c]
Malay	0 (0)	6 (14.0)	
Indian	1 (5.3)	1 (2.3)	
White	2 (10.5)	1 (2.3)	
Others	2 (10.5)	3 (7.0)	
Subtype			
Acral	8 (42.1)	16 (37.2)	0.830 [c]
Cutaneous	7 (36.8)	14 (32.6)	
Mucosal	4 (21.1)	13 (30.2)	
M category			
1a	2 (10.5)	9 (20.9)	0.570 [c]
1b	4 (21.1)	12 (27.9)	
1c	12 (63.2)	18 (41.9)	
1d	1 (5.3)	4 (9.3)	
BRAF status			
Wild type	9 (60.0)	27 (77.1)	0.304 [c]
Mutation	6 (40.0)	8 (22.9)	
cKIT status			
Wild type	7 (70.0)	26 (83.9)	0.378 [c]
Mutation	3 (30.0)	5 (16.1)	
Any administration of systemic non-PD1 therapy			
No	9 (47.7)	25 (58.1)	0.432 [b]
Yes	10 (52.6)	18 (41.9)	
Median overall survival, months (95% CI)	6 (5.07, 6.93)	21 (13.33, 28.67)	<0.001 [d]

[a] p-value calculated using Mann–Whitney U test. [b] p-value estimated using chi-squared test. [c] p-value estimated using Fisher's exact test. [d] p-value estimated using log-rank test. CI, confidence interval.

3.3. Cutaneous Adverse Reactions

There are limited data from Asia regarding the impact of cutaneous adverse reactions on overall survival. In this study, 11 patients who received PD1 inhibitors developed cutaneous adverse reactions whereas 32 patients did not. Comparing the two populations, patients who developed CARs had a greater median overall survival of 33 months (95% CI: 17.27, 48.73) compared to 15 months (95% CI: 9.20, 20.80; $p = 0.013$) for patients who did not develop CARs (HR 0.29; 95% CI: 0.098, 0.834; $p = 0.022$, Table 4, Figure 1b). A comparison of the two groups of patients showed that there was no difference in age, gender, ethnicity, melanoma subtype, M category, *BRAF* mutational status, *cKIT* mutational status and the use of non-PD1 inhibitor systemic therapies before or after PD1-inhibitor treatment (Table 4). Patients who developed CARs were predominantly ethnically Chinese, although this was not significant when compared with patients who did not develop CARs (Table 4).

Table 4. Comparing patients with cutaneous adverse reactions vs. no cutaneous adverse reactions to PD1 inhibitors.

Characteristics	No CAR (n = 32)	CAR (n = 11)	p-Value
Median age (range)	60.5 (31–76)	58 (33–74)	0.666 [a]
Gender			
Female	23 (71.9)	6 (54.5)	0.457 [b]
Male	9 (28.1)	5 (45.5)	
Ethnicity			
Chinese	22 (68.8)	10 (90.9)	0.757 [b]
Malay	5 (15.6)	1 (9.1)	
Indian	1 (3.1)	0 (0)	
White	1 (3.1)	0 (0)	
Others	3 (9.4)	0 (0)	
Subtype			
Acral	9 (28.1)	7 (63.6)	0.079 [b]
Cutaneous	13 (40.6)	1 (9.1)	
Mucosal	10 (31.3)	3 (27.3)	
M category			
1a	6 (18.8)	3 (27.2)	0.631 [b]
1b	8 (25.0)	4 (36.4)	
1c	14 (43.8)	4 (36.4)	
1d	4 (12.5)	0 (0)	
BRAF status			
Wild type	19 (70.4)	8 (100)	0.154 [b]
Mutation	8 (29.6)	0 (0)	
cKIT status			
Wild type	18 (85.7)	8 (80.0)	0.999 [b]
Mutation	3 (14.3)	2 (20.0)	
Any administration of systemic non-PD1 therapy			
No	17 (53.1)	8 (72.7)	0.309 [b]
Yes	15 (46.9)	3 (27.3)	
PD1 inhibitor line of treatment			
First line	24 (75)	9 (81.8)	0.999 [b]
Second line or later	8 (25)	2 (18.2)	
Median overall survival, months (95% CI)	15 (9.20, 20.80)	33 (17.27, 48.73)	0.013 [c]

CAR: Cutaneous adverse reaction. CI, confidence interval. [a] p-value calculated using Mann–Whitney U test. [b] p-value estimated using Fisher's exact test. [c] p-value estimated using log-rank test.

The commonest cutaneous adverse reaction to PD1 inhibitors was vitiligo (four patients), followed by eczema exacerbation (three patients), lichenoid dermatitis (two patients), psoriasiform eruption (one patient) and exanthem (one patient) (Table 5). One patient had both vitiligo and bullous pemphigoid. Skin biopsies for histological analyses were performed for patients presenting with bullae, lichenoid and psoriasiform eruptions, which all showed dermal eosinophils, supporting a drug-induced cause of the cutaneous manifestations (Table 5). Cutaneous adverse reactions developed following both pembrolizumab and nivolumab use, and in all melanoma subtypes, although there was an over-representation of acral melanoma cases. One patient had to discontinue PD1 inhibitor therapy due to pneumonitis and another patient discontinued PD1 inhibitor therapy due to extensive bullous pemphigoid, which was resolved with the use of topical corticosteroids and oral doxycycline.

Table 5. Cutaneous adverse reactions to PD1 inhibitors.

Cutaneous Adverse Reaction	No. of Patients	PD1 Inhibitor	Melanoma Subtype	Histology of Skin Reaction	Management
Vitiligo	3 (27.3%)	Pembrolizumab then nivolumab and ipilimumab	Mucosal	Not performed	Continue PD1 inhibitor
		Nivolumab	Mucosal	Not performed	Continue PD1 inhibitor
		Pembrolizumab	Acral	Not performed	Continue PD1 inhibitor
Vitiligo and bullous pemphigoid (BP)	1 (9.1%)	Nivolumab	Acral	Subepidermal blister with dermal lymphocytes, histiocytes and eosinophils	Topical corticosteroids, oral doxycycline. Stopped PD1 inhibitor (bullous pemphigoid)
Eczema exacerbation	3 (27.3%)	Pembrolizumab then nivolumab and ipilimumab	Cutaneous	Not performed	Topical corticosteroids, continue PD1 inhibitor
		Nivolumab	Acral	Not performed	Topical corticosteroids, continue PD1 inhibitor
		Nivolumab then pembrolizumab	Acral	Not performed	Topical corticosteroids, continue PD1 inhibitor
Lichenoid dermatitis	2 (18.1%)	Pembrolizumab then nivolumab	Acral	Interface dermatitis with subcorneal neutrophilic collections and perivascular dermal lymphocytic infiltrate with plasma cells and eosinophils	Topical corticosteroids, continue PD1 inhibitor
		Nivolumab	Acral	Irregular acanthosis and spongiosis with superficial dermal oedema and chronic inflammatory infiltrate with eosinophils	Topical corticosteroids, continue PD1 inhibitor
Psoriasiform eruption	1 (9.1%)	Nivolumab	Acral	Irregular psoriasiform hyperplasia with focal mild spongiosis where a small collection of neutrophils is seen in the upper epidermis. Superficial perivascular infiltrate of lymphocytes and eosinophils	Topical corticosteroids, stopped PD1 inhibitor (pneumonitis)
Exanthem	1 (9.1%)	Nivolumab	Mucosal	Not performed	Topical corticosteroids, continue PD1 inhibitor

4. Discussion

Given that the population in Asia has been projected to grow by 44% between 2000 and 2050 [24], the absolute number of melanoma cases can also be expected to increase, highlighting the need for more data on the treatment of melanoma in Asian populations. This study provides insight into the demographics and outcomes of metastatic melanoma in Singapore. Previous studies on melanoma have limited data on stage IV melanoma, and no data on PD1 inhibitor outcomes [25–28]. In this study, acral melanoma was the commonest subtype, whereas in previous studies, non-acral cutaneous melanoma was commonest when the study population predominantly consisted of stage I-III melanoma and mucosal, ocular and melanoma of unknown primary were included in the study population [26]. In other Singaporean studies of only cutaneous melanoma at predominantly stage I-III, acral lentiginous melanoma was the most common histological subtype [25,28,29]. In studies involving mainly white patients, non-acral cutaneous melanoma was the most common subtype in advanced melanoma [30], reinforcing the differences in melanoma subtypes between ethnicities.

In this study, the median overall survival of patients with PD1 inhibitors was 21 months (median follow-up 9.5 months), which is similar to studies in Japan (OS = 16.93 months, median follow-up unknown) [6] and China (OS = 16 months, median follow-up 11 months) [8]. Mucosal melanoma constituted the highest proportion of patients in the Japanese study [6], whereas acral melanoma was predominant in the Chinese study [8], similar to this study. In the landmark CheckMate 037 study, which consisted primarily of patients from Europe and America, the median overall survival of patients on nivolumab was 15.7 months with a median follow-up of 2 years, but the melanoma subtypes were not stated [5]. In terms of the long-term follow-up of results, the CheckMate 067 trial, which also consisted primarily of white patients from Europe and America, followed 945 patients for at least 5 years, and the median overall survival was more than 60 months for the nivolumab with ipilimumab group [3]. A small Japanese study of 24 patients with mainly acral melanoma treated with nivolumab showed an overall survival of 32.9 months with a median follow-up of 32.9 months and a longer overall survival than other Asian studies; this could be attributed to the longer follow-up time [7]. Larger studies of Asian melanoma patients with longer follow-up durations are required to compare longer-term results with PD1 inhibitors between Asian and white populations.

A subset of patients in this study developed cutaneous adverse reactions to PD1 inhibitors, and this was associated with an increased overall survival, similar to findings from a study in China [18] and some studies from Japan [6,17,19], but differing from other studies from Japan and Taiwan [20,22,31]. Larger studies are required for the generalisation to other Asian populations.

The pathophysiology underlying the association between CARs and overall survival has not been completely elucidated. There are several postulated mechanisms to explain the association between CARs due to PD1 inhibitors and overall survival. One possible mechanism involves shared antigens between melanocytes and melanoma cells, such as tyrosinase and related proteins TRP-1 and TRP-2, gp100 and Melan-A [32]. It is possible that the development of vitiligo indicates an immune reaction towards both normal melanocytes and melanoma cells following PD1 inhibitor administration. In addition, it has been demonstrated that PD1 blockade overcomes T cell exhaustion, leading to the activation of the T cell population both in the tumour microenvironment and systemically [33,34]. As eczema, psoriasis, lichenoid eruptions and vitiligo are T-cell-mediated processes [35], the development of such cutaneous reactions might indicate a robust anti-tumour response and thus improved outcomes.

A previous population-based epidemiological study showed that mucosal melanoma from different anatomical sites exhibited different survival outcomes, with localised pharyngeal, gastroesophageal and vaginal mucosal melanoma exhibiting outcomes that were as poor as metastatic disease, despite aggressive local therapy [36]. Our study included 17 cases of mucosal melanoma, which consisted of melanoma of the anorectum (4 cases), head and neck (6 cases), oesophagus (1 case) and vagina/vulva (6 cases) (Supplementary Table S1). Another study of mucosal melanoma in Chinese patients found genetic variation in mucosal melanoma samples across different body sites, with a reduced overall survival in oesophagus and small bowel melanoma cases [37]. The small number of cases in each site in our study precludes a similar analysis, which would be beneficial in future studies.

Our study has limitations. This was a retrospective study with inherent limitations of incomplete data collection, especially with regard to other epidemiological risk factors such as family history and lifetime sun exposure. Nine cases were lost to follow-up. The number of cases in our study was small, but this is a reflection of the low incidence of melanoma in our population.

5. Conclusions

In conclusion, this study adds to the growing body of evidence on the benefit of PD1 inhibitors in Asians. Our study also demonstrates that the development of cutaneous adverse reactions can be associated with an increased overall survival in some patients with metastatic melanoma. Future mechanistic studies would be helpful to tease out the specific pathophysiology underlying this association and aid the prognostication of response to PD1 inhibitors.

Supplementary Materials: The following supporting information can be downloaded at: https://www.mdpi.com/article/10.3390/diagnostics14151601/s1, Table S1: Sites of melanoma; Table S2: Histological details of cutaneous melanoma cases; Table S3: Analysis of factors affecting overall survival in patients receiving PD1 inhibitors using the multivariable Cox proportional hazard regression model (n = 43).

Author Contributions: Conceptualisation, A.Y.-L.L., J.Y.C. and C.C.O.; methodology, A.Y.-L.L., J.Y.C. and C.C.O.; formal analysis, A.Y.-L.L., J.Y.C. and C.C.O.; investigation, A.Y.-L.L., J.Y.C. and C.C.O.; writing—original draft preparation, A.Y.-L.L., J.Y.C. and C.C.O.; writing—review and editing, A.Y.-L.L., J.Y.C. and C.C.O.; visualisation, A.Y.-L.L.; funding acquisition, J.Y.C. and C.C.O. All authors have read and agreed to the published version of the manuscript.

Funding: This work was supported by the Singapore Ministry of Health's National Medical Research Council under its Transition Award (TA21jun-0005) and RTF Seed Fund (SEEDFD21jun-0002) (for J.Y.C.), and Transition Award (TA21jun-0002) and RTF Fund (RTF21nov-004) (for C.C.O.).

Institutional Review Board Statement: The study was conducted in accordance with the Declaration of Helsinki and approved by the Institutional Review Board of the National Cancer Centre Singapore (protocol code 2018/3065, approval date 05/02/2024).

Informed Consent Statement: Informed consent was obtained from all subjects involved in the study.

Data Availability Statement: The original contributions presented in the study are included in the article/Supplementary Materials; further inquiries can be directed to the corresponding authors.

Conflicts of Interest: The authors declare no conflicts of interest.

References

1. Ferlay, J.; Colombet, M.; Soerjomataram, I.; Mathers, C.; Parkin, D.M.; Piñeros, M.; Znaor, A.; Bray, F. Estimating the Global Cancer Incidence and Mortality in 2018: GLOBOCAN Sources and Methods. *Int. J. Cancer* **2019**, *144*, 1941–1953. [CrossRef] [PubMed]
2. Sanmamed, M.F.; Chen, L. A Paradigm Shift in Cancer Immunotherapy: From Enhancement to Normalization. *Cell* **2018**, *175*, 313–326. [CrossRef] [PubMed]
3. Larkin, J.; Chiarion-Sileni, V.; Gonzalez, R.; Grob, J.-J.; Rutkowski, P.; Lao, C.D.; Cowey, C.L.; Schadendorf, D.; Wagstaff, J.; Dummer, R.; et al. Five-Year Survival with Combined Nivolumab and Ipilimumab in Advanced Melanoma. *N. Engl. J. Med.* **2019**, *381*, 1535–1546. [CrossRef] [PubMed]
4. Larkin, J.; Chiarion-Sileni, V.; Gonzalez, R.; Grob, J.-J.; Cowey, C.L.; Lao, C.D.; Schadendorf, D.; Dummer, R.; Smylie, M.; Rutkowski, P.; et al. Combined Nivolumab and Ipilimumab or Monotherapy in Untreated Melanoma. *N. Engl. J. Med.* **2015**, *373*, 23–34. [CrossRef] [PubMed]
5. Larkin, J.; Minor, D.; D'Angelo, S.; Neyns, B.; Smylie, M.; Miller, W.H., Jr.; Gutzmer, R.; Linette, G.; Chmielowski, B.; Lao, C.D.; et al. Overall Survival in Patients with Advanced Melanoma Who Received Nivolumab Versus Investigator's Choice Chemotherapy in CheckMate 037: A Randomized, Controlled, Open-Label Phase III Trial. *J. Clin. Oncol.* **2017**, *36*, 383–390. [CrossRef]
6. Yamazaki, N.; Takenouchi, T.; Nakamura, Y.; Takahashi, A.; Namikawa, K.; Kitano, S.; Fujita, T.; Kubota, K.; Yamanaka, T.; Kawakami, Y. Prospective Observational Study of the Efficacy of Nivolumab in Japanese Patients with Advanced Melanoma (CREATIVE Study). *Jpn. J. Clin. Oncol.* **2021**, *51*, 1232–1241. [CrossRef] [PubMed]
7. Yamazaki, N.; Kiyohara, Y.; Uhara, H.; Uehara, J.; Fujisawa, Y.; Takenouchi, T.; Otsuka, M.; Uchi, H.; Ihn, H.; Hatsumichi, M.; et al. Long-term Follow up of Nivolumab in Previously Untreated Japanese Patients with Advanced or Recurrent Malignant Melanoma. *Cancer Sci.* **2019**, *110*, 1995–2003. [CrossRef] [PubMed]
8. Wen, X.; Ding, Y.; Li, J.; Zhao, J.; Peng, R.; Li, D.; Zhu, B.; Wang, Y.; Zhang, X.; Zhang, X. The Experience of Immune Checkpoint Inhibitors in Chinese Patients with Metastatic Melanoma: A Retrospective Case Series. *Cancer Immunol. Immunother.* **2017**, *66*, 1153–1162. [CrossRef] [PubMed]

9. Nakamura, Y.; Namikawa, K.; Yoshino, K.; Yoshikawa, S.; Uchi, H.; Goto, K.; Nakamura, Y.; Fukushima, S.; Kiniwa, Y.; Takenouchi, T.; et al. Anti-PD1 Checkpoint Inhibitor Therapy in Acral Melanoma: A Multicenter Study of 193 Japanese Patients. *Ann. Oncol.* 2020, *31*, 1198–1206. [CrossRef]
10. Zhao, L.; Yang, Y.; Ma, B.; Li, W.; Li, T.; Han, L.; Zhang, Y.; Shang, Y.-M.; Lin, H.; Gao, Q. Factors Influencing the Efficacy of Anti-PD-1 Therapy in Chinese Patients with Advanced Melanoma. *J. Oncol.* 2019, *2019*, 6454989. [CrossRef]
11. Bottlaender, L.; Amini-Adle, M.; Maucort-Boulch, D.; Robinson, P.; Thomas, L.; Dalle, S. Cutaneous Adverse Events: A Predictor of Tumour Response under Anti-PD-1 Therapy for Metastatic Melanoma, a Cohort Analysis of 189 Patients. *J. Eur. Acad. Dermatol. Venereol.* 2020, *34*, 2096–2105. [CrossRef] [PubMed]
12. Dousset, L.; Pacaud, A.; Barnetche, T.; Kostine, M.; Dutriaux, C.; Pham-Ledard, A.; Beylot-Barry, M.; Gérard, E.; Prey, S.; Andreu, N.; et al. Analysis of Tumor Response and Clinical Factors Associated with Vitiligo in Patients Receiving Anti–Programmed Cell Death-1 Therapies for Melanoma: A Cross-Sectional Study. *JAAD Int.* 2021, *5*, 112–120. [CrossRef]
13. Indini, A.; Guardo, L.D.; Cimminiello, C.; Prisciandaro, M.; Randon, G.; Braud, F.D.; Vecchio, M.D. Immune-Related Adverse Events Correlate with Improved Survival in Patients Undergoing Anti-PD1 Immunotherapy for Metastatic Melanoma. *J. Cancer Res. Clin.* 2019, *145*, 511–521. [CrossRef] [PubMed]
14. Villa-Crespo, L.; Podlipnik, S.; Anglada, N.; Izquierdo, C.; Giavedoni, P.; Iglesias, P.; Dominguez, M.; Aya, F.; Arance, A.; Malvehy, J.; et al. Timeline of Adverse Events during Immune Checkpoint Inhibitors for Advanced Melanoma and Their Impacts on Survival. *Cancers* 2022, *14*, 1237. [CrossRef] [PubMed]
15. Holstead, R.G.; Kartolo, B.A.; Hopman, W.M.; Baetz, T.D. Impact of the Development of Immune Related Adverse Events in Metastatic Melanoma Treated with PD-1 Inhibitors. *Melanoma Res.* 2021, *31*, 258–263. [CrossRef]
16. Freeman-Keller, M.; Kim, Y.; Cronin, H.; Richards, A.; Gibney, G.; Weber, J.S. Nivolumab in Resected and Unresectable Metastatic Melanoma: Characteristics of Immune-Related Adverse Events and Association with Outcomes. *Clin. Cancer Res.* 2016, *22*, 886–894. [CrossRef] [PubMed]
17. Nakamura, Y.; Tanaka, R.; Asami, Y.; Teramoto, Y.; Imamura, T.; Sato, S.; Maruyama, H.; Fujisawa, Y.; Matsuya, T.; Fujimoto, M.; et al. Correlation between Vitiligo Occurrence and Clinical Benefit in Advanced Melanoma Patients Treated with Nivolumab: A Multi-institutional Retrospective Study. *J. Dermatol.* 2017, *44*, 117–122. [CrossRef]
18. Zhao, J.-J.; Wen, X.-Z.; Ding, Y.; Li, D.-D.; Zhu, B.-Y.; Li, J.-J.; Weng, D.-S.; Zhang, X.; Zhang, X.-S. Association between Immune-Related Adverse Events and Efficacy of PD-1 Inhibitors in Chinese Patients with Advanced Melanoma. *Aging* 2020, *12*, 10663–10675. [CrossRef] [PubMed]
19. Yamazaki, N.; Kiyohara, Y.; Uhara, H.; Uehara, J.; Fujimoto, M.; Takenouchi, T.; Otsuka, M.; Uchi, H.; Ihn, H.; Minami, H. Efficacy and Safety of Nivolumab in Japanese Patients with Previously Untreated Advanced Melanoma: A Phase II Study. *Cancer Sci.* 2017, *108*, 1223–1230. [CrossRef]
20. Fujisawa, Y.; Yoshino, K.; Otsuka, A.; Funakoshi, T.; Uchi, H.; Fujimura, T.; Matsushita, S.; Hata, H.; Okuhira, H.; Tanaka, R.; et al. Retrospective Study of Advanced Melanoma Patients Treated with Ipilimumab after Nivolumab: Analysis of 60 Japanese Patients. *J. Dermatol. Sci.* 2018, *89*, 60–66. [CrossRef]
21. Wu, C.-E.; Yang, C.-K.; Peng, M.-T.; Huang, P.-W.; Lin, Y.-F.; Cheng, C.-Y.; Chang, Y.-Y.; Chen, H.-W.; Hsieh, J.-J.; Chang, J.W.-C. Immune Checkpoint Inhibitors for Advanced Melanoma: Experience at a Single Institution in Taiwan. *Front. Oncol.* 2020, *10*, 905. [CrossRef] [PubMed]
22. Kobayashi, T.; Iwama, S.; Yasuda, Y.; Okada, N.; Okuji, T.; Ito, M.; Onoue, T.; Goto, M.; Sugiyama, M.; Tsunekawa, T.; et al. Pituitary Dysfunction Induced by Immune Checkpoint Inhibitors Is Associated with Better Overall Survival in Both Malignant Melanoma and Non-Small Cell Lung Carcinoma: A Prospective Study. *J. Immunother. Cancer* 2020, *8*, e000779. [CrossRef] [PubMed]
23. Amin, M.B.; Edge, S.B.; Greene, F.L.; Byrd, D.R.; Brookland, R.K.; Washington, M.K.; Gershenwald, J.E.; Compton, C.C.; Hess, K.R.; Sullivan, D.C.; et al. *AJCC Cancer Staging Manual*, 8th ed.; Springer: Berlin/Heidelberg, Germany, 2017; ISBN 978-3-319-40617-6.
24. Chang, J.W.; Guo, J.; Hung, C.; Lu, S.; Shin, S.J.; Quek, R.; Ying, A.; Ho, G.F.; Nguyen, H.S.; Dhabhar, B.; et al. Sunrise in Melanoma Management: Time to Focus on Melanoma Burden in Asia. *Asia Pac. J. Clin. Oncol.* 2017, *13*, 423–427. [CrossRef] [PubMed]
25. Yeo, P.M.; Lim, Z.V.; Tan, W.D.V.; Zhao, X.; Chia, H.Y.; Tan, S.H.; Teo, M.C.C.; Tan, M.W.P. Melanoma in Singapore: A 20-Year Review of Disease and Treatment Outcomes. *Ann. Acad. Medicine Singap.* 2021, *50*, 456–466. [CrossRef] [PubMed]
26. Teh, Y.L.; Goh, W.L.; Tan, S.H.; Yong, G.; Sairi, A.N.H.; Soo, K.C.; Ong, J.; Chia, C.; Tan, G.; Soeharno, H.; et al. Treatment and Outcomes of Melanoma in Asia: Results from the National Cancer Centre Singapore. *Asia Pac. J. Clin. Oncol.* 2017, *14*, e95–e102. [CrossRef]
27. Tan, E.; Chua, S.H.; Lim, J.T.; Goh, C.L. Malignant Melanoma Seen in a Tertiary Dermatological Centre, Singapore. *Ann. Acad. Med. Singap.* 2001, *30*, 414–418.
28. Lee, H.Y.; Chay, W.Y.; Tang, M.B.; Chio, M.T.; Tan, S.H. Melanoma: Differences between Asian and Caucasian Patients. *Ann. Acad. Med. Singap.* 2012, *41*, 17–20. [CrossRef]
29. Lee, H.Y.; Oh, C.C. Melanoma in Singapore: Putting Our Best Foot Forward! *Ann. Acad. Med. Singap.* 2021, *50*, 454–455. [CrossRef]
30. Bai, X.; Shoushtari, A.N.; Warner, A.B.; Si, L.; Tang, B.; Cui, C.; Yang, X.; Wei, X.; Quach, H.T.; Cann, C.G.; et al. Benefit and Toxicity of Programmed Death-1 Blockade Vary by Ethnicity in Patients with Advanced Melanoma: An International Multicentre Observational Study*. *Brit. J. Dermatol.* 2022, *187*, 401–410. [CrossRef]

31. Wu, C.-E.; Yang, C.-K.; Peng, M.-T.; Huang, P.-W.; Chang, C.-F.; Yeh, K.-Y.; Chen, C.-B.; Wang, C.-L.; Hsu, C.-W.; Chen, I.-W.; et al. The Association between Immune-Related Adverse Events and Survival Outcomes in Asian Patients with Advanced Melanoma Receiving Anti-PD-1 Antibodies. *BMC Cancer* **2020**, *20*, 1018. [CrossRef]
32. Byrne, K.T.; Turk, M.J. New Perspectives on the Role of Vitiligo in Immune Responses to Melanoma. *Oncotarget* **2011**, *2*, 684–694. [CrossRef] [PubMed]
33. Taube, J.M.; Klein, A.; Brahmer, J.R.; Xu, H.; Pan, X.; Kim, J.H.; Chen, L.; Pardoll, D.M.; Topalian, S.L.; Anders, R.A. Association of PD-1, PD-1 Ligands, and Other Features of the Tumor Immune Microenvironment with Response to Anti–PD-1 Therapy. *Clin. Cancer Res.* **2014**, *20*, 5064–5074. [CrossRef] [PubMed]
34. Spitzer, M.H.; Carmi, Y.; Reticker-Flynn, N.E.; Kwek, S.S.; Madhireddy, D.; Martins, M.M.; Gherardini, P.F.; Prestwood, T.R.; Chabon, J.; Bendall, S.C.; et al. Systemic Immunity Is Required for Effective Cancer Immunotherapy. *Cell* **2017**, *168*, 487–502.e15. [CrossRef] [PubMed]
35. Eyerich, K.; Eyerich, S. Immune Response Patterns in Non-communicable Inflammatory Skin Diseases. *J. Eur. Acad. Dermatol. Venereol.* **2018**, *32*, 692–703. [CrossRef]
36. Bishop, K.D.; Olszewski, A.J. Epidemiology and Survival Outcomes of Ocular and Mucosal Melanomas: A Population-based Analysis. *Int. J. Cancer* **2014**, *134*, 2961–2971. [CrossRef]
37. Wang, H.-Y.; Liu, Y.; Deng, L.; Jiang, K.; Yang, X.-H.; Wu, X.-Y.; Guo, K.-H.; Wang, F. Clinical Significance of Genetic Profiling Based on Different Anatomic Sites in Patients with Mucosal Melanoma Who Received or Did Not Receive Immune Checkpoint Inhibitors. *Cancer Cell Int.* **2023**, *23*, 187. [CrossRef]

Disclaimer/Publisher's Note: The statements, opinions and data contained in all publications are solely those of the individual author(s) and contributor(s) and not of MDPI and/or the editor(s). MDPI and/or the editor(s) disclaim responsibility for any injury to people or property resulting from any ideas, methods, instructions or products referred to in the content.

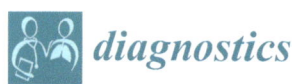 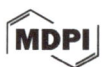

Article

Advancing Dermatological Diagnostics: Interpretable AI for Enhanced Skin Lesion Classification

Carlo Metta [1,*], Andrea Beretta [1], Riccardo Guidotti [2], Yuan Yin [3], Patrick Gallinari [3], Salvatore Rinzivillo [1] and Fosca Giannotti [4]

[1] Institute of Information Science and Technologies (ISTI-CNR), 56124 Pisa, Italy; andrea.beretta@isti.cnr.it (A.B.); rinzivillo@isti.cnr.it (S.R.)
[2] Department of Computer Science, Universitá di Pisa, 56124 Pisa, Italy; riccardo.guidotti@unipi.it
[3] Laboratoire d'Informatique de Paris 6, Sorbonne Université, 75005 Paris, Italy; yuan.yin@isir.upmc.fr (Y.Y.); patrick.gallinari@sorbonne-universite.fr (P.G.)
[4] Faculty of Sciences, Scuola Normale Superiore di Pisa, 56126 Paris, Italy; fosca.giannotti@sns.it
* Correspondence: carlo.metta@isti.cnr.it

Abstract: A crucial challenge in critical settings like medical diagnosis is making deep learning models used in decision-making systems interpretable. Efforts in Explainable Artificial Intelligence (XAI) are underway to address this challenge. Yet, many XAI methods are evaluated on broad classifiers and fail to address complex, real-world issues, such as medical diagnosis. In our study, we focus on enhancing user trust and confidence in automated AI decision-making systems, particularly for diagnosing skin lesions, by tailoring an XAI method to explain an AI model's ability to identify various skin lesion types. We generate explanations using synthetic images of skin lesions as examples and counterexamples, offering a method for practitioners to pinpoint the critical features influencing the classification outcome. A validation survey involving domain experts, novices, and laypersons has demonstrated that explanations increase trust and confidence in the automated decision system. Furthermore, our exploration of the model's latent space reveals clear separations among the most common skin lesion classes, a distinction that likely arises from the unique characteristics of each class and could assist in correcting frequent misdiagnoses by human professionals.

Keywords: Explainable Artificial Intelligence; skin image analysis; dermoscopic images; adversial autoecnoders; AI in healthcare

1. Introduction

Decision support systems powered by Artificial Intelligence (AI) have recently seen a significant surge in interest across various fields due to their impressive capabilities. Nonetheless, their application in sensitive areas, particularly those affecting human decisions such as in healthcare, has sparked ethical concerns regarding the opacity of AI-driven decisions [1,2]. There is an emerging consensus on the need for AI systems that not only augment the decision-making process of medical professionals with AI-generated insights and recommendations [3,4] but also ensure that the rationale behind AI decisions is transparent. This is especially pertinent in the context of skin image classification, where the lack of interpretability in the decision-making process of deep learning models complicates the interaction between the AI system and medical practitioners. It is, therefore, crucial to enhance existing classification models with explainability features that facilitate more insightful interactions and provide additional diagnostic tools [5]. This paper addresses these challenges within the scope of skin lesion diagnosis from images.

The flourishing field of Explainable AI (XAI) has thus gained considerable attention [2,6–8], with saliency maps being a prevalent form of explanation for image classifiers. These maps visually represent the contribution of each pixel toward the model's decision, offering a pixel-level insight into the decision-making process. Despite the array of approaches to generate saliency maps, they are often criticized for their lack of clarity in critical medical situations. Explanation methods vary, being classified as model-specific or model-agnostic based on their reliance on the inner workings of the AI model, and as global or local, indicating whether the explanation pertains to the model as a whole or to individual predictions [6,7]. Notable model-specific explainers like IntGrad [9], GradInput [10], and ε-LRP [11] specialize in deep neural networks and generate saliency maps. However, these maps can be fragmented and challenging to interpret in urgent medical scenarios. Conversely, model and data agnostic local explainers such as LIME [12] and SHAP [13] suffer from their reliance on image segmentation, which can compromise the plausibility of their explanations by reducing them to obscured versions of the original image, a practice that diminishes trust and utility in medical contexts [14].

Addressing these limitations, ABELE (Adversarial Black box Explainer generating Latent Exemplars), was proposed as a local, model-agnostic explainer tailored for image classifiers [15]. ABELE explains decisions by providing exemplar and counter-exemplar images—those classified similarly or differently from the input image, respectively—alongside a saliency map that underscores decision-critical areas.

This paper aims to build upon and refine the methodologies discussed in [3,15–17], exploring the application of an explanation method in a genuine medical context, specifically for diagnosing skin lesions from images. Utilizing the labeled dataset from the ISIC 2019 (International Skin Imaging Collaboration) challenge (https://challenge.isic-archive.com/data/, accessed on 1 September 2019), we train a cutting-edge deep learning classifier based on the ResNet architecture [18] and elucidate the model's decisions using ABELE [15]. This approach allows practitioners to interpret the model's reasoning through the provided exemplars and counter-exemplars. Our study evaluates the utility of these explanations through a user study with medical professionals, novices, and laypeople, aiming to gauge their impact on trust and confidence in the AI system.

The contributions of this paper are multifaceted. Firstly, it refines and evaluates ABELE within a real-world medical scenario. Secondly, it introduces a latent space analysis performed by the adversarial autoencoder in ABELE, providing insights that could aid in distinguishing between similar skin lesion types commonly confused by human diagnosticians. Thirdly, it develops a user interface for exploring ABELE's explanations. Lastly, through a comprehensive user study, it demonstrates that explanations enhance trust and confidence in AI decision systems, particularly among domain experts and highly educated individuals. This study also uncovers a persistent skepticism toward AI among older demographics, as well as a decrease in trust among experts following incorrect AI advice. Additionally, we observe that the saliency maps generated by ABELE are superior to those by other local explainers, such as LIME and LORE [19].

The remainder of this document is structured as follows: Section 3 outlines the methodology, Section 4 details the case study and introduces the visualization tool, Section 5 introduces the visual explanation outputted by the explainer, Section 6 presents the survey findings, Section 8 explores the latent space analysis, and Section 10 summarizes our findings and suggests avenues for future research.

2. Related Work

XAI has emerged as a focal point in medical imaging, aiming to shed light on the intricate workings and decisions of AI models in a clear and comprehensible manner. In the healthcare sector, the role of XAI is pivotal for enhancing the trust and confidence of both practitioners and patients toward AI-driven diagnostic and treatment approaches.

Numerous research efforts have delved into the application of XAI within medical imaging contexts, encompassing areas such as chest X-rays [20], CT scans [21], and MRI scans [22]. These studies have employed a range of XAI techniques, including but not limited to saliency maps, attribution maps, and decision trees. A landmark study by Jampani et al. [23] marked one of the initial attempts to utilize saliency map models across various medical imaging domains. Subsequent research has expanded upon this foundation, exploring decision trees and rule-based systems for articulating explanations behind AI-driven diagnoses in medical imaging. Notably, Seung et al. [24] demonstrated the effectiveness of decision trees in elucidating deep learning model predictions for chest X-ray analyses. This particular study underscored the capability of decision trees in offering transparent explanations regarding AI model decision-making processes.

Moreover, XAI has been rigorously evaluated in diagnostic scenarios involving breast cancer [25], lung nodules [26], and brain tumors [27], among others. Across these evaluations, a diversity of XAI methodologies—including saliency maps, decision trees, and attribution maps—have been leveraged to illuminate the decision-making mechanisms of AI models.

Within the field of medical imaging, deep learning has emerged as a pivotal force, particularly in the detection and segmentation of skin lesions [28]. Recent advancements in convolutional neural networks (CNNs) have significantly enhanced the accuracy and efficiency of diagnosing various skin conditions, including melanoma, one of the deadliest forms of skin cancer [29]. Studies such as that by Esteva et al. (2017) [30] have demonstrated the capability of deep learning models to match or even surpass the diagnostic accuracy of dermatologists. Moreover, the integration of deep learning techniques with dermatoscopic imaging has opened new avenues for automated analysis, enabling the detailed examination of skin lesion features with unprecedented precision [31]. These technologies not only aid in early detection but also play a crucial role in delineating the boundaries of lesions, facilitating accurate surgery and treatment planning.

Collectively, these investigations affirm the critical and innovative role of XAI in medical imaging, showcasing its potential to foster greater trust and confidence in AI-assisted diagnoses and to enhance the understanding of the AI models' operational dynamics.

Despite these advancements, XAI in medical imaging confronts several pressing challenges that warrant attention [32], such as issues related to trust, data bias, interpretability, privacy, and integration into clinical workflows, among others. Key challenges include:

- Building Trust: A significant hurdle lies in engendering trust toward AI systems and their outputs. Achieving a high level of system explainability is vital for fostering trust and facilitating clinical adoption.
- Addressing Data Bias and Interpretability: The presence of bias in medical imaging data and the complexities associated with data interpretation can exacerbate when AI algorithms are trained on such data, potentially leading to skewed outcomes.
- Ensuring Privacy: The sensitive nature of medical imaging data necessitates stringent protections. Concerns regarding the handling and storage of these data, alongside the risk of data breaches or misuse, are paramount.
- Overcoming Data Limitations: The scarcity of high-quality medical imaging data can impede the efficacy of XAI algorithms, posing challenges to model training and validation.
- Clinical Workflow Integration: Seamlessly incorporating XAI systems into existing clinical workflows demands a thorough assessment of algorithmic performance and limitations, as well as their potential impact on clinical decision-making processes.
- Compliance with Regulation and Standards: The XAI domain in medical imaging is governed by a complex web of regulations and standards. Ensuring compliance with these regulatory frameworks is both challenging and labor-intensive.

This work aims to develop a human-centric approach to tackle existing hurdles in Explainable Artificial Intelligence for medical imaging. Our goal is to facilitate the integration of these technologies into clinical settings by developing dependable and transparent decision-support tools that incorporate XAI techniques into the clinical workflow.

Our approach to XAI is categorized under generative explanation-based methods. This involves leveraging a generative mechanism to craft visual explanation. Specifically, the Contrastive Explanations Method (CEM) [33] is adept at generating explanations by identifying the minimal necessary or absent regions in an image for a particular classification decision. Concurrent research [34–36] has focused on generating explanations that highlight modifications needed to either amplify or diminish the classifier's confidence in its prediction, employing concepts such as prototypes or counterfactuals. The technique of Explanation by Progressive Exaggeration [37] introduces a novel way to elucidate the decisions of opaque classifiers by utilizing a generative adversarial network (GAN) [38]. It systematically alters the input in a manner that shifts the model's prediction, functioning in a model-agnostic fashion and relying solely on the predictor's values and its gradient relative to the input.

Our work aligns with these cutting-edge explorations; however, we opt for a distinctive architecture, the adversarial autoencoder (AAE). The AAE presents a key advantage over the GAN by offering a more nuanced manipulation of the latent space—the compact, lower-dimensional representation of data. This precision facilitates the production of samples more aligned with the actual data distribution, ensuring coherence and relevance in the generated outputs. Furthermore, unlike GANs, which are predicated on a min-max contest between the generator and discriminator, AAEs incorporate a reconstruction loss, enhancing the similarity between generated and input data.

Additionally, AAEs have utility in unsupervised representation learning, enabling them to distill a condensed representation of data useful for other tasks like classification. This capability stems from the encoder component of the AAE, which projects data into the latent space, and the decoder, which reconstructs data from this space back to its original form.

In summary, AAEs offer a more controlled and interpretable mechanism for data generation compared to GANs. This makes them a superior and more versatile instrument for XAI applications, particularly within the context of medical imaging.

3. Methods

In this section, we present the two main components of the methodology adopted to classify and explain the dataset. More details can be found in [3,15,18].

3.1. Black Box Classifier

To establish a robust classifier that excels in image classification tasks and supports subsequent learning phases, we opted for the ResNet architecture. Renowned for its proven efficacy across a number of complex datasets and challenges [18], ResNet stands out as our architecture of choice. Rather than training a ResNet model from scratch, we opt for a transfer learning set, utilizing a ResNet model pre-trained on the ImageNet dataset. This approach is particularly beneficial in scenarios where data availability is limited relative to the complexity of the network [39]. During the transfer learning process, we replaced the model's final fully connected layer with a new one, tailored to match the dataset's class count. Consequently, this classification layer undergoes training from the beginning, while the remaining parts of the ResNet model are fine-tuned. We adopted binary cross entropy loss for each class, framing the task as a series of one-vs-rest binary classification challenges.

3.2. Adversarial Autoencoders

A key concern when utilizing synthetic examples for black box explanation development is ensuring consistency with the original examples' distribution. Addressed in [15], this challenge is met through the deployment of adversarial autoencoders (AAEs) [40], a hybrid model that combines the principles of generative adversarial networks (GANs) [38] with autoencoder-based representation learning.

AAEs, as probabilistic autoencoders, are designed to generate new items that closely resemble the input training data. They achieve this by aligning the aggregated posterior distribution of input data's latent representation with a chosen prior distribution. The AAE model encompasses an *encoder* mapping from $\mathbb{R}^n$ to $\mathbb{R}^k$, a *decoder* mapping back, and a *discriminator* assessing the authenticity of the latent features, where n is the image pixel count and k represents the latent feature count. Within this framework, x represents an instance of training data, with z denoting its latent representation derived via the *encoder*. The AAE is characterized by various distributions, including the prior $p(z)$, the data $p_d(x)$, the model $p(x)$, and the encoding and decoding functions $q(z|x)$ and $p(x|z)$. The goal is for the aggregated posterior $q(z)$, obtained through encoding, to mirror the prior distribution $p(z)$, ensuring fidelity in the generated examples while minimizing reconstruction errors. Through this process, the AAE model successfully confuses the *discriminator*, making it challenging to distinguish between genuine and generated latent instances (see Figure 1).

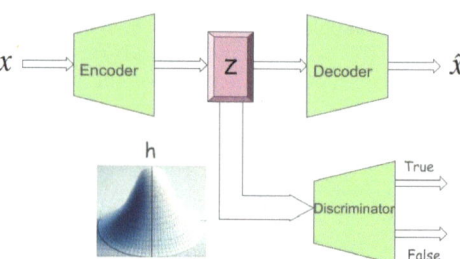

Figure 1. Adversarial autoencoder architecture.

The AAE training process encompasses two stages: Reconstruction, focusing on minimizing the loss between encoded and decoded data, and Regularization, which fine-tunes the *discriminator* using both real training data and encoded values. Upon completion, the decoder acts as a generative model, bridging the prior distribution $p(z)$ with the data distribution $p_d(x)$.

3.3. ABELE Explainer

ABELE (Adversarial Black box Explainer generating Latent Exemplars) is a local, model-agnostic explainer tailored for image classifiers [15]. For a given image x, ABELE gives explanations comprising sets of exemplars and counter-exemplars, as well as a saliency map. These exemplars and counter-exemplars are images classified identically or differently to x, respectively, offering insights into the classification rationale. The saliency map further delineates regions influencing the image's classification. ABELE initiates the explanation process by generating a latent feature space neighborhood via an adversarial autoencoder (AAE) [40], followed by learning a decision tree to provide local decision-making and counterfactual rules [41]. This process involves selecting and decoding exemplars and counter-exemplars conforming to these rules to produce a saliency map.

3.3.1. Encoding

The image x in question is encoded through the AAE, with the *encoder* yielding a latent representation $z \in \mathbb{R}^k$, utilizing k latent features, where k is significantly less than n, the dimensionality of x.

3.3.2. Neighborhood Generation

ABELE generates a set H comprising N latent feature space instances, resembling z's characteristics. This neighborhood, inclusive of instances mirroring $b(x)$'s decision ($H_=$) and those diverging ($H_{\neq}$), aims to replicate b's local behavior. The generation of H may follow diverse strategies, with our experiments favoring a genetic algorithm to optimize a fitness function [41]. Post-generation, each $h \in H$ undergoes validation and decoding through the *disde* module, subsequently being classified by the black box model b to ascertain its class y.

3.3.3. Local Classifier Rule Extraction

With the local neighborhood H established, ABELE constructs a decision tree classifier c, training it on H labeled according to $b(\widetilde{H})$. This surrogate model seeks to closely emulate

b's behavior within the defined neighborhood, extracting rules and counterfactual rules. This method, illustrated in Figure 2, encapsulates the journey from the initial image to the derivation of the decision tree, highlighting the extraction of pivotal rules. This process is denoted as LLORE, a latent variant of LORE [41].

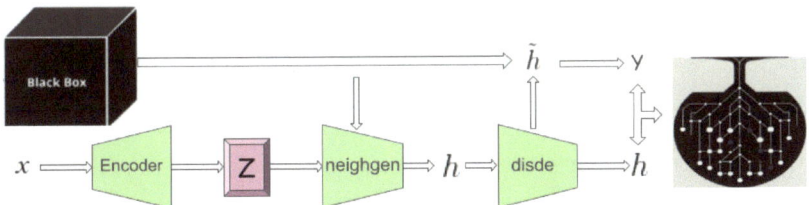

Figure 2. Latent local rules extractor (LLORE) module.

3.3.4. Explanation Extraction

In contexts such as medical or managerial decision-making, explanations often revolve around referring to exemplars with similar (or differing) decision outcomes. ABELE adopts this rationale, modeling the explanation of an image x as a triple $e = \langle \widetilde{H}_e, \widetilde{H}_c, s \rangle$, comprising exemplars $\widetilde{H}_e$, counter-exemplars $\widetilde{H}_c$, and a saliency map s. Exemplars and counter-exemplars represent images with outcomes that match or differ from $b(x)$, respectively. ABELE generates these through the *eg* module (Figure 3-left), initially producing a set of latent instances H that fulfill the decision rule r or counter-factual rules Φ, as depicted in Figure 2. Subsequently, it validates and decodes these into exemplars $\widetilde{H}_e$ or counter-exemplars $\widetilde{H}_c$ via the *disde* module (see Figure 4). The saliency map s underscores regions in x influencing its classification or steering it toward a different category. This map is derived using the *se* module (Figure 3-right), which calculates the pixel-to-pixel difference between x and each exemplar in $\widetilde{H}_e$, assigning the median of these differences to each pixel in s. Formally, for each pixel i in the saliency map s, it is defined as $s[i] = median_{\forall \widetilde{h}_e \in \widetilde{H}_e}(x[i] - \widetilde{h}_e[i])$.

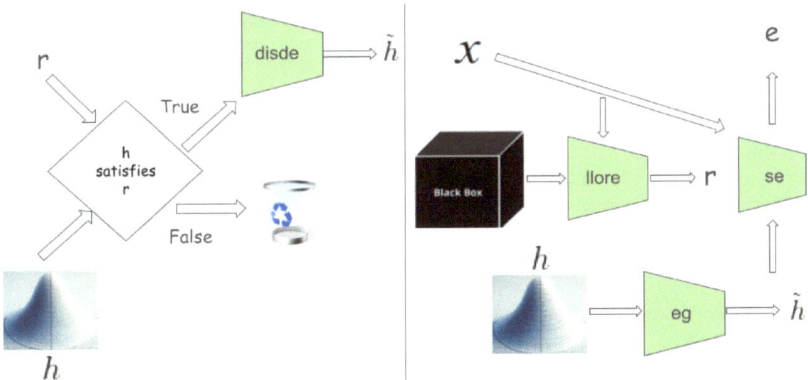

Figure 3. (**Left**): Exemplar generator (*eg*) module. (**Right**): ABELE architecture.

The efficacy of ABELE heavily relies on the quality of the encoder and decoder functions used; the more effective the autoencoder, the more realistic and valuable the explanations become. The following section delves into the autoencoder's structural nuances necessary to achieve reliable outcomes for the ISIC dataset.

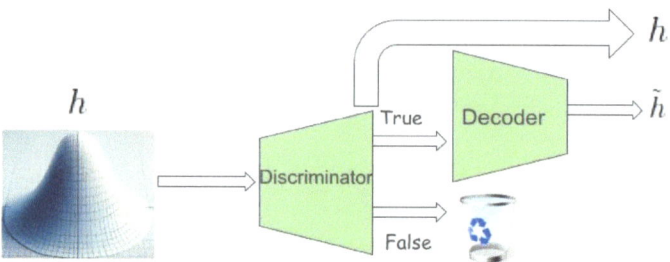

Figure 4. Discriminator and Decoder (disde) modules.

3.4. Progressively Growing Adversarial Autoencoder

We detail here the customization of ABELE we conducted in order to make it usable for complex image classification tasks.

3.4.1. Challenges of Generative Models

Training generative adversarial models presents significant challenges, often marred by various common failures such as convergence issues and the well-documented Mode Collapse [42]—a situation where the generator produces a limited variety of outputs. These issues stem from the adversarial training dynamic, where the generator and discriminator are trained simultaneously in a zero-sum game, making equilibrium elusive. As the generator improves, the discriminator's performance may deteriorate, leading to less meaningful feedback and potentially causing the generator's performance to falter if training continues beyond this point.

Moreover, real-world datasets, particularly in healthcare, compound these difficulties with issues like fragmentation, imbalance, and data scarcity, which hamper the efficiency and accuracy of machine learning models, especially fragile generative models.

A standard training approach for an AAE on the ISIC dataset, without addressing these issues, led to subpar performance, primarily due to mode collapse. To mitigate these generative failures and dataset limitations, we implemented a suite of cutting-edge techniques capable of addressing these challenges and enabling successful AAE training with satisfactory performance.

3.4.2. Addressing Mode Collapse in Generative Models

A diverse output range is desirable for generative models; however, the generator's tendency to favor outputs that appear most plausible to the discriminator can lead to repetitive generation of a single or a limited set of outputs, known as mode collapse. Various techniques, such as Mini Batch Discrimination [43], Wasserstein Loss [44], Unrolled GANs [45], and Conditional AAE [46], have been proposed to alleviate mode collapse by either implementing empirical fixes or adjusting the training scheme's internal structure.

The exact causes of mode collapse and other failures are not fully understood, with such phenomena becoming more frequent in the health domain, likely due to challenges like limited data, the necessity for high-resolution image processing, and unbalanced datasets. To successfully train an AAE and avoid these pitfalls, we adopted a combination of techniques tailored to address these specific challenges.

3.4.3. Progressively Growing Adversarial Autoencoder

Progressively Growing GANs, as introduced in [47], extend the GAN training process to foster more stable generative model training for high-resolution images. This technique begins training with low-resolution images, gradually increasing resolution by adding layers to both the generator and discriminator models until reaching the target size.

In typical GAN setups, the discriminator evaluates the generator's output directly. However, in an AAE framework, the discriminator assesses the encoded latent space rather than the reconstructed image. To harness the benefits of progressive growth in this context, we designed the Progressively Growing Adversarial Autoencoder (PGAAE). This approach starts with a basic convolutional layer block in both the encoder and decoder to reconstruct low-resolution images (7 × 7 pixels). Incrementally, we add more blocks, enhancing the network's capacity to process the desired image size (224 × 224 pixels), while keeping the latent space dimensions constant. This ensures that the discriminator consistently receives inputs of the same size. While fixing the discriminator's network may seem advantageous, we discovered that gradually expanding its width allows for processing increasingly complex information more effectively. Conversely, deepening the discriminator tends to destabilize training, leading to various failures, including performance degradation and catastrophic forgetting [42].

The rationale behind this methodology stems from the training instability caused by complex, high-dimensional data. Generating high-fidelity images challenges generative models to replicate both structural complexity and fine details, where high resolution exacerbates discrepancies, undermining training stability. Additionally, large images necessitate significant memory, reducing the feasible batch size and introducing further training instability.

Layer-by-layer learning enables the model to initially grasp broad structural aspects before refining focus on detailed textures. This progressive layer introduction acts as a sophisticated form of regularization across both encoder and decoder networks, smoothing the parameter space to mitigate issues like mode collapse.

The PGAAE network paradigm is reported in Figure 5. The structure begins with a simple AAE, focusing on 7 × 7 pixel images, progressively advancing through six stages to achieve 224 × 224 pixel image reproduction. To enhance the discriminator's capability at each stage, its architecture broadens, incorporating two dense layers that progressively expand from 500 to 3000 neurons. Each convolutional block consists of a `conv2d` layer followed by batch normalization and a ReLu activation, with either `max pooling` or `up sampling` depending on the encoder or decoder role.

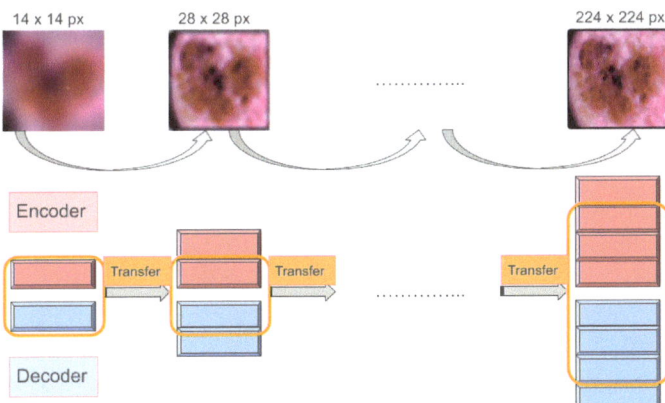

Figure 5. A Progressively Growing AAE. At each step, an autoencoder is trained to generate an image that is twice the size of the previous one, starting from an image of 14 × 14 pixels and gradually increasing to an image of 224 × 224 pixels. The learned features from one autoencoder are then transferred to the next. To handle the growing image size, both the encoder and decoder networks are expanded by adding one convolutional block at each step. The transfer learning is confined to the shared network architecture.

3.4.4. Denoising Autoencoder

A significant challenge in training generative models is their tendency to learn the identity function, particularly when hidden layers surpass input nodes, allowing simple data replication without meaningful representation learning.

Denoising autoencoders, as described in [48], introduce stochasticity to combat this by corrupting input images, which the model then strives to reconstruct. This process not only deters the model from identity mapping but also fosters the learning of robust representations.

Introducing noise to the discriminator's inputs [49] further enhances generalization, mitigates the vanishing gradient issue, and fosters better convergence. Combining denoising techniques with noise injection into the discriminator enhances the model, particularly noticeable in achieving high-quality reconstructions in latent spaces with 256 features. Gaussian noise with a standard deviation of $\sigma = 0.1$ proved effective, with little benefit observed beyond this range.

3.4.5. Mini Batch Discrimination

Mini Batch Discrimination, as detailed in [43], was introduced to prevent the generator network from collapsing. This technique discriminates across entire minibatches of samples within generative adversarial networks, rather than evaluating individual samples.

The principle behind this approach is for the discriminator to assess batches of data in their entirety, rather than single data points. This strategy significantly simplifies the identification of mode collapse, as the discriminator can recognize when samples within a batch are excessively similar and thus should be deemed inauthentic. Consequently, this compels the generator to diversify its output within each batch. An L_1 penalty norm is integrated with the input and directed toward the penultimate layer of the discriminator, quantifying the similarity among samples within the same batch. This penalization prompts the discriminator to reject batches that exhibit high internal similarity. Coupled with the progressive growth of the network, this technique has proven effective in averting mode collapse in batches of moderate size (16–64), albeit at the expense of a slight increase in discriminator complexity. Training with smaller batch sizes, necessitated by hardware constraints due to the processing of high-resolution images and managing a high-dimensional latent space, inherently raises the risk of mode collapse.

As per [43], the fine-tuning of two hyperparameters, designated as B and C, is required for the minibatch discrimination layer. These parameters determine the number of discrimination kernels and the dimensionality of the space for calculating sample closeness, respectively. Theoretically, larger values of B and C enhance performance but at the cost of computational efficiency. An optimal balance between accuracy and computational speed was found with $B = 16$ and $C = 5$.

3.4.6. Performance

Following an extensive optimization of the encoder, decoder, and discriminator architectures, our PGAAE equipped with 256 latent features achieved a reconstruction error, quantified by the RMSE, ranging from 0.08 to 0.24. This variance is contingent upon whether the data pertain to the most prevalent or the rarest class of skin lesions. Employing data augmentation was crucial for addressing the dataset's limitations regarding scarcity and imbalance. This strategy substantially mitigated mode collapse, enabling the generation of diverse and high-quality skin lesion images. Consequently, the ABELE explainer is now proficient in producing coherent and meaningful explanations.

It is important to underscore that the ABELE framework operates effectively irrespective of the classifier employed. Naturally, different classifiers yield distinct explanations, highlighting the flexibility and adaptability of the ABELE system.

4. Case Study

This section outlines our case study, including the characteristics of the training dataset and the methodologies employed for training both the black box classifier and the autoencoder.

4.1. Dataset

The International Skin Imaging Collaboration (ISIC), under the auspices of the International Society for Digital Imaging of the Skin (ISDIS), launched the Skin Lesion Analysis toward Melanoma Detection Challenge aiming to bolster global efforts in melanoma diagnosis (https://challenge2019.isic-archive.com/, accessed on 1 September 2019). This challenge focuses on developing a classifier capable of distinguishing among nine distinct diagnostic categories of skin cancer: MEL (melanoma), NV (melanocytic nevus), BCC (basal cell carcinoma), AK (actinic keratosis), BKL (benign keratosis), DF (dermatofibroma), VASC (vascular lesion), SCC (squamous cell carcinoma), and UNK (unknown, none of the others/out-of-distribution), see Figure 6. The provided dataset comprises a training set with 25,331 images of skin lesions labeled by category and a test set containing 8238 images, the labels of which are not publicly accessible.

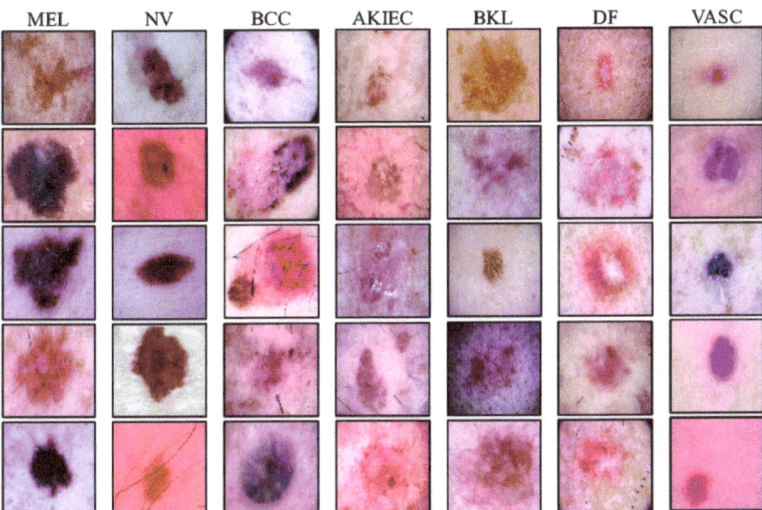

Figure 6. Dermoscopic images sampled from ISIC 2019 dataset.

4.2. Black Box Training

From the training set, we allocated 80% of the samples for training and the remaining 20% for validation purposes. The UNK category was excluded from our training focus since it is not present in the training set, aligning with our objective to develop a diagnostic classifier. The necessity for a reliable classifier to assist medical practitioners influenced this decision, endorsing a model capable of rejecting UNK samples when confidence in classification is low. This capability is crucial from a diagnostic accuracy perspective, preferring a cautious rejection of out-of-distribution samples over potentially erroneous labeling. Due to varying image resolutions, we employed specific preprocessing techniques:

- For training, images undergo random scaling, rotation, and cropping to fit the network input, ensuring the lesions remain undistorted. The processed images are resized to 224 × 224.
- Validation and test images are first scaled to 256 × 256 based on the shorter edge, then centrally cropped to 224 × 224.

Evaluation followed the original challenge's metric system, utilizing normalized multi-class accuracy as the performance measure. This metric, defined as the average recall across all classes, ensures equal importance across categories, preventing biased performance toward dominant ones. The optimized ResNet model, selected based on validation set performance, achieved a balanced multi-class accuracy of 0.838 on the test set (see Table 1 for the full performance description). Given the controlled conditions under which images were captured, ensuring minimal distributional shifts between training and validation sets, cross-validation was deemed unnecessary. To circumvent overfitting given the dataset's size, we fine-tuned a pre-selected pre-trained ResNet model, basing our architectural choice on its historical efficacy and computational feasibility rather than dataset-specific performance. The learning rate was fine-tuned to 10^{-4}, optimizing both convergence speed and validation accuracy, with the best-performing model on the validation set being retained for further use.

Table 1. Detailed Black Box performance on each skin lesion category.

Metrics	Diagnosis Categories							
	SCC	MEL	NV	BCC	AK	BKL	DF	VASC
Recall	0.836	0.818	0.927	0.942	0.890	0.847	0.963	0.886
Specificity	0.969	0.926	0.882	0.960	0.964	0.955	0.988	0.996
Accuracy	0.966	0.906	0.906	0.958	0.961	0.944	0.987	0.995
F1	0.505	0.763	0.910	0.845	0.624	0.753	0.630	0.772
PPV	0.362	0.716	0.894	0.766	0.480	0.678	0.469	0.684
NPV	0.996	0.957	0.918	0.991	0.995	0.982	0.999	0.999
AUC	0.978	0.948	0.967	0.990	0.980	0.966	0.996	0.997
AUC80	0.967	0.907	0.940	0.984	0.970	0.946	0.996	0.997
AP	0.810	0.844	0.967	0.941	0.802	0.848	0.910	0.917

The 50-layer ResNet architecture comprises 18 sequential modules, including one conv1 module (7 × 7, 64 filters, stride 2), three conv2 modules, four conv3 modules, six conv4 modules, three conv5 modules, and a final fully connected module fc. Each conv2 to conv5 module constitutes a residual block with three convolutional layers, where the block's output is a sum of its input and the convolutional output. Spatial reduction occurs only in the first layer of conv3, conv4, and conv5 modules, with the fc module serving as the classification layer. The fc module integrates average pooling followed by a 9-output fully connected layer with sigmoid activation to make predictions across the different diagnostic categories. The innovative structure of ResNet, particularly through its residual blocks, facilitates the training of deeper networks by addressing vanishing gradients. This architecture ensures that the network can learn complex patterns associated with various skin lesion types while maintaining computational efficiency.

Each residual block within the conv2 to conv5 modules consists of a specific sequence of convolutional layers designed to process and enhance the feature representation of the input images. These blocks employ a combination of 1 × 1 and 3 × 3 convolutional filters, allowing the network to capture both the detailed and abstract features of skin lesions effectively. By strategically increasing the number of filters and adjusting the stride in these blocks, the network progressively refines its feature maps, leading to a more discriminative representation suitable for classification tasks.

The decision to incorporate a newly trained prediction layer (fc module) at the end of the network underscores our commitment to tailoring the model to the specific requirements of skin lesion classification. This approach allows for fine-grained tuning and adaptation to the unique characteristics of the ISIC dataset, ensuring that the model is well-equipped to handle the variability and complexity inherent in dermatological imaging.

In summary, the deployment of a 50-layer ResNet architecture, coupled with thoughtful preprocessing and strategic model tuning, forms the cornerstone of our approach to tackling the challenge of skin lesion analysis toward melanoma detection. By leveraging the robustness and depth of ResNet, alongside a dataset-specific training regimen, we aim to push the boundaries of automated medical diagnosis, offering a tool that augments the capabilities of healthcare professionals in their fight against skin cancer.

4.3. PGAAE Training

Adapting ABELE for the sophisticated image classification task tackled by the ResNet black box classifier necessitated specific customizations. These adjustments are detailed in [3]. After extensive optimization across all three network components (encoder, decoder, and discriminator), our Progressively Growing Adversarial Autoencoder (PGAAE) with 256 latent features attained a root mean square error (RMSE) spanning from 0.08 to 0.24. This range reflects variability in error based on the frequency of occurrence of the skin lesion classes under consideration. The choice of 256 latent features was determined through initial testing, revealing it as the optimal balance between achieving satisfactory reconstruction accuracy, maintaining high image resolution, and conserving computational resources. Within the context of processing images of the targeted 224 × 224 resolution, a latent feature count ranging between 64 and 512 is typically advocated in the literature.

Data augmentation played a crucial role in addressing the challenges posed by dataset scarcity and imbalance. This strategy significantly diminished the occurrence of mode collapse, enabling the generation of diverse and high-quality skin lesion images (Figure 7). Equipped with PGAAE, ABELE demonstrates its capability to furnish insightful explanations, as verified through a participant survey discussed in the subsequent section.

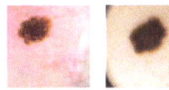 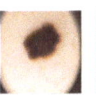 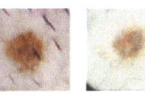 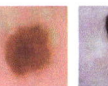 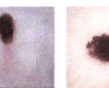 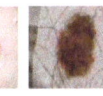 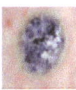

Figure 7. Synthetic skin lesion samples generated by ABELE and classified as melanocytic nevus by the ResNet black box, except for the upper-right image classified as actinic keratosis.

4.4. User Visualization Module

This segment introduces the innovative visualization module for interpreting explanations rendered by ABELE. The module elucidates the black box model's recommendations alongside the explanations generated by ABELE. A screenshot from a dedicated web application (https://kdd.isti.cnr.it/isic_viz/, accessed on 1 March 2023) illustrates the module's functionality, displaying the analyzed image, the black box's classification, and a synthetically generated counter-exemplar by ABELE in the upper section of the interface. For instance, an image of melanoma and its counter-exemplar, classified as melanocytic nevus, are showcased in Figure 8.

The lower part of the application presents a collection of images akin to the analyzed instance, bearing the same classification. This neighborhood, curated by ABELE and depicted as a list, offers insights into the latent space's variance surrounding the examined image. The counter-exemplar—distinguished from the original instance by its different classification—is chosen from this collection based on its minimal Euclidean distance to the original image in the latent space, yet with a maximized prediction for an alternate label. Additionally, the module's bottom section exhibits four exemplars; these are images ABELE generated, all sharing the black box's assigned label to the original image.

The ABELE visualization module, developed in JavaScript as a web application, interfaces with a backend through a RESTful API, enabling interaction with the black box and ABELE. A demonstrator version was created, allowing users to select from a predefined set of instances for exploration, rather than uploading new ones. This demonstrator served as a foundation for conducting the survey highlighted in the following discussion.

– Choose one of the case studies we selected using the menu below

id:156 - class:Melanoma

Image to explain (predicted class)

Melanoma

Neighborhood:
- Melanoma 7
- Melanocytic nevus 488
- Basal cell carcinoma 181
- Actinic keratosis 32
- Dermatofibroma 194
- Vascular lesion 98

Counter example image (class)

Melanocytic nevus

Prototype images

The following images are generated syntethically and they are classified with class **Melanoma** by the blackbox

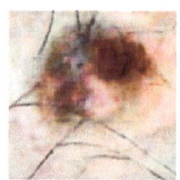 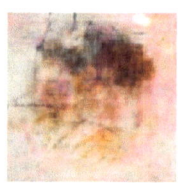 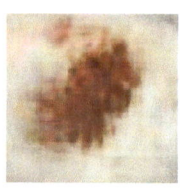 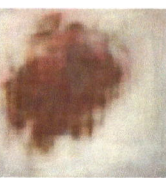

Figure 8. User visualization module to present the classification and the corresponding explanation. The upper part presents the input instance and a counter-exemplar. The lower part shows four exemplars that share the same class as the input.

5. Explanation

The interface designed to convey the outcomes of both the classifier and the explanator to users features a streamlined visual layout organized into four distinct sections: (1) the original image analyzed by the CNN, alongside the classification it was assigned; (2) a highlight section that underscores specific areas of the image that positively (depicted in brown) or negatively (depicted in green) influenced the classification decision; (3) a collection of synthetic prototypes created by the AAE that share the same classification as the input image; (4) a counter-exemplar, which is a synthetic image representing a prototype assigned a different classification by the CNN compared to the input image.

An illustrative example presented in Figure 9 depicts an image classified as Melanocytic nevus. The highlighted section allows users to discern which portions of the image were deemed significant by the CNN for its classification. This result is further elucidated by showcasing four prototypes: images synthesized by the AAE, designed to bolster the user's confidence in the black box's decision by facilitating a comparison between the original image and the exemplars. The counter-exemplar serves to challenge the black box's conclusion by offering an image akin to the input yet classified under a different category by the CNN.

ABELE compiles statistics related to the input's neighboring instances within the latent space. These data aid in understanding how the CNN's model space segments around the specific input, providing insights into the range of classifications the black box associates with the given instance. For the instance illustrated in Figure 9, the latent space statistics and rules are encapsulated as follows:

$$\text{Neighborhood}\{NV : 41, BCC : 18, AK : 4, BKL : 26, DF : 11\}$$

$$e = \begin{cases} \text{rules} = \{7 > -1.01, 99 \leq 0.07, 225 > -0.75, 255 \leq -0.02, \\ \quad\quad\quad\quad 238 > 0.15, 137 \leq -0.14\} \to \{\text{class: NV}\}, \\ \text{counter-rules} = \{\{7 \leq -1.01\} \to \{\text{class: BCC}\}\} \end{cases}$$

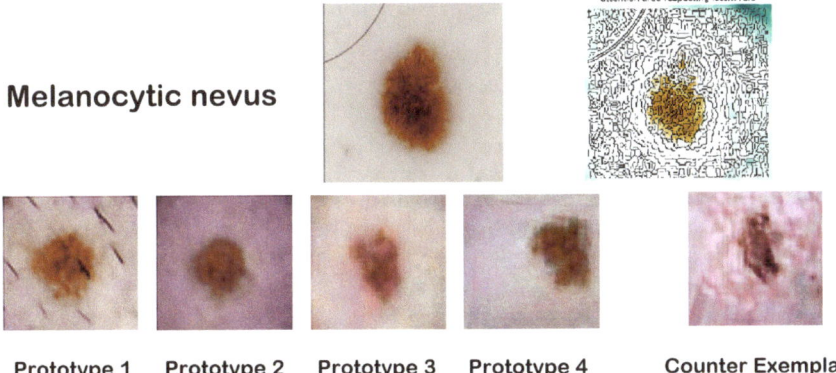

Figure 9. ABELE graphic explanation for a melanocytic nevus.

Here, the Neighborhood section outlines the distribution of synthetic latent instances produced by the AAE. Rules and counter-rules are delineated in relation to the ordinal positions within the latent space. While this format is primarily for internal purposes and does not directly inform the user, it serves as a foundation for the visual interface to facilitate an interactive enhancement of the provided explanation.

Another explanation, showcased in Figure 10, refers to a basal cell carcinoma case. A counter-exemplar depicting a vascular lesion (VASC) is crafted in alignment with a local counterfactual rule derived from the decision tree.

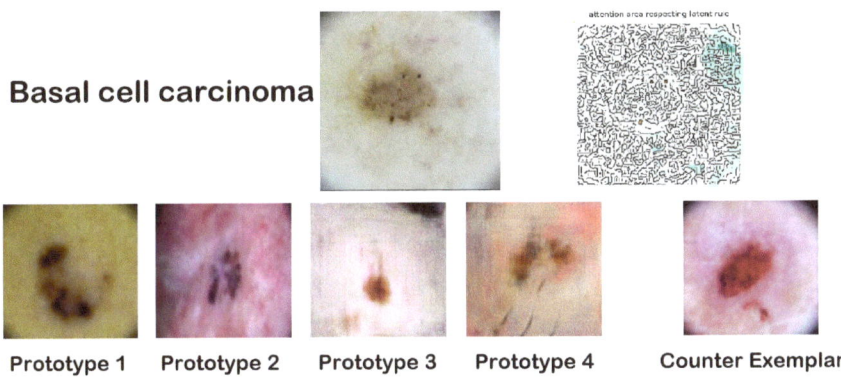

Figure 10. ABELE graphic explanation for a basal cell carcinoma.

The comprehensive breakdown of latent rules for this case is as follows:

$$\text{Neighborhood}\{NV : 34, BCC : 24, DF : 28, VASC : 14\}$$

$$e = \begin{cases} r = \{7 \leq 0.81, 187 \leq 0.46, 224 \leq -0.10, 219 \leq 0.07, \\ \qquad 242 > -0.25\} \rightarrow \{\text{class: BCC}\}, \\ c = \{219 > 0.07\} \rightarrow \{\text{class: VASC}\} \end{cases}$$

6. Validation and Assessment

This study presents a method designed to evaluate the effectiveness of ABELE explanations in the context of skin lesion diagnosis. Our primary objective was to ascertain the value of these explanations in aiding physicians and healthcare professionals in the diagnosis and treatment of skin cancers. Additionally, we sought to gauge their confidence in diagnosis models based on opaque algorithms and the clarity of the explanations offered by the explainer tool.

6.1. Survey Design and Methodological Approach

The survey was structured around ten questions, each associated with a distinct medical case image. The format for each question was uniform across all cases, consisting of four segments. The study protocol commenced with participants enrolling online and giving their informed consent. They were then provided with a concise overview of the task at hand. The method of manipulation was direct, aligning with methodologies adopted in prior studies [50,51]. Through this research, our goal is to deepen the understanding of the dynamics influencing the preference for automated guidance in medical contexts. Furthermore, we aim to build upon the existing literature by examining the potential repercussions of suboptimal automated advice and its impact on system trust. Unless otherwise noted, each segment presented a new image x to the participants. Each question was identified by a sequential number, denoted as Q_i, where i ranges from 1 to 10. Each question, from Q1 to Q10, incorporates the same four points, from P1 to P4, as detailed subsequently.

Point 1 (P1). Participants were shown an unlabeled skin lesion image randomly selected from the dataset, alongside its ABELE-generated explanation, as displayed by the visualization module. Specifically, two exemplars and two counter-exemplars from another lesion class were shown to the participants. They were then asked to categorize the image into one of two predefined classes using the explanation as a guide. This segment is aimed at determining whether the explanations provided by ABELE significantly aid in differentiating between images, even for those without expert knowledge. From another perspective, this serves as a practical assessment of the usefulness metric, which has been theoretically evaluated in [15].

Point 2 (P2). Participants were shown a labeled image and were requested to assess their confidence in the classification made by the opaque algorithm (using a 0–100 slider).

Point 3 (P3). The same labeled image from P2 was presented again, but this time accompanied by the explanation generated by ABELE. Participants were asked to re-evaluate their confidence after reviewing the explanation. The purpose of P2 and P3 is to ascertain whether exposure to an explanation leads to a change in confidence in the AI's capabilities.

Point 4 (P4). Participants were asked to evaluate the extent to which the exemplars and counter-exemplars assisted them in aligning their classification with the AI's decision, and their trust in the explanations produced by ABELE.

Throughout the survey, participants were not made aware of the accuracy of their predictions nor were they allowed to revise their prior responses or explanations upon receiving new information. To examine how participants react to incorrect advice, question six (Q6) intentionally included a misclassification (P2), followed by misleading advice regarding exemplars and counter-exemplars (P3). The remaining nine cases featured images that were correctly classified. Each survey question, encompassing the points described above, was designed to evaluate different facets of the participant's interaction with the AI-generated explanations, assessing the four segments across all ten questions.

6.2. Hypotheses and Goals

The research framework was structured around specific hypotheses aimed at evaluating the impact of ABELE explanations on skin lesion classification tasks. These hypotheses are as follows:

- H1: The explanations provided by ABELE facilitate the classification task for the users, particularly for domain experts, who are expected to achieve higher classification accuracy (assessed implicitly through P1).
- H2: The explanations generated by ABELE enhance users' trust and confidence in the classifications made by the black box model (assessed implicitly through P2 and P3, and explicitly through P4).

- H3: Participants exhibit a significant decrease in confidence and trust in the model after being presented with incorrect advice (assessed implicitly through the deliberate introduction of an error).

6.3. Results and Discussion

The survey was completed by 156 participants. These individuals enrolled in the survey via an online platform, after which they digitally acknowledged a consent form, completed a demographic questionnaire, and received an overview of various types of skin cancers involved in the study. To ensure meaningful data analysis, only responses from participants who completed at least one entire question (10% of the questionnaire), covering all four points, were considered. The collective demographic profile of the participants is illustrated in Figure 11. Notably, 94% of the participants came from a scientific background, with 27% having educational achievements in medicine or dermatology.

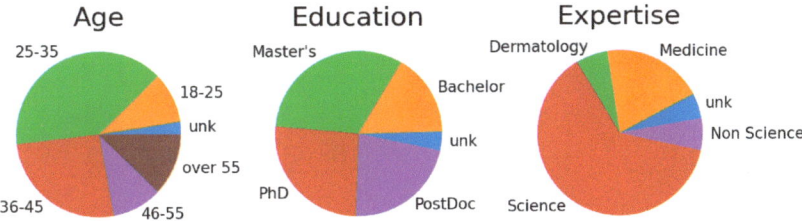

Figure 11. Demographic statistics of the survey participants.

Initially, we evaluated the participants' ability to classify skin lesion images using the explanations by assigning scores based on their performance in P1. Participants were categorized into two groups: Sub-sample A, consisting of those who correctly classified at least 70% of the images, and Sub-sample B, comprising the remainder. Alternative thresholds within the [60–90%] range were considered but ultimately not used, as they did not significantly alter the statistical outcomes. The overall average performance was impressive (82.02%), including among those without specialized knowledge in the domain (78.67%), and was even more pronounced among those with a medical or dermatology specialization (91.26%). An analysis using the one-way ANOVA on ranks (Kruskal–Wallis H test) [52] between sub-samples A and B revealed that educational level or age did not significantly affect classification performance. However, there was a notable difference ($F = 4.061$, $p = 0.043$) based on the participants' fields of specialization—those with a medical or dermatology background were more prevalent in sub-sample A, supporting H1 for domain experts and highlighting commendable performance among participants from other fields.

Figure 12 displays the change in participants' confidence in the black box classification before and after exposure to ABELE explanations, reflecting responses from P2 and P3. An increase in trust after viewing exemplars and counter-exemplars was observed in all questions except Q3 and Q9, indicating that explanations generally bolster model trust. Notably, the anomaly in Q3 suggests that non-medical experts influenced this particular outcome. A significant boost in confidence from 67.69% to 77.12%, peaking for Q6 (+21.95%), was noted—Q6 being uniquely misclassified by the black box model and showing the lowest pre-explanation confidence at 53.08%. This trend may indicate a resistance to incorrect advice, where consistent erroneous suggestions actually restore confidence levels. Participants are initially resistant to incorrect advice, but consistency in such advice resets their perception. This observation aligns with prior studies in the field of algorithm aversion [50,51,53].

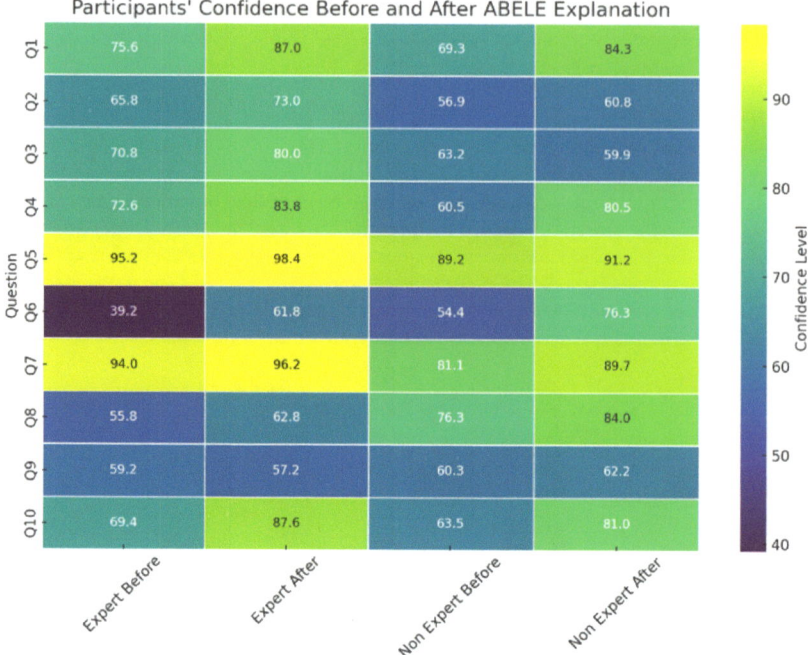

Figure 12. Participants' confidence in the classification of the black box before and after receiving the explanation of ABELE.

Confidence increases were not uniform across demographics. Figure 13 highlights several insights: an observable rise in confidence across all age groups except those over 55, whose confidence is inherently low and diminishes further post-explanation, possibly due to a generational distrust in AI technology. Educational level inversely correlates with initial confidence levels, yet post-explanation confidence surges, particularly among the more educated—a hint at the Dunning–Kruger effect [54]. Predictably, individuals with medical backgrounds expressed greater confidence than their counterparts from other scientific or non-scientific fields.

Specifically designed to explore H3, Q6 focused on responses to misclassifications by the black-box model. Data indicate a modest skepticism toward the black box's sixth classification, with no significant drop in confidence after incorrect advice (68.75% for Q1 to Q5, 60.03% for Q6, and 66.71% for Q7 to Q10). Yet, a more focused analysis on medical experts reveals a 14% confidence decline following incorrect advice (78.04% for Q1 to Q5, 56.19% for Q6, and 63.95% for Q7 to Q10), corroborating H3: domain experts' trust and confidence in the model diminish after encountering inaccurate advice.

Figure 14 condenses the impact of exemplars and counter-exemplars on the recognition of lesion classes as perceived by participants in P4. Consistent with confidence trends observed around Q6, both experts and non-experts reported a drop in confidence in the assistance provided by exemplars and counter-exemplars. Notably, ABELE's explanations were found to be more beneficial for medical experts than the general population, with exemplars proving more influential than counter-exemplars for all groups. This effect could stem from the task's classification complexity, where the relevance of exemplars escalates with the number of classes, diverging from binary classification tasks where exemplars and counter-exemplars may hold similar weight.

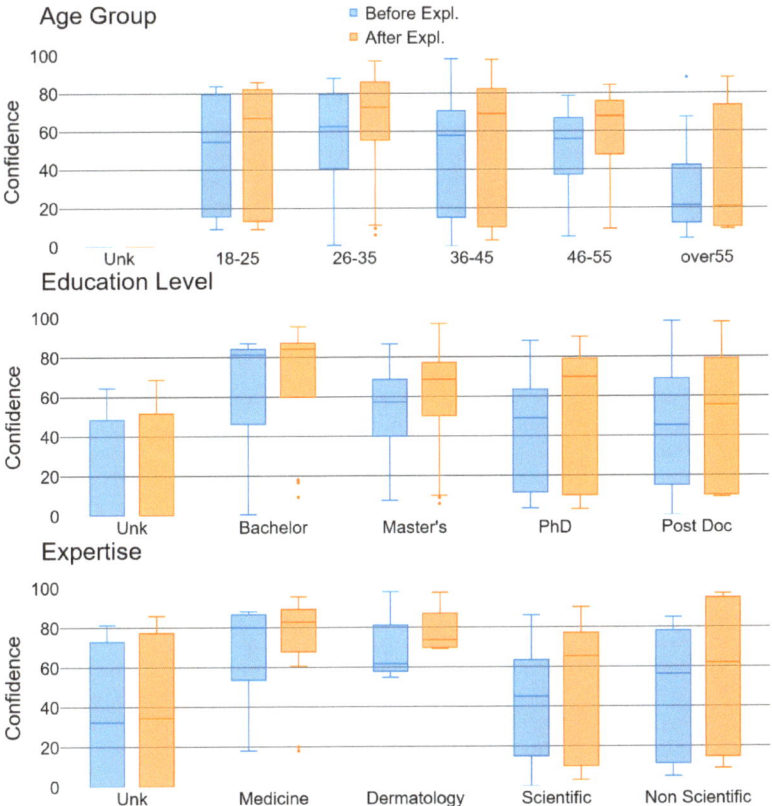

Figure 13. Participants' confidence among different age groups (**top**), education level (**center**), domains (**bottom**), before and after explanations (from [17]).

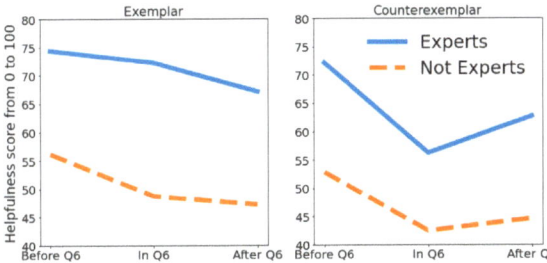

Figure 14. How much exemplars and counter-exemplars helped according to the participants' responses, divided between groups of experts and non-experts (from [17]).

The validation survey, encompassing a diverse demographic of participants, has unearthed intriguing findings that both reinforce and extend the existing literature in the field. Notably, our observations align with the discourse in recent studies like that of Ribeiro et al. [12] on model-agnostic interpretations and that of Lundberg and Lee [13] on SHAP values, which advocate for the customization of explanations to suit the user's expertise. A particularly compelling observation from our survey was the differential impact of explanations on diagnostic confidence across varying levels of expertise. Prior work, such as that by Holzinger et al. [55], emphasized the importance of XAI in enhancing user trust and understanding; our findings introduce a nuanced perspective where the specificity and nature of explanations may significantly influence user responses. Specifically, while domain experts showed increased confidence when provided with detailed, technical explanations, laypersons and novices were more positively influenced by simplified, visually driven explanations. This dichotomy underscores the necessity of adapting explanation models to the user's background, echoing the sentiments of Gunning and Aha [56] regarding the adaptability of XAI systems. Such insights advocate for the development of adaptive XAI systems capable of dynamically adjusting the complexity and format of explanations based on user profiles, leveraging user feedback to optimize explanatory output. This advancement could pave the way for personalized explanation frameworks, as discussed by Caruana et al. [57], enhancing the interpretability and accessibility of AI-assisted diagnostics for a wider audience, thus marking a significant stride toward democratizing medical diagnostic tools through AI.

7. Explaining via Saliency Map

In Figure 9, we present an example of ABELE's explanation mechanism. Synthetic exemplars and counter-exemplars provided by ABELE prove to be significantly more informative than traditional saliency maps. These maps allow for a comparison with those generated by established explanatory frameworks such as LIME and LORE. The saliency maps depicted in Figure 15 yield deletion AUC (Area Under Curve) scores of 0.888 for LIME, 0.785 for LORE, and 0.593 for ABELE. The deletion metric evaluates the decline in the probability of the designated class as crucial pixels, as identified by the saliency map, are incrementally removed from the image. A lower AUC score suggests a more effective explanation. This metric was calculated across a dataset of 200 images, with the average scores indicating that segmentation-based methods (LIME: 0.736 mean AUC score, LORE: 0.711 mean AUC score) tend to underperform in generating meaningful saliency maps, whereas ABELE excels by producing more detailed maps (0.461 mean AUC score). In Figure 16 (Top), we outline the deletion curves, represented as the mean AUC of accuracy versus the percentage of pixels removed for 200 sample images. Notably, ABELE's curve descends more swiftly and begins at an earlier point relative to the percentage of pixels removed, indicating a more refined and detailed saliency map.

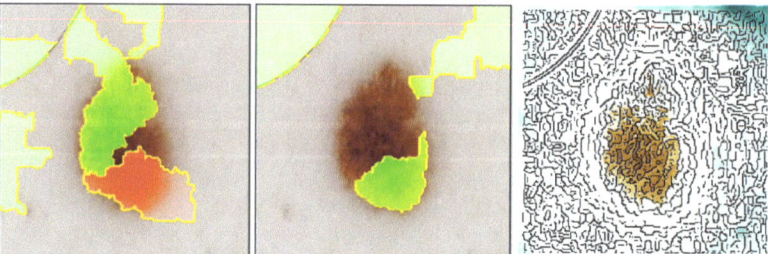

Figure 15. Saliency maps for LIME (**left**), LORE (**center**), and ABELE (**right**). LIME and LORE highlight the macro-regions of the image that contribute positively (green) or negatively (red) to the prediction while ABELE provides a more fine-grained level of information with a divergent color scale, from relevant areas (dark orange) to marginally significant areas (green/cyan) (from [17]).

A parallel observation is made when analyzing the insertion metric, which adopts an opposite strategy by incrementally adding each pixel according to its ascending importance. This process expects an improvement in the black box prediction as more features are incorporated, leading to a stepwise increase in model performance. A larger AUC indicates a superior explanation. Figure 16 (Bottom) illustrates that ABELE achieves consistently higher insertion scores across an average of 200 samples (0.417 for LIME, 0.471 for LORE, and 0.748 for ABELE). The rapid ascent in ABELE's insertion curve signifies that its saliency map more accurately identifies the image segments most critical to the classifier's decision-making process.

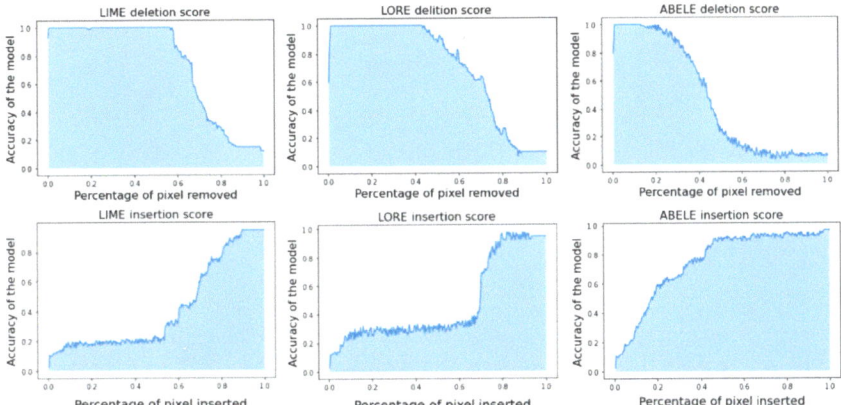

Figure 16. Deletion (**Top**) and Insertion (**Bottom**) metrics expressed as mean AUC of accuracy vs. percentage of removed or inserted pixels for 200 sample images. ABELE deletion curve drops earlier and faster relative to the percentage of removed pixels, signaling finer and more granular maps. ABELE insertion curve grows much earlier with respect to LIME and LORE (from [17]).

8. Explaining through Latent Space Analysis

The PGAAE model employed by ABELE maps the ISIC dataset into a 256-dimensional latent space, exhibiting a structured posterior distribution. This feature, as highlighted in [15], enables the use of latent space for visualizing the proximity among individual data instances, offering valuable insights. Such visualizations can assist medical experts and data scientists in better comprehending the distinctive characteristics of various skin cancers, thereby enhancing classification accuracy or trust in the explainer.

Employing multidimensional scaling (MDS) [58] for dimensionality reduction, we translate the latent space information into a two-dimensional visual representation. This process converts the 256-dimensional latent space into a 2D visual field. Figure 17 visualizes the latent encoding of eight skin cancer classes, revealing that primary features of skin lesions can also be discerned in this 2D projection. Notably, all classes except melanoma distribute around the perimeter, avoiding the center, whereas melanomas predominantly occupy the central region of the plot.

This distribution pattern suggests a similarity hierarchy among the skin cancer types. As noted in [59], Benign Keratosis is often misdiagnosed as melanoma, with misidentification rates ranging from 7.7% to 31.0% across different studies. To further explore differentiation capabilities among skin lesion classes, a Random Forest (RF) classifier with 500 trees was trained on the 2D MDS space. This classifier successfully distinguishes Melanoma from Benign Keratosis with 85.60% accuracy (see Figure 18-left), providing a visual tool for distinguishing between lesion types with performance comparable to that of the original complex model. Melanocytic Nevus also exhibits unique characteristics, with a significant proportion of samples centralized in the plot, reflecting the clinical observation that a considerable number of melanomas, especially in younger patients, evolve from benign nevi [60]. The RF classifier demonstrates a 78.53% accuracy in distinguishing Melanoma from Melanocytic Nevus (see Figure 18-right), paralleling the accuracy of state-of-the-art classification techniques.

Our study extends beyond the traditional two-dimensional latent space analysis, introducing a novel application of multidimensional scaling (MDS) in three dimensions. This enhancement is not merely a technical increment but a strategic move to unlock deeper insights into the complex nature of skin lesions. By transitioning from a 2D to a 3D latent space representation, we aim to explore the nuanced interplay between various lesion types, potentially uncovering hidden patterns and relationships that were previously obscured.

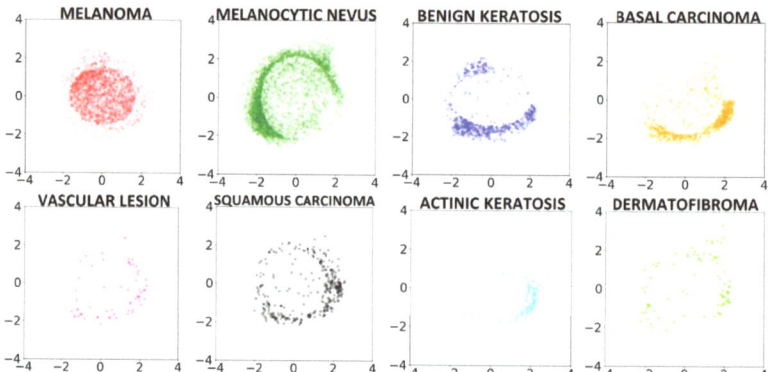

Figure 17. Training set represented in two dimensions through an MDS applied on the latent space learned by the PGAAE (from [17]).

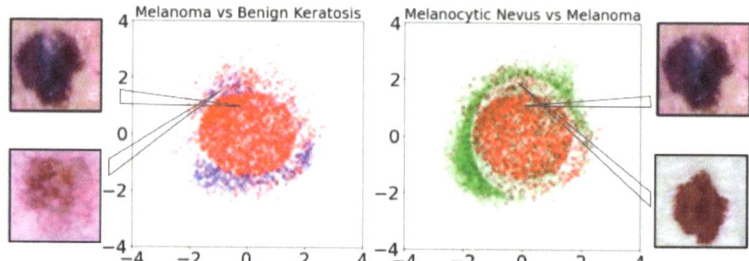

Figure 18. Visual separation between melanoma and benign keratosis (**Left**) and melanocytic nevus (**Right**).

Our exploration revealed a distinct spatial distribution of two prevalent skin lesion classes—melanoma and melanocytic nevus—when modeled in this enriched three-dimensional space. Specifically, we observed once again a robust separation between these classes, with melanomas predominantly located within a spherical region, marked by red dots, and melanocytic nevi, denoted by green dots, primarily positioned outside this spherical boundary (see Figure 19). This spatial arrangement not only validates the model's capability to distinguish between these clinically significant categories but also suggests a deeper, perhaps previously unexplored, biomarker-based differentiation between them.

Moreover, the 3D mapping facilitated a more intuitive and comprehensive visualization of the data, offering a tangible, three-dimensional landscape for medical practitioners to navigate. This approach could significantly enhance diagnostic accuracy by providing clinicians with a more detailed, spatially nuanced understanding of the lesions under examination. Importantly, this method allows for the identification of outliers or atypical presentations, which are often crucial in early-stage melanoma detection.

To further enrich this diagnostic landscape, in future works we will propose the integration of exemplars and counter-exemplars within this 3D model. By zooming into specific data points—individual lesions in this context—we can offer detailed comparative analyses between similar lesion types. This not only aids in the immediate diagnostic process but also serves as an educational tool, enabling practitioners to refine their diagnostic criteria based on visual and spatial comparisons of lesion characteristics in the latent space.

Given the intense focus on melanoma detection within oncological research, accurately predicting the transformation of a nevus into malignant melanoma remains a significant challenge. Future studies should consider the temporal evolution of oncological data.

Our methodologies and discoveries could aid clinicians in more precisely evaluating the potential malignancy of benign skin lesions.

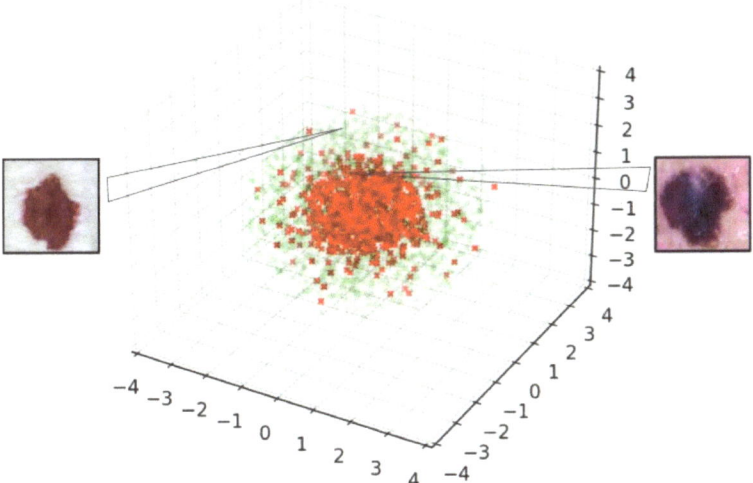

Figure 19. Visual 3d separation between melanoma (red) and melanocytic nevus (green).

9. Discussion and Future Work

In light of the significant advancements made in the field of dermatological diagnostics through interpretable AI, this section outlines new challenges and proposes practical experiments to further the research direction initiated by this study. Our objective is to bridge existing gaps and pave the way for groundbreaking solutions in the realm of medical diagnostics.

Despite the successes achieved, a challenge remains in generating high-fidelity explanations for complex or rare skin lesion cases where the model's confidence is low. To address this, we propose an experiment involving the creation of a more diverse and challenging dataset that includes underrepresented skin lesion types. This dataset will be used to train and evaluate an enhanced version of ABELE, focusing on its ability to generate meaningful explanations for these complex cases.

Another promising direction involves the exploration of cross-modal explanation methods that not only leverage visual explanations but also incorporate textual descriptions generated through natural language processing techniques. This experiment aims to develop a multimodal explanation framework that provides clinicians with a holistic understanding of the AI's decision-making process.

- Experiment 1a: Integrate ABELE with a language model capable of generating descriptive explanations for the visual exemplars and counter-exemplars.
- Experiment 1b: Conduct user studies with medical professionals to assess the impact of multimodal explanations on their trust and understanding of AI-based diagnostics.

To further enhance the practical utility of AI in dermatology, we propose the development of a real-time interactive explanation system. This system may allow users to interactively query the AI model about specific regions of interest in the skin lesion images and receive instant visual and textual explanations.

The rapid evolution of deep learning architectures offers opportunities to improve the accuracy and interpretability of skin lesion classification models. We propose an experiment to explore the application of novel neural network architectures, such as Transformer models, in the context of dermatological image analysis.

- Experiment 2a: Evaluate the performance of Transformer-based models on the ISIC dataset and compare it with the ResNet-based approach.
- Experiment 2b: Investigate the integration of Transformer models with ABELE to assess the impact on explanation quality and user trust.

Finally, we advocate for a longitudinal study to monitor the adoption and impact of AI and XAI tools in dermatological practice over time. This study may focus on understanding the evolving needs of healthcare professionals and how AI tools can be adapted to meet these requirements.

The proposed challenges and experiments aim to push the boundaries of current research in interpretable AI for skin lesion classification. By addressing these challenges, we hope to unlock new possibilities for AI-assisted diagnostics that are more trustworthy, paving the way for broader acceptance and utilization in clinical settings. Exploring novel architectures, multimodal explanations, and real-time interaction systems promises to enhance the diagnostic process, enabling clinicians to make more informed decisions with greater confidence in the AI's recommendations. Through the proposed longitudinal study, we can gain valuable insights into the long-term effects of AI integration in dermatology, identifying areas for improvement and adaptation to ensure that AI tools remain relevant and beneficial in the face of evolving medical practices and patient needs.

10. Conclusions

This paper demonstrates the application of classification and post hoc explanation methodologies in the context of skin lesion detection. It has been established that ABELE, following meticulous customization and training, can generate insightful explanations that significantly benefit medical practitioners, offering superior qualitative value over traditional local explainers. The primary challenge lies in the generative model's training phase. Latent space analysis reveals an intriguing distribution of images within the latent space, potentially aiding in the differentiation of commonly misclassified skin lesions (benign versus malignant). Furthermore, a survey involving experts and non-experts in skin cancer and healthcare sectors corroborated the hypothesis that unvalidated explanation methods lack utility. Future research avenues include applying ABELE to various diseases and health domains, particularly those reliant solely on raw images or scans of specific body parts. In skin cancer diagnosis, tactile feedback plays a crucial role alongside visual analysis. Enhancements to the user visualization module to support real-time explanation generation would necessitate substantial efforts and resources, as explanation extraction currently depends on the complexity of the image.

Despite the advancements presented in our study, it faces certain limitations that provide avenues for future research. One primary limitation is the reliance on a predefined dataset, which may not fully represent the diversity of skin lesions and different shades of skin color encountered in clinical practice. This can potentially lead to biases in model training and explanation generation. To address this, future work could focus on expanding the dataset to include a wider variety of lesion types, stages, and patient demographics, ensuring a more comprehensive and inclusive model training process. Lastly, this study predominantly focuses on the model's ability to generate explanations for medical practitioners, with less emphasis on patient comprehension. Developing patient-friendly explanation modules that translate complex diagnostic information into understandable insights could enhance patient engagement and satisfaction, paving the way for a more patient-centric approach in AI-assisted diagnostics.

Author Contributions: Conceptualization, C.M., R.G., P.G., S.R. and F.G.; Data curation, A.B.; Funding acquisition, P.G. and F.G.; Methodology, C.M., R.G. and S.R.; Software, C.M., R.G., Y.Y. and S.R.; Validation, C.M., A.B., R.G., Y.Y. and S.R.; Visualization, C.M., R.G. and S.R. All authors have read and agreed to the published version of the manuscript.

Funding: This work is supported by the European Community under the Horizon 2020 programme: G.A. 871042 *SoBigData++*, G.A. 952026 *HumanE AI Net*, G.A. 101092749 *CREXDATA*, ERC-2018-

ADG G.A. 834756 *XAI*, G.A. 952215 *TAILOR*, and the NextGenerationEU programme under the funding schemes PNRR-PE-AI scheme (M4C2, investment 1.3, line on AI) FAIR (Future Artificial Intelligence Research), and "SoBigData.it—Strengthening the Italian RI for Social Mining and Big Data Analytics"—Prot. IR0000013.

Institutional Review Board Statement: This study was conducted in accordance with the Declaration of Helsinki and approved by the Institutional Ethics Committee of Istituto di Scienza e Tecnologie dell'Informazione "A. Faedo" (ISTI-CNR) 6 April 2022—prot. n. 0026692/2022.

Informed Consent Statement: Informed consent was obtained from all subjects involved in the study.

Data Availability Statement: ISIC 2019 dataset is publicly available at https://challenge.isic-archive.com/data (accessed on 1 September 2019).

Conflicts of Interest: The authors declare no conflicts of interest. The funders had no role in the design of the study; in the collection, analyses, or interpretation of data; in the writing of the manuscript; or in the decision to publish the results.

References

1. Pedreschi, D.; Giannotti, F.; Guidotti, R.; Monreale, A.; Ruggieri, S.; Turini, F. Meaningful Explanations of Black Box AI Decision Systems. *AAAI Conf. Artif. Intell.* **2019**, *33*, 9780–9784. [CrossRef]
2. Miller, T. Explanation in artificial intelligence: Insights from the social sciences. *Artif. Intell.* **2019**, *267*, 1–38. [CrossRef]
3. Metta, C.; Guidotti, R.; Yin, Y.; Gallinari, P.; Rinzivillo, S. Exemplars and Counterexemplars Explanations for Image Classifiers, Targeting Skin Lesion Labeling. In Proceedings of the 2021 IEEE Symposium on Computers and Communications (ISCC), Athens, Greece, 5–8 September 2021.
4. Panigutti, C.; Perotti, A.; Pedreschi, D. Doctor XAI: An ontology-based approach to black-box sequential data classification explanations. In Proceedings of the 2020 Conference on Fairness, Accountability, and Transparency, Barcelona, Spain, 27–30 January 2020; pp. 629–639.
5. Markus, A.F.; Kors, J.A.; Rijnbeek, P.R. The role of explainability in creating trustworthy artificial intelligence for health care: A comprehensive survey of the terminology, design choices, and evaluation strategies. *J. Biomed. Inform.* **2021**, *113*, 103655. [CrossRef]
6. Adadi, A.; Berrada, M. Peeking Inside the Black-Box: A Survey on Explainable Artificial Intelligence (XAI). *IEEE Access* **2018**, *6*, 52138–52160. [CrossRef]
7. Guidotti, R.; Monreale, A.; Ruggieri, S.; Turini, F.; Giannotti, F.; Pedreschi, D. A Survey of Methods for Explaining Black Box Models. *ACM Comput. Surv.* **2019**, *51*, 93:1–93:42. [CrossRef]
8. Arrieta, A.B.; Díaz-Rodríguez, N.; Ser, J.D.; Bennetot, A.; Tabik, S.; Barbado, A.; Garcia, S.; Gil-Lopez, S.; Molina, D.; Benjamins, R.; et al. Explainable Artificial Intelligence (XAI): Concepts, taxonomies, opportunities and challenges toward responsible AI. *Inf. Fusion* **2020**, *58*, 82–115. [CrossRef]
9. Sundararajan, M. Axiomatic attribution for DNN. In Proceedings of the ICML, Sydney, Australia, 6–11 August 2017.
10. Shrikumar, A.; Greenside, P.; Shcherbina, A.; Kundaje, A. Not Just a Black Box: Learning Important Features through Propagating Activation Differences. *arXiv* **2016**, arXiv:1605.01713.
11. Bach, S.; Binder, A.; Montavon, G.; Klauschen, F.; Müller, K.R.; Samek, W. On pixel-wise explanations for non-linear classifier decisions by layer-wise relevance propagation. *PLoS ONE* **2015**, *10*, e0130140. [CrossRef] [PubMed]
12. Ribeiro, M.T.; Singh, S.; Guestrin, C. "Why Should I Trust You?": Explaining the Predictions of Any Classifier. In Proceedings of the 22nd ACM SIGKDD International Conference on Knowledge Discovery and Data Mining, San Francisco, CA, USA, 13–17 August 2016; pp. 1135–1144.
13. Lundberg, S.M.; Lee, S. A Unified Approach to Interpreting Model Predictions. In Proceedings of the NIPS, Long Beach, CA, USA, 4–9 December 2017; pp. 4765–4774.
14. Aurangzeb, A.M.; Ankur, T.; Carly, E. Interpretable Machine Learning in Healthcare. In Proceedings of the 2018 IEEE International Conference on Healthcare Informatics (ICHI), New York, NY, USA, 4–7 June 2018; p. 447.
15. Guidotti, R.; Monreale, A.; Matwin, S.; Pedreschi, D. Black Box Explanation by Learning Image Exemplars in the Latent Feature Space. In Proceedings of the ECML/PKDD (1), Würzburg, Germany, 16–20 September 2019; Lecture Notes in Computer Science; Springer: Cham, Switzerland, 2019; Volume 11906, pp. 189–205.
16. Metta, C.; Guidotti, R.; Yin, Y.; Gallinari, P.; Rinzivillo, S. Exemplars and Counterexemplars Explanations for Skin Lesion Classifiers. *Front. Artif. Intell. Appl.* **2022**, *354*, 258–260.
17. Metta, C.; Beretta, A.; Guidotti, R.; Yin, Y.; Gallinari, P.; Rinzivillo, S.; Giannotti, F. Improving trust and confidence in medical skin lesion diagnosis through explainable deep learning. *Int. J. Data Sci. Anal.* **2023**. [CrossRef]
18. He, K.; Zhang, X.; Ren, S.; Sun, J. Deep Residual Learning for Image Recognition. In Proceedings of the IEEE Conference on Computer Vision and Pattern Recognition, Las Vegas, NV, USA, 27–30 June 2016; pp. 770–778.
19. Guidotti, R.; Monreale, A.; Ruggieri, S.; Pedreschi, D.; Turini, F.; Giannotti, F. Local Rule-Based Explanations of Black Box Decision Systems. *arXiv* **2018**, arXiv:1805.10820.

20. Ozer, C.; Oksuz, I. Explainable Image Quality Analysis of Chest X-rays. In Proceedings of the Medical Imaging with Deep Learning, Lübeck, Germany, 7–9 July 2021; Volume 143, pp. 567–580.
21. Boutorh, A.; Rahim, H.; Bendoumia, Y. Explainable AI Models for COVID-19 Diagnosis Using CT-Scan Images and Clinical Data. In *International Meeting on Computational Intelligence Methods for Bioinformatics and Biostatistics*; Springer: Cham, Switzerland, 2022; pp. 185–199.
22. Farahani, F.V.; Fiok, K.; Lahijanian, B.; Karwowski, W.; Douglas, P.K. Explainable AI: A review of applications to neuroimaging data. *Front. Neurosci.* **2022**, *16*, 906290. [CrossRef] [PubMed]
23. Jampani, V.; Ujjwal, Sivaswamy, J.; Vaidya, V. Assessment of computational visual attention models on medical images. In Proceedings of the Eighth Indian Conference on Computer Vision, Graphics and Image Processing, Mumbai, India, 16–19 December 2012; Volume 80, pp. 1–8.
24. Yoo, S.H.; Geng, H.; Chiu, T.L.; Yu, S.K.; Cho, D.C.; Heo, J.; Choi, M.S.; Choi, I.H.; Cung Van, C.; Nhung, N.V.; et al. Deep Learning-Based Decision-Tree Classifier for COVID-19 Diagnosis from Chest X-ray Imaging. *Front. Med.* **2020**, *7*, 427. [CrossRef] [PubMed]
25. Papanastasopoulos, Z.; Samala, R.K.; Chan, H.P.; Hadjiiski, L.; Paramagul, C.; Helvie, M.A.; Neal, C.H. Explainable AI for medical imaging: Deep-learning CNN ensemble for classification of estrogen receptor status from breast MRI. In Proceedings of the Medical Imaging 2020: Computer-Aided Diagnosis, Houston, TX, USA, 16–19 February 2020; Volume 11314.
26. Wang, C.; Liu, Y.; Wang, F.; Zhang, C.; Wang, Y.; Yuan, M.; Yang, G. Towards Reliable and Explainable AI Model for Solid Pulmonary Nodule Diagnosis. *arXiv* **2022**, arXiv:2204.04219.
27. Wang, C.; Liu, Y.; Wang, F.; Zhang, C.; Wang, Y.; Yuan, M.; Yang, G. Explainability of deep neural networks for MRI analysis of brain tumors. *Int. J. Comput. Assist. Radiol. Surg.* **2022**, *17*, 1673–1683.
28. Mirikharaji, Z.; Abhishek, K.; Bissoto, A.; Barata, C.; Avila, S.; Valle, E.; Celebi, M.E.; Hamarneh, G. A survey on deep learning for skin lesion segmentation. *Med. Image Anal.* **2023**, *88*, 102863. [CrossRef] [PubMed]
29. Acosta, M.F.J.; Tovar, L.Y.C.; Garcia-Zapirain, M.B.; Percybrooks, W.S. Melanoma diagnosis using deep learning techniques on dermatoscopic images. *BMC Med. Imaging* **2021**, *21*, 6. [CrossRef] [PubMed]
30. Esteva, A.; Kuprel, B.; Novoa, R.A.; Ko, J.; Swetter, S.M.; Blau, H.M.; Thrun, S. Dermatologist-level classification of skin cancer with deep neural networks. *Nature* **2017**, *542*, 115–118. [CrossRef]
31. Gouda, W.; Sama, N.U.; Al-Waakid, G.; Humayun, M.; Jhanjhi, N.Z. Detection of Skin Cancer Based on Skin Lesion Images Using Deep Learning. *Healthcare* **2022**, *10*, 1183. [CrossRef]
32. Chen, H.; Gomez, C.; Huang, C. Explainable medical imaging AI needs human-centered design: Guidelines and evidence from a systematic review. *NPJ Digit. Med* **2022**, *5*, 156. [CrossRef]
33. Dhurandhar, A.; Chen, P.Y.; Luss, R.; Tu, C.C.; Ting, P.; Shanmugam, K.; Das, P. Explanations based on the missing: Towards contrastive explanations with pertinent negatives. *Adv. Neural Inf. Process. Syst.* **2018**, *31*, 592–603.
34. Liu, S.; Kailkhura, B.; Loveland, D.; Han, Y. Generative Counterfactual Introspection for Explainable Deep Learning. In Proceedings of the IEEE Global Conference on Signal and Information Processing, Ottawa, ON, Canada, 11–14 November 2019.
35. Joshi, S.; Koyejo, O.; Vijitbenjaronk, W.; Kim, B.; Ghosh, J. Towards Realistic Individual Recourse and Actionable Explanations in Black-Box Decision Making Systems. *arXiv* **2019**, arXiv:1907.09615.
36. Samangouei, P.; Saeedi, A.; Nakagawa, L.; Silberman, N. Model explanation via decision boundary crossing transformations. In Proceedings of the European Conference on Computer Vision (ECCV), Munich, Germany, 8–14 September 2018; pp. 666–681.
37. Singla, S.; Pollack, B.; Chen, J.; Batmanghelich, K. Explanation by Progressive Exaggeration. In Proceedings of the International Conference on Learning Representations, Addis Ababa, Ethiopia, 26–30 April 2020.
38. Goodfellow, I.; Pouget-Abadie, J.; Mirza, M.; Xu, B.; Warde-Farley, D.; Ozair, S.; Courville, A.; Bengio, Y. Generative Adversarial Nets. In Proceedings of the NeurIPS Proceedings, Montreal, QC, Canada, 8–13 December 2014.
39. Pan, S.J.; Yang, Q. A Survey on Transfer Learning. *IEEE Trans. Knowl. Data Eng.* **2010**, *22*, 1345–1359. [CrossRef]
40. Makhzani, A.; Shlens, J.; Jaitly, N.; Goodfellow, I.J. Adversarial Autoencoders. *arXiv* **2015**, arXiv:1511.05644.
41. Guidotti, R.; Monreale, A.; Giannotti, F.; Pedreschi, D.; Ruggieri, S.; Turini, F. Factual and Counterfactual Explanations for Black Box Decision Making. *IEEE Intell. Syst.* **2019**, *34*, 14–23. [CrossRef]
42. Thanh-Tung, H.; Tran, T. Catastrophic forgetting and mode collapse in GANs. In Proceedings of the 2020 International Joint Conference on Neural Networks (IJCNN), Glasgow, UK, 19–24 July 2020.
43. Salimans, T.; Goodfellow, I.; Zaremba, W.; Cheung, V.; Radford, A.; Chen, X. Improved Techniques for Training GANs. In Proceedings of the NIPS, Barcelona, Spain, 5–10 December 2016.
44. Dukler, Y.; Li, W.; Lin, A.; Montufar, G. Wasserstein of Wasserstein Loss for Learning Generative Models. In Proceedings of the 36th International Conference on Machine Learning, Long Beach, CA, USA, 9–15 June 2019.
45. Metz, L.; Poole, B.; Pfau, D.; Sohl-Dickstein, J. Unrolled Generative Adversarial Networks. In Proceedings of the International Conference on Learning Representations, Toulon, France, 24–26 April 2017.
46. Zhang, Z.; Song, Y.; Qi, H. Age Progression/Regression by Conditional Adversarial Autoencoder. In Proceedings of the IEEE Conference on Computer Vision and Pattern Recognition, Honolulu, HI, USA, 21–26 July 2017.
47. Karras, T.; Aila, T.; Laine, S.; Lehtinen, J. Progressive Growing of GANs for Improved Quality, Stability, and Variation. In Proceedings of the International Conference on Learning Representations, Vancouver, BC, Canada, 30 April–3 May 2018.

48. Vincent, P.; Larochelle, H.; Bengio, Y.; Manzagol, P.A. Extracting and composing robust features with denoising autoencoders. In Proceedings of the 25th International Conference on Machine Learning, Helsinki, Finland, 5–9 July 2008.
49. Arjovsky, M.; Bottou, L. Towards Principled Methods for Training Generative Adversarial Networks. In Proceedings of the International Conference on Learning Representations, Toulon, France, 24–26 April 2017.
50. Prahl, A.; Van Swol, L. Understanding Algorithm Aversion: When Is Advice from Automation Discounted? *J. Forecast.* **2017**, *36*, 691–702. [CrossRef]
51. Dzindolet, M.T.; Pierce, L.G.; Beck, H.P.; Dawe, L.A. The Perceived Utility of Human and Automated Aids in a Visual Detection Task. *Hum. Factors* **2002**, *44*, 79–94. [CrossRef] [PubMed]
52. Kruskal, W.H.; Wallis, W.A. Use of ranks in one-criterion variance analysis. *Arch. Dermatol.* **2002**, *138*, 1562–1566.
53. Beretta, A.; Zancanaro, M.; Lepri, B. Following wrong suggestions: Self-blame in human and computer scenarios. In Proceedings of the IFIP Conference on Human-Computer Interaction, Paphos, Cyprus, 2–6 September 2019; Springer: Cham, Switzerland, 2019; pp. 542–550.
54. Kruger, J.; Dunning, D. Unskilled and unaware of it: How difficulties in recognizing one's own incompetence lead to inflated self-assessments. *Pers. Soc. Psychol.* **1999**, *77*, 1121–1134. [CrossRef]
55. Holzinger, A.; Langs, G.; Denk, H.; Zatloukal, K.; Müller, H. Causability and explainability of artificial intelligence in medicine. *Wiley Interdiscip. Rev. Data Min. Knowl. Discov.* **2019**, *9*, e1312. [CrossRef]
56. Gunning, D.; Aha, D. DARPA's Explainable Artificial Intelligence (XAI) Program. *AI Mag.* **2019**, *40*, 44–58. [CrossRef]
57. Caruana, R.; Lou, Y.; Gehrke, J.; Koch, P.; Sturm, M.; Elhadad, N. Intelligible Models for HealthCare: Predicting Pneumonia Risk and Hospital 30-day Readmission. In Proceedings of the 21th ACM SIGKDD International Conference on Knowledge Discovery and Data Mining, Sydney, Australia, 10–13 August 2015; pp. 1721–1730.
58. Kruskal, J.B. Multidimensional scaling by optimizing goodness of fit to a nonmetric hypothesis. *Psychometrika* **1964**, *29*, 1–27. [CrossRef]
59. Izikson, L.; Sober, A.J.; Mihm, M.C.; Zembowicz, A. Prevalence of Melanoma Clinically Resembling Seborrheic Keratosis: Analysis of 9204 Cases. *J. Am. Stat. Assoc.* **1952**, *47*, 583–621. [CrossRef]
60. Sondermann, W.; Utikal, J.S.; Enk, A.H.; Schadendorf, D.; Klode, J.; Hauschild, A.; Weichenthal, M.; French, L.E.; Berking, C.; Schilling, B.; et al. Prediction of melanoma evolution in melanocytic nevi via artificial intelligence: A call for prospective data. *EJC Eur. J. Cancer* **2019**, *119*, 30–34. [CrossRef]

Disclaimer/Publisher's Note: The statements, opinions and data contained in all publications are solely those of the individual author(s) and contributor(s) and not of MDPI and/or the editor(s). MDPI and/or the editor(s) disclaim responsibility for any injury to people or property resulting from any ideas, methods, instructions or products referred to in the content.

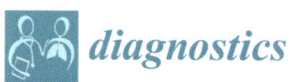 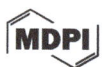

Article

Advancing Differentiation of Hepatic Metastases in Malignant Melanoma through Dual-Energy Computed Tomography Rho/Z Maps

Ibrahim Yel, Vitali Koch, Leon D. Gruenewald, Scherwin Mahmoudi, Leona S. Alizadeh, Aynur Goekduman, Katrin Eichler, Thomas J. Vogl, Mirela Dimitrova *,† and Christian Booz †

Clinic for Radiology and Nuclear Medicine, University Hospital Frankfurt, Goethe University Frankfurt, 60590 Frankfurt am Main, Germany; dr.ibrahimyel@gmail.com (I.Y.); vitali-koch@gmx.de (V.K.); gruenewald.leon@me.com (L.D.G.); scherwin.mahmoudi@gmail.com (S.M.); leona.alizadeh@outlook.de (L.S.A.); aynur.goekduman@med.uni-frankfurt.de (A.G.); k.eichler@em.uni-frankfurt.de (K.E.); t.vogl@em.uni-frankfurt.de (T.J.V.); boozchristian@gmail.com (C.B.)
* Correspondence: dmtr.a.mirela@gmail.com
† These authors contributed equally to this work.

Abstract: Objectives: The aim of this study is to evaluate the diagnostic accuracy of dual-energy computed tomography (DECT)-based Rho/Z maps in differentiating between metastases and benign liver lesions in patients diagnosed with malignant melanoma compared to conventional CT value measurements. Methods: This retrospective study included 73 patients (mean age, 70 ± 13 years; 43 m/30 w) suffering from malignant melanoma who had undergone third-generation DECT as part of tumor staging between December 2017 and December 2021. For this study, we measured Rho (electron density) and Z (effective atomic number) values as well as Hounsfield units (HUs) in hypodense liver lesions. Values were compared, and diagnostic accuracy for differentiation was computed using receiver operating characteristic (ROC) curve analyses. Additional performed MRI or biopsies served as a standard of reference. Results: A total of 136 lesions (51 metastases, 71 cysts, and 14 hemangiomas) in contrast-enhanced DECT images were evaluated. The most notable discrepancy ($p < 0.001$) between measured values and the highest diagnostic accuracy for distinguishing melanoma metastases from benign cysts was observed for the Z (0.992; 95% CI, 0.956–1) parameters, followed by Rho (0.908; 95% CI, 0.842–0.953) and finally HU_{120kV} (0.829; 95% CI, 0.751–0.891). Conversely, when discriminating between liver metastases and hemangiomas, the HU_{120kV} parameters showed the most significant difference ($p < 0.001$) and yielded the highest values for diagnostic accuracy (0.859; 95% CI, 0.740–0.937), followed by the Z parameters (0.790; 95% CI, 0.681–0.876) and finally the Rho values (0.621; 95% CI, 0.501–0.730). Conclusions: Rho and Z measurements derived from DECT allow for improved differentiation of liver metastases and benign liver cysts in patients with malignant melanoma compared to conventional CT value measurements. In contrast, in differentiation between liver hemangiomas and metastases, Rho/Z maps show inferior diagnostic accuracy. Therefore, differentiation between these two lesions remains a challenge for CT imaging.

Keywords: malignant melanoma; metastasis; dual-energy CT; Rho/Z; HU

1. Introduction

Cutaneous malignant melanoma, while representing only 4% of all skin tumors, is responsible for approximately 80% of all skin cancer deaths. It represents one of the most aggressive and dangerous skin tumors and is often associated with a poor prognosis [1]. The incidence is increasing, especially in fair-skinned people, on a global scale. Australia has the highest melanoma incidence rates worldwide. In Europe, the melanoma incidence is highest in the northern regions and lowest in the southern regions [2]. In 2020, 325,000 new cases of melanoma were estimated globally, while 57,000 people died of the disease [3]. The number of new cases in Germany has increased more than fivefold in the last 50 years [4]. Nowadays, malignant melanoma is considered to be a multi-factorial disease. In evaluating risk factors, exogenous and endogenous factors are distinguished. The most crucial external melanoma risk is increased ultraviolet exposure, especially in early childhood [5]. In adults, both artificial and natural UV radiation increase the risk of developing melanoma. Even when compared, spending time in a solarium is significantly more dangerous than bathing outside in the sun when it comes to developing skin cancer. The average age of diagnosis is 60 years for women and 68 years for men. Furthermore, malignant melanoma can occur on any part of the body. In women, malignant melanoma is most commonly found on the lower legs, whereas in men, the head and trunk are most commonly affected.

Malignant melanoma in the advanced, metastatic stage almost always has a lethal outcome with a short survival time. Therefore, early and highly accurate tumor staging is crucial for treatment decisions and prognosis [6]. Current guidelines recommend staging CT scans of the chest and abdomen as a standard imaging modality due to its widespread availability [7,8]. CT imaging, while instrumental in diagnosing various medical conditions, often encounters challenges in confidently distinguishing between malignant and benign lesions. One of the primary limitations lies in the inherent nature of CT scans, which primarily provide anatomical information with limited tissue characterization capabilities. Consequently, subtle differences in the imaging characteristics of malignant and benign lesions may not always be discernible with CT images alone. Additionally, certain benign lesions can manifest with features that mimic malignancy, further complicating the diagnostic process. Moreover, the reliance on morphological criteria, such as lesion size and enhancement patterns, for differentiation may lead to inaccuracies, as these features can overlap between benign and malignant entities. For instance, cysts, hemangiomas, and metastases may share similar CT values due to factors like low vascularity and necrosis within metastatic lesions, contributing to diagnostic uncertainty [9,10]. Moreover, it is worth noting that liver metastases may occasionally present with high attenuation due to hemorrhagic content, which can pose challenges in differentiating them from hemangiomas [11]. The differentiation of cysts can also pose challenges, especially when presenting with septations, nodularities, or hemorrhagic contents. In addition, small, hypodense metastases may be difficult to differentiate from benign hepatic lesions. Small lesions (<1 cm) are rarely malignant in patients without a known primary disease. However, it is important to note that in patients with known primary tumors, lesions meeting this criterion have up to a 30% chance of being malignant [12,13]. As a result, CT imaging may necessitate supplementary diagnostic modalities or clinical correlation to enhance diagnostic confidence in distinguishing between the malignant and the benign. MRI or biopsies are often for used for accurate differentiation. Nevertheless, limited MRI availability, specific contraindications, and the invasive character of biopsies with potential complication risks are critical in some patients. Furthermore, compared to computed tomography, MRI examinations are also significantly more complex, time-consuming, and associated with higher costs. As previously noted, CT imaging has its limitations. In this study, our primary focus lies in enhancing the capabilities of CT imaging, specifically aiming to overcome some of these limitations.

Over the past few years, technological advancements in CT have improved image quality, reduced scan times, and even provided additional information to improve diagnostic accuracy. In this context, dual-energy CT (DECT) has been proven to be a highly accurate method for tumor assessment due to its shown improved material characterization and differentiation compared to conventional single-energy CT [14,15]. In this context, DECT postprocessing provides a variety of additional quantitative parameters of tumor characteristics, including atomic number maps (Rho/Z) showing the Rho and Z of lesions [16,17]. Numerous studies have assessed DECT advantages, especially in oncology [14,18–22]. However, this technique has not been evaluated to differentiate liver metastases and benign lesions in patients with malignant melanoma. Therefore, this study aimed to investigate and compare the diagnostic accuracy of DECT-based Rho and Z values and conventional HU measurements for the differentiation of MRI- or biopsy-proven hypodense liver metastases and benign lesions in patients suffering from malignant melanoma.

Until now, hypodense liver lesions in patients with malignant melanoma could only be detected in computed tomographic staging using image morphological elements. With the dual-energy CT technology routinely used at our institute in recent years, better material differentiation is now possible due to the tube voltage discrepancies in the two X-ray tubes. The aim of this work is to improve the detection of malignant melanoma metastases in the liver using dual-energy computed tomography in combination with special computer software. It was investigated to what extent patients with diagnosed malignant melanoma can be distinguished between benign liver lesions and liver metastases on the basis of electron density and effective atomic numbers. This could result in an additional method of CT diagnosis, of metastases of malignant melanoma, to HU measurement.

2. Materials and Methods

The institutional review board approved this retrospective study. The requirement to obtain written informed consent was waived.

2.1. Study Population

A total of 2154 patients (patient age > 18 years) with histologically confirmed malignant melanoma who had undergone routine third-generation dual-source DECT malignant melanoma staging between December 2017 and December 2021 were considered for inclusion in this retrospective study. The exclusion criteria were amelanotic melanoma (n = 9 patients), scans without contrast media application (n = 862 patients), and patients with neither malignant melanoma metastases nor benign cysts in the liver (n = 1210 patients). The final study population consisted of 73 patients. Figure 1 illustrates the patient selection process in this study.

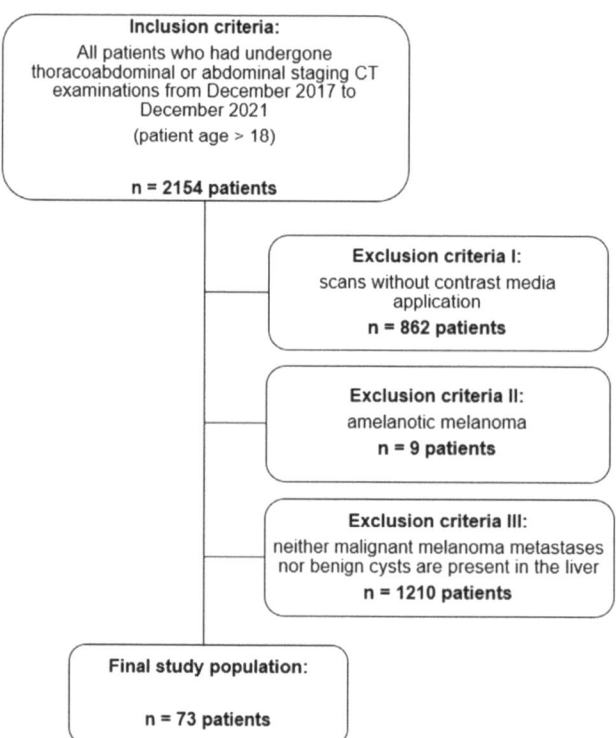

Figure 1. Flow chart showing the selection process in this study.

2.2. Dual-Energy CT Scan Protocol

Routine chest–abdominal staging CT scans were performed with third-generation dual-source DECT (Somatom Force, Siemens Healthineers, Forchheim, Germany) with the intravenous administration of a contrast agent after an 85 s delay. Contrast media (Imeron 400 mgI/mL, Bracco, Milan, Italy) were intravenously injected at a dose of 1.3 mL per kilogram of body weight and a flow rate of 3 mL/s through a superficial vein of the forearm. The CT examinations were all performed in the craniocaudal scan direction using DE mode, in which two X-ray tubes were operated at two different voltage levels (tube A: 100 kV and tube B: Sn150 kV with a tin filter). The rotation time was 0.5 s, collimation width 128 × 0.6 mm, and pitch 0.6 mm.

2.3. CT Image Reconstruction

In each CT scan, three different image sets were acquired, 100 kVp, Sn150 kVp, and the calculated weighted average (ratio 0.5:0.5), to resemble the image properties of a single-energy 120 kVp scan [21]. Standard reconstructions (axial, coronal, and sagittal; section thickness, 1 mm; increment, 0.75 mm) were generated using a dual-energy medium-soft convolution kernel (Qr40, advanced model-based iterative reconstruction [ADMIRE] level of 3) for the high- and low-kilovolt series. All reconstructions were transferred to the picture archiving and communication system (PACS) for image evaluation.

2.4. CT Measurements

DECT image series were postprocessed on a dedicated DECT workstation (syngo.via, version VB10B; Siemens Healthineers, Erlangen, Germany) using the Rho/z map algorithm to achieve tissue differentiation based on Rho and Z. The calculation parameters of the generated data were selected as follows: resolution, 10; minimum HU_{120kV} threshold, 40; maximum HU_{120kV} threshold, 50.

Circular regions of interest (ROIs) were placed in malignant melanoma liver metastases and liver cysts to obtain Rho/z and HU_{120kV} data, avoiding lesion margins, large blood vessels, and surrounding artifacts. Each lesion was measured ten times, and the average was calculated.

2.5. Reference Standard

MRI or biopsy served as a standard reference in this study for lesion definition. The MRI scan protocols included T1-weighted imaging before and after intravenous injection, T2-weighted sequences with and without fat saturation, diffusion-weighted images, and corresponding apparent diffusion coefficient (ADC) maps. MRI interpretation, as well as the identification of lesions in cases where biopsy served as reference, were performed by one board-certified radiologist (blinded) with 31 years of experience in liver imaging.

2.6. Statistical Analysis

Statistical analysis was performed using commercially available software (MedCalc for Windows, version 13, and GraphPad Prism for Windows, version 7). The Kolmogorov–Smirnov test was used for analyzing the normality of data. Variables were given as means ± standard deviations and analyzed with the Wilcoxon matched-pairs test. $p < 0.05$ was considered to show a statistically significant difference.

For better visualization of the data variance, we recalculated the mean differences (MDs) between melanoma liver metastases and benign lesions into percentage differences, as the Z values were measured with a different unit than Rho and HU_{120kV}. The calculations were made with the following equation:

$$\text{Percentage difference} = \frac{MD_{\text{metastases}} - MD_{\text{benign lesion}}}{(MD_{\text{metastases}} + MD_{\text{benign lesion}})/2} \times 100$$

For the quantitative image analysis, ROC curve analysis and the area under the curve (AUC) were applied to define optimal cut-off values for the differentiation of liver lesions. For these optimal cut-off values, sensitivity and specificity values were calculated. The values of overall sensitivity, specificity, positive predictive value (PPV), and negative predictive value (NPV) were given as means. Finally, AUC values were compared to demonstrate significant differences and to calculate the standard error using the DeLong test.

3. Results

A total of 136 lesions (51 metastases, 38%; 71 cysts, 52%; and 14 hemangiomas, 10%) were evaluated in 73 patients (70 ± 13 years; range, 39–92) consisting of 30 women (41%; 69 ± 15 years; range, 39–90) and 43 men (59%; 70 ± 12 years; range, 47–92). An average of one lesion per patient was reported, ranging from one to three. The characteristics of the study population are presented in Table 1.

Table 1. Characterization of the study population (n = 73).

Characteristics	Value
Number of patients	73
Mean age ± SD, range	70 ± 13, 39–92
Men	43/73 (0.59)
Mean age of men ± SD, range	70 ± 12, 47–92
Women	30/79 (0.41)
Mean age of women ± SD, range	69 ± 15, 39–90
Average number of lesions per patient, range	1, 1–3

The Z and Rho values showed a significant difference ($p < 0.001$) between malignant melanoma metastases and benign liver cysts (Z, MD, 1.613 ± 0.0921; percentage difference (PD), 110%; and Rho, MD, 34.71 ± 3.318 and PD, 88%). The HU_{120kV} measurements (MD, 22.46 ± 3.007; PD, 63%) also demonstrated a significant difference ($p < 0.001$) for metastases and cysts. However, the Z parameters showed the greatest difference in measured values, followed by Rho and finally HU_{120kV}. When comparing hemangiomas and metastases, the most pronounced dissimilarity ($p < 0.001$) was observed in the HU_{120kV} values (MD, 21.62 ± 7.45; PD, 37%), with secondary distinctions noted in the Z (MD, 0.60 ± 0.12; PD, 23%) and Rho (MD, 11.27 ± 5.12, PD, 21%) parameters. The quantitative parameters for the Rho, Z, and HU_{120kV} parameters are summarized in Table 2.

Table 2. Rho/Z and HU_{120kV} mean values for malignant melanoma metastasis, cysts, and hemangiomas.

Parameters	Cyst (n = 71)	Metastasis (n = 51)	Hemangioma (n = 14)
Rho	21.89 ± 16.24	56.60 ± 20.36	45.43 ± 12.76
Z	0.63 ± 0.33	2.26 ± 0.96	2.87 ± 0.30
HU_{120kV}	24.27 ± 1.957	46.73 ± 16.23	68.35 ± 10.87

The ROC curve demonstrated that the Rho and Z parameters have high diagnostic accuracy for differentiating malignant melanoma liver metastases and benign cysts. The Z values indicated the highest AUC value (0.992; 95% CI, 0.956–1), followed by Rho (0.908; 95% CI, 0.842–0.953). In both measurements, the sensitivity ranged from 98.04% (95% CI, 89.6–100) for Z and 96.08% (95% CI, 86.5–99.5) for Rho, while the specificity was 95.77 (95% CI, 88.1–99.1) for Z and 74.65% (95% CI, 62.9–84.2) for Rho. In comparison, the HU_{120kV} parameters showed a lower AUC value (0.829; 95% CI, 0.751–0.891) as well as lower sensitivity (86.27%; 95% CI, 73.7–94.3) and specificity (63.38%; 95% CI, 51.1–74.5).

To visualize the measurement differences between benign lesions and metastases, box-and-whisker plots (Figure 2) are used to show the data distribution through their quartiles.

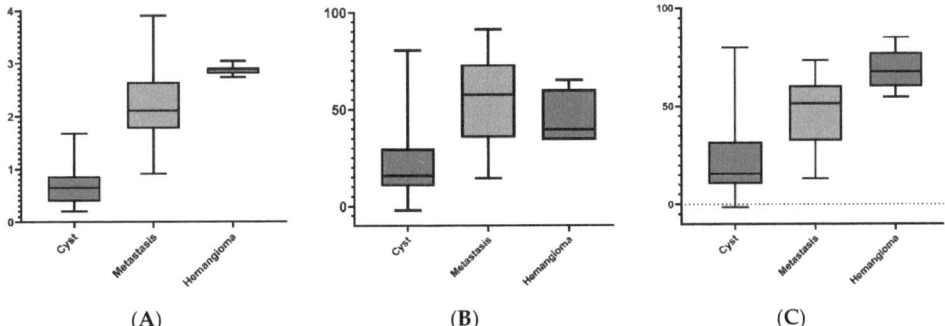

(A) (B) (C)

Figure 2. Box-and-whisker plots visualize the comparison of region-based mean Z values (**A**), Rho values (**B**), and CT numbers for 120 kV in HUs (**C**) between benign cysts, malignant melanoma metastases, and hemangiomas. Overall, the most significant disparity between cysts and metastases is observed in the Z and Rho values, whereas for hemangiomas and metastases, the most significant differentiation is observed in the HU_{120kV} parameters, followed by the Z values.

In a comparative analysis, the ROC curve for distinguishing hemangioma versus metastasis exhibited the highest AUC value with the HU_{120kV} parameters (0.859; 95% CI, 0.740–0.937), followed by the Z parameters (0.790; 95% CI, 0.681–0.876). Conversely, the Rho parameters demonstrated the lowest AUC value in this context (0.621; 95% CI, 0.501–0.730). Notably, the Z and Rho parameters (Z, 95.83%; 95% CI, 78.9–99.9 and Rho, 95.83%; 95% CI, 78.9–99.9) demonstrated superior specificity in comparison to the HU_{120kV} parameters (80%; 95% CI, 28.40–99.50). The AUC values, along with their corresponding 95% CI, sensitivities, specificities, PPVs, and NPVs for each lesion and parameter, are presented in Tables 3 and 4.

Table 3. Diagnostic accuracy of Rho, Z, and HU_{120kV} in differentiating benign liver cysts and melanoma metastases.

Parameters	AUC	Sensitivity (%)	Specificity (%)	PPV (%)	NPV (%)
Rho	0.908 (0.842–0.953)	96.08 (86.5–99.50)	74.65 (62.9–84.20)	73.1 (64.5–80.30)	96.4 (87.1–99)
Z	0.992 (0.956–1)	98.04 (89.6–100)	95.77 (88.1–99.1)	94.3 (84.6–98.10)	98.6 (90.7–99.80)
HU_{120kV}	0.829 (0.751–0.891)	86.27 (73.7–94.30)	63.38 (51.1–74.50)	62.9 (55–70.10)	86.5 (76–92.90)

Table 4. Diagnostic accuracy of Rho, Z, and HU_{120kV} in differentiating liver hemangiomas and melanoma metastases.

Parameters	AUC	Sensitivity (%)	Specificity (%)	PPV (%)	NPV (%)
Rho	0.621 (0.501–0.730)	39.20 (25.8–53.9)	95.83 (78.9–99.9)	95.2 (74.0–99.3)	42.6 (37.0–48.4)
Z	0.790 (0.681–0.876)	70.59 (56.2–82.5)	95.83 (78.9–99.9)	97.30 (84.0–99.6)	60.5 (49.9–70.3)
HU_{120kV}	0.859 (0.740–0.937)	82.35 (69.1–91.6)	80.00 (28.4–99.5)	91.1 (80.9–96.1)	61.5 (46.8–74.4)

The diagnostic performances of Rho, Z, and HU_{120kV} in differentiating liver lesions are displayed as ROC curves in Figures 3 and 4.

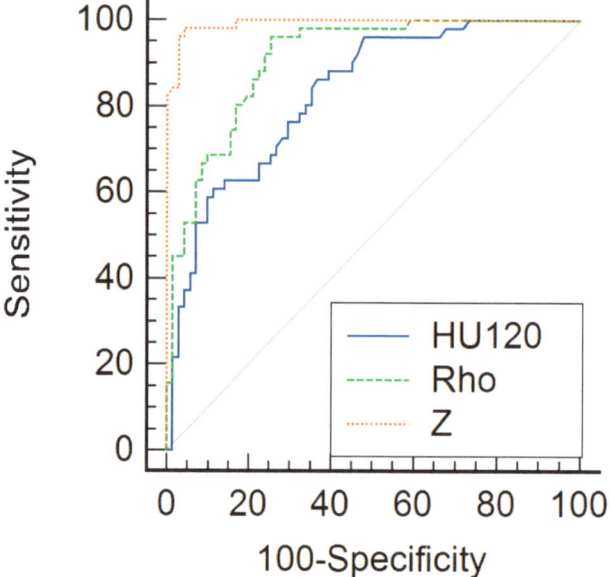

Figure 3. Comparison of representative ROC curves of Z values (orange line), Rho values (green line), and CT numbers for 120 kV in HUs (blue line) for differentiation between benign cysts and malignant melanoma metastases. The Z (area under the curve [AUC] = 0.992) and Rho (AUC = 0.908) parameters yielded significantly higher diagnostic accuracy for the differentiation between cysts and metastases compared to the HU_{120kV} measurements (AUC = 0.829).

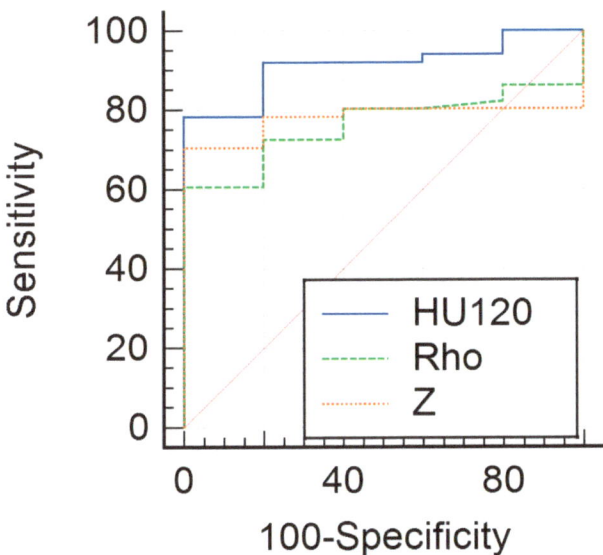

Figure 4. Comparison of representative ROC curves of Z values (orange line), Rho values (green line), and HU_{120kV} parameters (blue line) for differentiation between hemangioma and malignant melanoma metastases. The HU_{120kV} measurements (AUC = 0.859) and Z (AUC = 0.790) parameters yielded significantly higher diagnostic accuracy for the differentiation between hemangioma and metastases compared to Rho (AUC = 0.621).

In Figure 5, an exemplary CT scan of a patient reveals multiple hypodense liver lesions in the context of malignant melanoma. Despite the acquisition of HU measurements, distinguishing between these lesions proved challenging. Nevertheless, a clear diagnosis remained challenging, which is why Rho/Z maps were derived.

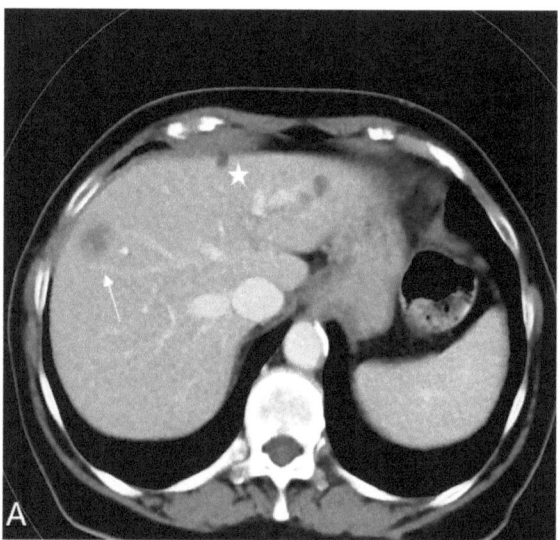
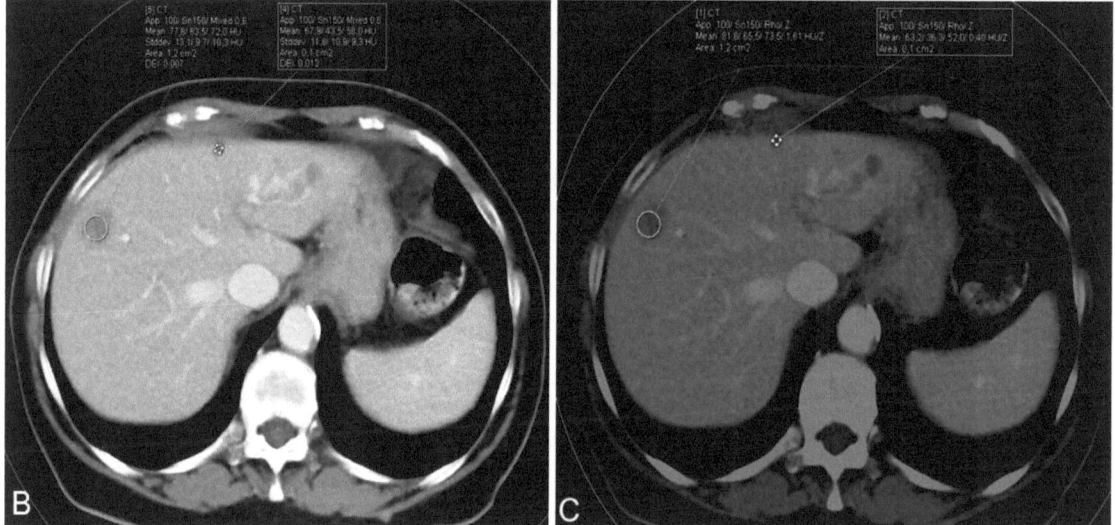

Figure 5. Axial contrast-enhanced CT scan in a 54-year-old female suffering from malignant melanoma. The scan showed multiple hypodense liver lesions in different segments, including a biopsy-confirmed liver metastasis in segment 8 (arrow) and an MRI-confirmed subcapsular liver cyst in segment 4 (star) (**A**). Conventional CT value measurements (**B**) demonstrated surprisingly high mean CT values for both lesions (72.0 and 58.0, respectively), while the mean Rho and Z values (**C**) showed greater differences for both lesions (Rho, 79.5 and 51.9; Z, 1.53 and 0.40, respectively) facilitating CT-based differentiation between metastases and cysts.

4. Discussion

The results of this retrospective study demonstrate the improved diagnostic accuracy of Rho/Z maps and corresponding measurements reconstructed from DECT data in differentiating malignant from benign liver lesions in patients with malignant melanoma compared to conventional CT value measurements. In summary, when discriminating between metastases and cysts, the Z values (AUC, 0.992; 95% CI, 0.956–1) and Rho values

(AUC, 0.908; 95% CI, 0.842–0.953) showed superior diagnostic accuracy measures than the HU_{120kV} parameters (AUC, 0.829; 95% CI, 0.751–0.891), indicating the beneficial potential of DECT in assessing hypodense liver lesions in patients with malignant melanoma undergoing staging CT examinations. Conversely, when discriminating between metastases and hemangiomas, the HU_{120kV} parameters yielded higher diagnostic accuracy values (0.859; 95% CI, 0.740–0.937), followed by the Z values (0.790; 95% CI, 0.681–0.876) and finally the Rho values (0.621; 95% CI, 0.501–0.730). However, the Rho and Z parameters (Rho, 95.83%; 95% CI, 78.90–99-9 and Z, 95.83%; 95% CI, 78.90–99.9) exhibited higher specificity compared to HU_{120kV} (80%; 95% CI, 28.40–99.50), indicating that while differentiation between metastases and hemangiomas in CT scans remains challenging when relying solely on visual characteristics and standard HU values, the use of Rho/Z maps can enhance diagnostic confidence in differentiating between liver metastases and benign cysts. This is crucial for patient outcomes because metastases are the leading cause of death associated with melanoma, with a 5-year survival rate of 23% for patients with metastases at the time of diagnosis [23]. The extent of the disease and the location of distant metastases determine what kind of therapy is required. Generally, as soon as distant metastases occur, therapy is only palliative. However, recent studies have shown that targeted immunotherapies can prolong survival. Nevertheless, the outcome of the treatment is dependent heavily on a patient's immunological status and the stage of the tumor [23,24]. In this context, numerous patients present with incidental benign liver lesions, with cysts being the most prevalent. Given the potential consequences of misdiagnosing a benign liver lesion as a metastasis, avoiding inappropriate treatment decisions is paramount. Therefore, achieving highly accurate staging that includes the liver is essential to promptly initiate optimal treatment and ultimately improve patient outcomes.

CT-based differentiation between liver lesions remains a challenge. The appearance of liver metastases in CT images may vary based on factors such as blood supply, hemorrhage, cellular differentiation, fibrosis, and necrosis, posing challenges in differentiation, particularly from hemangiomas. In addition, simple benign cysts can become complex if they are infected, hemorrhaged, or ruptured, increasing the HU value above the average value (0–20 HUs). Consequently, benign liver cysts may exhibit HU values similar to liver metastases in certain instances [25,26]. Furthermore, small lesions (<1 cm) pose difficulties in diagnosis. Therefore, accurate assessment of these liver lesions often necessitates biopsy or additional MRI evaluation [27,28]. However, limited MRI availability, specific contraindications, and the invasive nature of biopsy may introduce potential complications for some patients. As a result, staging melanoma patients can be particularly challenging in certain scenarios.

In recent years, DECT has become one of the main focuses of interest in CT-based oncological imaging owing to its many advantages, including better material characterization and differentiation. DECT is based on the principle that the attenuation of X-rays in tissue (expressed as the CT attenuation number in HUs) depends on the tissue density but also on the Z of the specific tissue and on the energy of the photon beam. Thus, DECT can thereby also quantify lesion iodine content. Various postprocessing techniques provide additional information to distinguish lesions by analyzing these parameters. Former studies have demonstrated DECT's advantage in distinguishing benign lesions from malignant ones compared to conventional single-energy CT [14,18,29–31]. However, there are insufficient studies that performed multiparametric analysis based on the Z and Rho of each tissue type using the application class of special postprocessing software (Rho/Z maps), especially in patients with malignant melanoma.

Different postprocessing techniques on dedicated software, for example, syngo.via (our software of choice), provide additional information for more accurate diagnosis of lesions by analyzing their electron density, effective atomic number, and iodine concentration. There have been a few previous studies that have shown the value of Rho/Z maps as an accurate addition to CT oncological diagnostics. Mileto et al. have shown that non-enhancing renal cysts, including hyperattenuating cysts, can be distinguished from enhancing masses on effective atomic number maps derived from dual-energy CT. In this study, the analysis showed an AUC for Z of greater than 0.9 (0.92; 95% CI, 0.89–0.94) for the evaluation of renal masses, indicating high diagnostic accuracy [32]. DECT-based Rho/Z maps were also used by Chijie Xu et al. to better distinguish osteoblastic metastases from bone islands (AUC for Z, 0.91; AUC for Rho, 0.88). Our findings are in accordance with the studies by Mileto et al. and Chijie Xu et al. and emphasize the value of DECT in abdominal oncologic imaging. Further studies have shown similar results for DECT Rho/Z measurements for other body regions, such as head and neck imaging, when differentiating benign from malignant thyroid nodules and T1 stage nasopharyngeal carcinoma from benign hyperplasia [33,34].

Current diagnostic techniques for identifying liver lesions and staging in melanoma patients involve a multifaceted approach utilizing various imaging modalities. Ultrasound, a widely accessible, non-invasive, and inexpensive tool, serves as an initial screening method due to its ability to detect hepatic lesions. However, its effectiveness may be limited by factors such as operator skill, patient cooperation, and the presence of bowel gas interference [35]. PET-CT has emerged as a key diagnostic tool for detecting liver lesions. This imaging modality combines the functional information obtained from PET, which highlights metabolic activity within tissues, with the anatomical details provided by CT imaging. PET-CT offers several advantages in the evaluation of liver lesions, including its ability to detect lesions with high metabolic activity indicative of malignancy, thereby aiding in the differentiation between benign and malignant lesions. However, despite its utility, PET-CT does have limitations. Notably, it presents a comparatively lower spatial resolution compared to MRI, potentially impacting the delineation of fine anatomical details. Additionally, concerns regarding accessibility and ionizing radiation exposure persist, with PET-CT's availability being less widespread than other imaging modalities and its utilization carrying a heightened risk of radiation exposure. MRI presents another crucial modality in liver lesion diagnostics, with superior soft tissue contrast resolution. Its capacity to detect nuanced alterations in liver tissue renders it highly adept at identifying small lesions and characterizing tumors. However, MRI does present limitations, primarily its lower availability compared to other imaging modalities. Furthermore, challenges arise in cases of patient non-cooperation, potentially leading to suboptimal study outcomes. Additionally, MRI may be contraindicated in patients with metal implants or those experiencing claustrophobia [36]. In contrast, DECT data facilitate rapid reconstruction of Rho/Z maps, with measurements easily accessible, making it a time-efficient and valuable additional clinical tool. This postprocessing tool is particularly beneficial for patients with MRI contraindications or coagulopathies prohibiting biopsy. Additionally, CT scans are readily available during on-call periods, unlike MRI or biopsy, potentially expediting diagnosis and treatment in specific cases. This highlights the potential of DECT-based Rho/Z maps as a versatile and efficient tool in clinical practice, particularly for patients with limitations to other imaging modalities or invasive procedures.

This study has limitations that need to be discussed. First, the present study is a single-center retrospective study, which may limit the generalizability of its findings. Second, our research was limited to a vendor-specific CT system and may not be applicable to other DECT technologies. Third, the scope of our analysis was limited to benign cysts, hemangiomas, and metastases in the liver, which are indeed the predominant liver lesions encountered in clinical practice. Further, our study is limited by a relatively small sample size of only 73 patients. Increasing the sample size would provide a broader understanding of our research and strengthen the reliability of our findings. Additionally, the limited number of participants may impede the detection of subtle yet clinically significant associations or effects within the patient population. Moving forward, it is essential for subsequent research efforts to replicate our study in larger cohorts to ensure the validity and generalizability of our findings. Nevertheless, future studies should aim to investigate the extent to which the Rho/Z values of cysts, hemangiomas, and metastases differ from other liver lesions, thus providing deeper insights into lesion differentiation. In addition, it should be noted that our research focused primarily on contrast-enhanced CT images. Therefore, there is a need for future investigations to assess the utility of non-contrast DECT images in this context. Further, the results of this study are specific to melanoma metastases and cannot be generalized to staging studies in the settings of other cancers.

Another limitation in the present study is that the impact of DECT on clinical outcomes was not investigated. While our study focused on evaluating the diagnostic accuracy of DECT-derived parameters in distinguishing between liver metastases and benign liver lesions in patients with melanoma, the broader implications of DECT on patient management and treatment outcomes were not explored. Further research is needed to assess the potential clinical benefits of DECT in influencing patient outcomes and guiding therapeutic decisions. Nonetheless, our findings suggest the potential applicability of Rho/Z maps to other malignancies featuring liver metastases and benign liver lesions, thereby warranting further investigation.

5. Conclusions

In conclusion, DECT-based Rho and Z measurements offer enhanced differentiation between liver metastases and benign liver cysts in patients with malignant melanoma compared to conventional CT measurements. Improved detection and characterization of lesions by DECT could expedite the diagnostic process and improve staging accuracy in patients with malignant melanoma, a critical factor for guiding treatment decisions. Nevertheless, patients with contraindications for other imaging modalities and diagnostic methods may particularly benefit from DECT-based Rho and Z measurements. This highlights the importance of considering DECT as a valuable additional tool in the staging of liver metastases in patients with malignant melanoma. Thus, if technically possible, Rho/Z maps and corresponding measurements should be applied in the context of tumor staging in patients with malignant melanoma and the presence of hypodense liver lesions.

In contrast, in the differentiation between hemangiomas and liver metastases, Rho/Z maps show inferior diagnostic accuracy compared to HU measurements. Therefore, differentiation between these two lesion types remains a challenge in CT imaging.

Author Contributions: Conceptualization, I.Y., V.K., L.D.G., S.M., L.S.A., A.G., K.E., M.D. and C.B.; Methodology, I.Y., V.K., L.D.G., S.M., L.S.A., A.G., M.D. and C.B.; Software, I.Y., M.D. and C.B.; Validation, I.Y., V.K., M.D. and C.B.; Formal analysis, I.Y., V.K., L.D.G., S.M., L.S.A., M.D. and C.B.; Investigation, I.Y., S.M., A.G., M.D. and C.B.; Resources, T.J.V.; Data curation, I.Y., L.D.G., M.D. and C.B.; Writing—original draft, I.Y., M.D. and C.B.; Writing—review & editing, I.Y., V.K., L.D.G., S.M., L.S.A., A.G., K.E., T.J.V., M.D. and C.B.; Visualization, I.Y., M.D. and C.B.; Supervision, I.Y., K.E., T.J.V., M.D. and C.B.; Project administration, I.Y., K.E., T.J.V., M.D. and C.B.; Funding acquisition, T.J.V. All authors have read and agreed to the published version of the manuscript.

Funding: This research received no external funding.

Institutional Review Board Statement: The study was conducted in accordance with the Declaration of Helsinki, and approved by the Institutional Review Board (or Ethics Committee) of Goethe University Frankfurt (protocol code 2023-1216 and 17.03.2023).

Informed Consent Statement: Patient consent was waived due to the retrospective nature of the study. All data were obtained in clinical routine.

Data Availability Statement: The data presented in this study are available on request from the corresponding author The data are not publicly available due to data protection.

Conflicts of Interest: Ibrahim Yel received speaker's fees from Siemens Healthineers. Christian Booz received speaker's fees from Siemens Healthineers. The authors declare no conflict of interest.

Abbreviations

ADC	Apparent diffusion coefficient	
AUC	Area under the curve	
DECT	Dual-energy CT	
MD	Mean difference	
NPV	Negative predictive value	
PACS	Picture archiving and communication system	
PPV	Positive predictive value	
Rho	Electron density	
ROI	Circular regions of interest	
ROC	Receiver operating characteristic	
SD	Standard deviation	
CI	Confidence interval	
Z	Effective atomic number	

References

1. Arnold, M.; Holterhues, C.; Hollestein, L.; Coebergh, J.; Nijsten, T.; Pukkala, E.; Holleczek, B.; Tryggvadóttir, L.; Comber, H.; Bento, M.; et al. Trends in incidence and predictions of cutaneous melanoma across Europe up to 2015. *J. Eur. Acad. Dermatol. Venereol.* **2014**, *28*, 1170–1178. [CrossRef] [PubMed]
2. Raimondi, S.; Suppa, M.; Gandini, S. Melanoma Epidemiology and Sun Exposure. *Acta Derm.-Venereol.* **2020**, *100*, adv00136. [CrossRef] [PubMed]
3. Arnold, M.; Singh, D.; Laversanne, M.; Vignat, J.; Vaccarella, S.; Meheus, F.; Cust, A.E.; de Vries, E.; Whiteman, D.C.; Bray, F. Global Burden of Cutaneous Melanoma in 2020 and Projections to 2040. *JAMA Dermatol.* **2022**, *158*, 495–503. [CrossRef] [PubMed]
4. Robert Koch-Institut. Krebs in Deutschland 2015/2016, 64. Available online: https://edoc.rki.de/bitstream/handle/176904/6012.3/krebs_in_deutschland_2019_2.pdf?sequence=6&isAllowed=y (accessed on 28 August 2023).
5. Rastrelli, M.; Tropea, S.; Rossi, C.R.; Alaibac, M. Melanoma: Epidemiology, risk factors, pathogenesis, diagnosis and classification. *In Vivo* **2014**, *28*, 1005–1011. [PubMed]
6. Moll, I. (Ed.) *Dermatologie*, 8th ed.; Thieme: Stuttgart, Germany, 2016.
7. Mohr, P.; Eggermont, A.M.M.; Hauschild, A.; Buzaid, A. Staging of cutaneous melanoma. *Ann. Oncol. Off. J. Eur. Soc. Med. Oncol.* **2009**, *20* (Suppl. 6), vi14–vi21. [CrossRef] [PubMed]
8. Patel, P.R.; Jesus, O.D. *CT Scan*; StatPearls: Treasure Island, FL, USA, 2022.
9. Ozaki, K.; Higuchi, S.; Kimura, H.; Gabata, T. Liver Metastases: Correlation between Imaging Features and Pathomolecular Environments. *Radiographics* **2022**, *42*, 1994–2013. [CrossRef] [PubMed]
10. Elbanna, K.Y.; Kielar, A.Z. Computed Tomography Versus Magnetic Resonance Imaging for Hepatic Lesion Characterization/Diagnosis. *Clin. Liver Dis.* **2021**, *17*, 159–164. [CrossRef] [PubMed]
11. Matos, A.P.; Altun, E.; Ramalho, M.; Velloni, F.; AlObaidy, M.; Semelka, R.C. An overview of imaging techniques for liver metastases management. *Expert Rev. Gastroenterol. Hepatol.* **2015**, *9*, 1561–1576. [CrossRef]
12. Schwartz, L.H.; Gandras, E.J.; Colangelo, S.M.; Ercolani, M.C.; Panicek, D.M. Prevalence and importance of small hepatic lesions found at CT in patients with cancer. *Radiology* **1999**, *210*, 71–74. [CrossRef]
13. Jones, E.C.; Chezmar, J.L.; Nelson, R.C.; Bernardino, M.E. The frequency and significance of small (less than or equal to 15 mm) hepatic lesions detected by CT. *Am. J. Roentgenol.* **1992**, *158*, 535–539. [CrossRef]
14. De Cecco, C.N.; Darnell, A.; Rengo, M.; Muscogiuri, G.; Bellini, D.; Ayuso, C.; Laghi, A. Dual-energy CT: Oncologic applications. *AJR. Am. J. Roentgenol.* **2012**, *199* (Suppl. 5), S98–S105. [CrossRef] [PubMed]
15. Seidensticker, P.R.; Hofmann, L.K. (Eds.) *Dual Source CT Imaging: With 52 Tables*; Springer Medizin: Berlin/Heidelberg, Germany, 2008.
16. Singh, T.; Gupta, P. Role of Dual-Energy Computed Tomography in Gallbladder Disease: A Review. *J. Gastroint. Abdom. Radiol.* **2022**, *5*, 107–113. [CrossRef]
17. Pascart, T.; Falgayrac, G.; Norberciak, L.; Lalanne, C.; Legrand, J.; Houvenagel, E.; Ea, H.-K.; Becce, F.; Budzik, J.-F. Dual-energy computed-tomography-based discrimination between basic calcium phosphate and calcium pyrophosphate crystal deposition in vivo. *Ther. Adv. Musculoskelet. Dis.* **2020**, *12*, 1759720X20936060. [CrossRef] [PubMed]
18. Agrawal, M.D.; Pinho, D.F.; Kulkarni, N.M.; Hahn, P.F.; Guimaraes, A.R.; Sahani, D.V. Oncologic applications of dual-energy CT in the abdomen. *Radiographics* **2014**, *34*, 589–612. [CrossRef] [PubMed]
19. George, E.; Wortman, J.R.; Fulwadhva, U.P.; Uyeda, J.W.; Sodickson, A.D. Dual energy CT applications in pancreatic pathologies. *Br. J. Radiol.* **2017**, *90*, 20170411. [CrossRef] [PubMed]
20. Wang, X.; Liu, D.; Zeng, X.; Jiang, S.; Li, L.; Yu, T.; Zhang, J. Dual-energy CT quantitative parameters for the differentiation of benign from malignant lesions and the prediction of histopathological and molecular subtypes in breast cancer. *Quant. Imaging Med. Surg.* **2021**, *11*, 1946–1957. [CrossRef] [PubMed]
21. Booz, C.; Nöske, J.; Martin, S.S.; Albrecht, M.H.; Yel, I.; Lenga, L.; Gruber-Rouh, T.; Eichler, K.; D'angelo, T.; Vogl, T.J.; et al. Virtual Noncalcium Dual-Energy CT: Detection of Lumbar Disk Herniation in Comparison with Standard Gray-scale CT. *Radiology* **2019**, *290*, 446–455. [CrossRef] [PubMed]

22. Booz, C.; Nöske, J.; Lenga, L.; Martin, S.S.; Yel, I.; Eichler, K.; Gruber-Rouh, T.; Huizinga, N.; Albrecht, M.H.; Vogl, T.J.; et al. Color-coded virtual non-calcium dual-energy CT for the depiction of bone marrow edema in patients with acute knee trauma: A multireader diagnostic accuracy study. *Eur. Radiol.* **2020**, *30*, 141–150. [CrossRef] [PubMed]
23. Ralli, M.; Botticelli, A.; Visconti, I.C.; Angeletti, D.; Fiore, M.; Marchetti, P.; Lambiase, A.; de Vincentiis, M.; Greco, A. Immunotherapy in the Treatment of Metastatic Melanoma: Current Knowledge and Future Directions. *J. Immunol. Res.* **2020**, *2020*, 9235638. [CrossRef]
24. Knackstedt, T.; Knackstedt, R.W.; Couto, R.; Gastman, B. Malignant Melanoma: Diagnostic and Management Update. *Plast. Reconstr. Surg.* **2018**, *142*, 202e–216e. [CrossRef]
25. Gore, R.M.; Thakrar, K.H.; Wenzke, D.R.; Newmark, G.M.; Mehta, U.K.; Berlin, J.W. That liver lesion on MDCT in the oncology patient: Is it important? *Cancer Imaging* **2012**, *12*, 373–384. [CrossRef] [PubMed]
26. Chenin, M.; Paisant, A.; Lebigot, J.; Bazeries, P.; Debbi, K.; Ronot, M.; Laurent, V.; Aubé, C. Cystic liver lesions: A pictorial review. *Insights Imaging* **2022**, *13*, 116. [CrossRef] [PubMed]
27. Park, J.H.; Kim, J.H. Pathologic differential diagnosis of metastatic carcinoma in the liver. *Clin. Mol. Hepatol.* **2019**, *25*, 12–20. [CrossRef] [PubMed]
28. Coenegrachts, K. Magnetic resonance imaging of the liver: New imaging strategies for evaluating focal liver lesions. *World J. Radiol.* **2009**, *1*, 72–85. [CrossRef] [PubMed]
29. Wang, Q.; Shi, G.; Qi, X.; Fan, X.; Wang, L. Quantitative analysis of the dual-energy CT virtual spectral curve for focal liver lesions characterization. *Eur. J. Radiol.* **2014**, *83*, 1759–1764. [CrossRef] [PubMed]
30. Ascenti, G.; Mileto, A.; Krauss, B.; Gaeta, M.; Blandino, A.; Scribano, E.; Settineri, N.; Mazziotti, S. Distinguishing enhancing from nonenhancing renal masses with dual-source dual-energy CT: Iodine quantification versus standard enhancement measurements. *Eur. Radiol.* **2013**, *23*, 2288–2295. [CrossRef] [PubMed]
31. Kaza, R.K.; Caoili, E.M.; Cohan, R.H.; Platt, J.F. Distinguishing enhancing from nonenhancing renal lesions with fast kilovoltage-switching dual-energy CT. *AJR Am. J. Roentgenol.* **2011**, *197*, 1375–1381. [CrossRef] [PubMed]
32. Mileto, A.; Allen, B.C.; Pietryga, J.A.; Farjat, A.E.; Zarzour, J.G.; Bellini, D.; Ebner, L.; Morgan, D.E. Characterization of Incidental Renal Mass With Dual-Energy CT: Diagnostic Accuracy of Effective Atomic Number Maps for Discriminating Nonenhancing Cysts From Enhancing Masses. *AJR Am. J. Roentgenol.* **2017**, *209*, W221–W230. [CrossRef]
33. Jiang, L.; Liu, D.; Long, L.; Chen, J.; Lan, X.; Zhang, J. Dual-source dual-energy computed tomography-derived quantitative parameters combined with machine learning for the differential diagnosis of benign and malignant thyroid nodules. *Quant. Imaging Med. Surg.* **2022**, *12*, 967–978. [CrossRef]
34. Shen, H.; Yuan, X.; Liu, D.; Tu, C.; Wang, X.; Liu, R.; Wang, X.; Lan, X.; Fu, K.; Zhang, J. Multiparametric dual-energy CT to differentiate stage T1 nasopharyngeal carcinoma from benign hyperplasia. *Quant. Imaging Med. Surg.* **2021**, *11*, 4004–4015. [CrossRef]
35. Cantisani, V.; Grazhdani, H.; Fioravanti, C.; Rosignuolo, M.; Calliada, F.; Messineo, D.; Bernieri, M.G.; Redler, A.; Catalano, C.; D'ambrosio, F. Liver metastases: Contrast-enhanced ultrasound compared with computed tomography and magnetic resonance. *World J. Gastroenterol.* **2014**, *20*, 9998–10007. [CrossRef] [PubMed]
36. Freitas, P.S.; Janicas, C.; Veiga, J.; Matos, A.P.; Herédia, V.; Ramalho, M. Imaging evaluation of the liver in oncology patients: A comparison of techniques. *World J. Hepatol.* **2021**, *13*, 1936–1955. [CrossRef] [PubMed]

Disclaimer/Publisher's Note: The statements, opinions and data contained in all publications are solely those of the individual author(s) and contributor(s) and not of MDPI and/or the editor(s). MDPI and/or the editor(s) disclaim responsibility for any injury to people or property resulting from any ideas, methods, instructions or products referred to in the content.

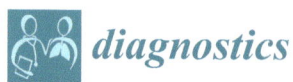 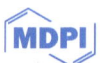

Article

A European Multicentric Investigation of Atypical Melanocytic Skin Lesions of Palms and Soles: The *iDScore-PalmoPlantar* Database

Linda Tognetti [1,*], Alessandra Cartocci [1], Aimilios Lallas [2], Elvira Moscarella [3], Ignazio Stanganelli [4,5], Gianluca Nazzaro [6], John Paoli [7,8], Maria Concetta Fargnoli [9], Paolo Broganelli [10], Harald Kittler [11], Jean-Luc Perrot [12], Gennaro Cataldo [13], Gabriele Cevenini [13], Sofia Lo Conte [1], Leonardelli Simone [1], Elisa Cinotti [1] and Pietro Rubegni [1]

[1] Dermatology Unit, Department of Medical, Surgical and Neurosciences, University of Siena, 53100 Siena, Italy
[2] First Department of Dermatology, Aristotle University, 54124 Thessaloniki, Greece
[3] Dermatology Unit, University of Campania Luigi Vanvitelli, 81100 Naples, Italy
[4] Skin Cancer Unit, Scientific Institute of Romagna for the Study of Cancer, Istituti di Ricovero e Cura a Carattere Scientifico (IRCCS), Istituto Tumori della Romagna (IRST), 47014 Meldola, Italy
[5] Department of Dermatology, University of Parma, 43121 Parma, Italy
[6] Fondazione IRCCS Ca' Granda Ospedale Maggiore Policlinico, 20122 Milan, Italy
[7] Department of Dermatology and Venereology, Institute of Clinical Sciences, Sahlgrenska Academy, University of Gothenburg, 41390 Gothenburg, Sweden; john.paoli@gu.se
[8] Department of Dermatology and Venereology, Region Västra Götaland, Sahlgrenska University Hospital, 41345 Gothenburg, Sweden
[9] Dermatology Unit, University of L'Aquila, 67100 L'Aquila, Italy
[10] Dermatology Unit, University Hospital of Torino, 4020 Torino, Italy
[11] Department of Dermatology, Medical University of Vienna, 1090 Vienna, Austria
[12] Dermatology Unit, University Hospital of St-Etienne, 42270 Saint Etienne, France
[13] Department of Medical Biotechnologies, University of Siena, 53100 Siena, Italy
* Correspondence: linda.tognetti@dbm.unisi.it; Tel.: +39-0577-585426; Fax: +39-0577-585420

Abstract: Background: The differential diagnosis of atypical melanocytic palmoplantar skin lesions (aMPLs) represents a diagnostic challenge, including atypical nevi (AN) and early melanomas (MMs) that display overlapping clinical and dermoscopic features. We aimed to set up a multicentric dataset of aMPL dermoscopic cases paired with multiple anamnestic risk factors and demographic and morphologic data. **Methods:** Each aMPL case was paired with a dermoscopic and clinical picture and a series of lesion-related data (maximum diameter value; location on the palm/sole in 17 areas; histologic diagnosis; and patient-related data (age, sex, family history of melanoma/sunburns, phototype, pheomelanin, eye/hair color, multiple/dysplastic body nevi, and traumatism on palms/soles). **Results:** A total of 542 aMPL cases—113 MM and 429 AN—were collected from 195 males and 347 females. No sex prevalence was found for melanomas, while women were found to have relatively more nevi. Melanomas were prevalent on the heel, plantar arch, and fingers in patients aged 65.3 on average, with an average diameter of 17 mm. Atypical nevi were prevalent on the plantar arch and palmar area of patients aged 41.33 on average, with an average diameter of 7 mm. **Conclusions:** Keeping in mind the risk profile of an aMPL patient can help obtain a timely differentiation between malignant/benign cases, thus avoiding delayed and inappropriate excision, respectively, with the latter often causing discomfort/dysfunctional scarring, especially at acral sites.

Keywords: acral melanoma; acral nevi; dermoscopy; integrated dataset; web registry; atypical pigmented palmoplantar lesions

1. Introduction

Acral-pigmented lesions are still less investigated by dermoscopy than facial or body-pigmented lesions, and the referring terminology is otherwise rather confused [1–5]. To

22. Booz, C.; Nöske, J.; Lenga, L.; Martin, S.S.; Yel, I.; Eichler, K.; Gruber-Rouh, T.; Huizinga, N.; Albrecht, M.H.; Vogl, T.J.; et al. Color-coded virtual non-calcium dual-energy CT for the depiction of bone marrow edema in patients with acute knee trauma: A multireader diagnostic accuracy study. *Eur. Radiol.* **2020**, *30*, 141–150. [CrossRef] [PubMed]
23. Ralli, M.; Botticelli, A.; Visconti, I.C.; Angeletti, D.; Fiore, M.; Marchetti, P.; Lambiase, A.; de Vincentiis, M.; Greco, A. Immunotherapy in the Treatment of Metastatic Melanoma: Current Knowledge and Future Directions. *J. Immunol. Res.* **2020**, *2020*, 9235638. [CrossRef]
24. Knackstedt, T.; Knackstedt, R.W.; Couto, R.; Gastman, B. Malignant Melanoma: Diagnostic and Management Update. *Plast. Reconstr. Surg.* **2018**, *142*, 202e–216e. [CrossRef]
25. Gore, R.M.; Thakrar, K.H.; Wenzke, D.R.; Newmark, G.M.; Mehta, U.K.; Berlin, J.W. That liver lesion on MDCT in the oncology patient: Is it important? *Cancer Imaging* **2012**, *12*, 373–384. [CrossRef] [PubMed]
26. Chenin, M.; Paisant, A.; Lebigot, J.; Bazeries, P.; Debbi, K.; Ronot, M.; Laurent, V.; Aubé, C. Cystic liver lesions: A pictorial review. *Insights Imaging* **2022**, *13*, 116. [CrossRef] [PubMed]
27. Park, J.H.; Kim, J.H. Pathologic differential diagnosis of metastatic carcinoma in the liver. *Clin. Mol. Hepatol.* **2019**, *25*, 12–20. [CrossRef] [PubMed]
28. Coenegrachts, K. Magnetic resonance imaging of the liver: New imaging strategies for evaluating focal liver lesions. *World J. Radiol.* **2009**, *1*, 72–85. [CrossRef] [PubMed]
29. Wang, Q.; Shi, G.; Qi, X.; Fan, X.; Wang, L. Quantitative analysis of the dual-energy CT virtual spectral curve for focal liver lesions characterization. *Eur. J. Radiol.* **2014**, *83*, 1759–1764. [CrossRef] [PubMed]
30. Ascenti, G.; Mileto, A.; Krauss, B.; Gaeta, M.; Blandino, A.; Scribano, E.; Settineri, N.; Mazziotti, S. Distinguishing enhancing from nonenhancing renal masses with dual-source dual-energy CT: Iodine quantification versus standard enhancement measurements. *Eur. Radiol.* **2013**, *23*, 2288–2295. [CrossRef] [PubMed]
31. Kaza, R.K.; Caoili, E.M.; Cohan, R.H.; Platt, J.F. Distinguishing enhancing from nonenhancing renal lesions with fast kilovoltage-switching dual-energy CT. *AJR Am. J. Roentgenol.* **2011**, *197*, 1375–1381. [CrossRef] [PubMed]
32. Mileto, A.; Allen, B.C.; Pietryga, J.A.; Farjat, A.E.; Zarzour, J.G.; Bellini, D.; Ebner, L.; Morgan, D.E. Characterization of Incidental Renal Mass With Dual-Energy CT: Diagnostic Accuracy of Effective Atomic Number Maps for Discriminating Nonenhancing Cysts From Enhancing Masses. *AJR Am. J. Roentgenol.* **2017**, *209*, W221–W230. [CrossRef]
33. Jiang, L.; Liu, D.; Long, L.; Chen, J.; Lan, X.; Zhang, J. Dual-source dual-energy computed tomography-derived quantitative parameters combined with machine learning for the differential diagnosis of benign and malignant thyroid nodules. *Quant. Imaging Med. Surg.* **2022**, *12*, 967–978. [CrossRef]
34. Shen, H.; Yuan, X.; Liu, D.; Tu, C.; Wang, X.; Liu, R.; Wang, X.; Lan, X.; Fu, K.; Zhang, J. Multiparametric dual-energy differentiate stage T1 nasopharyngeal carcinoma from benign hyperplasia. *Quant. Imaging Med. Surg.* **2021**, *11*, 400 [CrossRef]
35. Cantisani, V.; Grazhdani, H.; Fioravanti, C.; Rosignuolo, M.; Calliada, F.; Messineo, D.; Bernieri, M.G.; Redler, A.; Ca' D'ambrosio, F. Liver metastases: Contrast-enhanced ultrasound compared with computed tomography and magnetic *World J. Gastroenterol.* **2014**, *20*, 9998–10007. [CrossRef] [PubMed]
36. Freitas, P.S.; Janicas, C.; Veiga, J.; Matos, A.P.; Herédia, V.; Ramalho, M. Imaging evaluation of the liver in oncol A comparison of techniques. *World J. Hepatol.* **2021**, *13*, 1936–1955. [CrossRef] [PubMed]

Disclaimer/Publisher's Note: The statements, opinions and data contained in all publications are solely those author(s) and contributor(s) and not of MDPI and/or the editor(s). MDPI and/or the editor(s) disclaim responsibili people or property resulting from any ideas, methods, instructions or products referred to in the content.

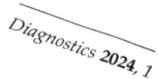

date, the term "acral" has been used to define melanocytic lesions localized not only on volar glabrous skin surfaces of the extremities but also on the nail apparatus and subungual region—especially in reference to acral lentiginous melanoma (MM) [1–5]. Moreover, in many different studies to date, the terms "acquired acral nevi", "congenital acral nevi", "acral melanocytic lesions", and "acral lentiginous melanoma" have been vaguely employed, without specifying if the lesions were on palms/soles or subungual region/nail. However, the acral glabrous skin, which is anatomically limited to the palms of the hands and soles of the feet, distally to the Wallace's line, significantly differs from other body sites skin areas, both clinically and dermoscopically, due to the presence of dermatoglyphics [1–7]. To avoid confusion, in this study we preferred naming the melanocytic lesion on glabrous acral skin as "melanocytic (M) palmoplantar (PP) lesions (Ls)" (MPPLs). This definition encompasses the spectrum of histologically benign MPPLs (with no/mild/moderate/severe atypia), histologically malignant MPPLs, and the grey zone of borderline provisional entities such as nevi MELTUMP/SAMPU/THIUMP/IAMPUS lesions [6].

The prevalence of MPPLs varies greatly according to populations, countries, and study groups, and it is essentially in line with that of benign MPPLs, ranging from 36–42% in dark phototypes and 18–23% in Caucasians [4–7]. This may also explain why studies focused on large datasets of acral nevi in Europe are scarce [8,9]. Interestingly, in dark skin types and Asiatic populations, the number of PP nevi is relatively high compared with other body sites and in a globally low total-body nevus count, while the trend is opposite in European and North American populations [1–7]. In parallel, the current bulk of knowledge from PP melanoma greatly derives from studies carried out in Asiatic countries (e.g., Japan, China, Taiwan) in the last 30 years [10–13], where this form accounts for nearly 50% of all MM cases. On the contrary, PP melanoma is traditionally considered rare in Caucasians, accounting for 3% of all MMs in North America and about 1–2% in Europe [1,3,9,11]. There is currently no univocal hypothesis to explain these discrepancies of both benign and malignant MPPLs among different populations: genetic predisposition is known to play a role, but genetic studies recently highlighted that PP nevi exhibit a mutational spectrum comparable to that of nevi arising on low cumulative sun-damaged skin [1,14,15]. Currently, PP melanoma is regarded as a non-UV-related tumor and represents a higher proportion of cases in countries with a lower incidence of melanoma overall [1]. External mechanisms and risk factors such as trauma, physical stress, and friction have been hypothesized to have a role in its development, but no conclusive data have been produced to date [16–18]. Additionally, other factors have been addressed such as the rarely examined location (sole melanoma), the atypical appearance (palm melanoma), and the lack of pigment (PP melanoma) [19,20].

Dermoscopic examination was shown to help increase the diagnostic accuracy of MPPLs, especially in differentiating malignant from benign cases [21,22] and in clear-cut lesions. Indeed, considering clear-cut PP nevi and PP melanomas, a series of specific dermoscopic patterns were first described by Japanese study groups and included benign-related features (parallel furrow pattern, lattice-like, fibrillar, globular, and homogenous) and malignancy-related features (parallel-ridge pattern, irregular diffuse pigmentation, and multicomponent pattern) [7,9,11,23–25]. We have otherwise to keep in mind that there are atypical MPPLs (aMPPLs) that exhibit equivocal clinical and dermoscopic features, including PP nevi mimicking PP melanomas (e.g., asymmetrical, maculopapular, and with non-homogenous pigmentation) and, vice versa, featureless or doubtful early melanoma [1,10,13,26]. In this subset of difficult "borderline" lesions, dermoscopy alone cannot reach adequate diagnostic accuracy, and further parameters should be taken into account to assess the risk of that lesion being malignant [24–26]. It has been widely demonstrated that the Bayesian scoring classifier models are reliable tools able to efficiently select and combine a series of patient and lesion objective parameters with dermoscopic data, with the final aim of developing a risk scoring model dedicated to a specific subset of lesions [27–33]. In particular, our group previously created and tested four different risk scoring models, named "integrated clinic-dermoscopic scores" (*iDScore*) for difficult-to-diagnose melanocytic skin lesions of the body (i.e., early melanomas and atypical nevi (AN) [28,29], for regressing nevi and melanomas with regression [30], and for atypical pigmented lesions of the face (i.e., lentigo maligna and benign simulators—pigmented actinic keratosis, solar lentigo, seborrheic keratosis, lichen planus-like keratosis, and atypical nevi) [31]. The development of an *iDScore* model relies, at first, on the preparation of a large detailed and standardized dataset of the lesions of interest. A dataset of 1700 cases of atypical melanocytic lesions of the body [32] and about 2000 cases of atypical pigmented lesions of the face [29] was developed, with each case integrated with multiple data of the patient and lesion and further subjected to pattern analysis and complex statistical analysis [28–33].

On these premises, we aimed to create, for the first time, a large international web registry able to provide a detailed characterization of aMPPLs (including early PP melanomas and atypical and/or dysplastic PP nevi) in terms of morphology (clinical and dermoscopic), epidemiology, patient risk factors, and anamnestic data.

In this study, we describe the development and implementation of a European multicenter database specifically dedicated to aMPPLs, the *iDScore-PalmoPlantar* dataset.

2. Materials and Methods

Ethics. This study was carried out in compliance with the Helsinki Declaration. Approval was obtained by the local ethical committee of Siena Hospital (Azienda Ospedaliero-Universitaria Senese, Siena, Italy, Study Protocol No. 16801) and was then shared with the participating centers. All data were de-identified before use and are kept in accordance with the EU General Data Protection Regulations (GDPR) on the processing of personal data and the protection of privacy in electronic communication (2016/679/EU) [34].

Study design. The development of the international clinical–dermoscopic database dedicated to aMPPLs was promoted as part of the *iDScore-PalmoPlantar* project by dermatologists (LT, PR, and EC) and technical figures (bioengineer: GC, biostatisticians: AC and SLC, and data manager: GC) of Siena University Hospital and extended to the Teledermoscopy Working Group (AL, MCF, IS, GN, PB, JP, HK, JLP, EM, FL, CL, ED, MS, and EC) under the Teledermatology Task Force of the European Academy of Dermatology and Venereology (EADV). The *iDScore-PalmoPlantar* project is devoted to the study of difficult-to-diagnose melanocytic skin lesions from a clinical and dermoscopic point of view. In particular, the *iDScore-PalmoPlantar* database was designed for educational and training purposes, through a tele-dermoscopic setting, accessible to all European dermatologists; thus, the database is currently hosted on a dedicated website, www.iDScore.net (accessed on 16 February 2023).

Center participation. A center was enrolled in the *iDScore-PalmoPlantar* project if it could provide at least 60 cases (up to a maximum of 110) of clinically and dermoscopically challenging aMPPLs excised in the suspect of malignancy. Thus, each center was required to provide a minimum of 20 malignant cases (up to 30) and a minimum of 40 benign cases (up to 80). Participation in the study was open to any European dermatology center actively working in skin cancer screening as a second-level referring center. The data were collected both retrospectively and prospectively: the collection phase lasted from September 2020 to March 2023. Since data were collected during routine consultation activity, there were neither costs nor financial compensation to participate. Each center designated one Site Investigator as responsible for the whole selection and submission process. Site Investigators were required to sign in to a web platform—hosted at www.iDScore.net—through secure access with personal credentials. Site Investigators were enabled to upload their cases from between October 2020 to June 2023 by using a "Contribution form" specifically created for the project and hosted on the website: the form was designed to record a total of 14 parameters (5 mandatory and 9 optional) along with 2 standardized image files. The assessment of the specific palmar or plantar location was mandatory; thus, site investigators were guided to select only one site per image among 9 areas of the palms or only one among 8 areas of the soles.

Inclusion criteria. In order to avoid repetition of clinical/anamnestic data and thus bias affecting the analysis, each lesion had to be derived from one patient only. Each aMPPL case must be composed of one dermoscopic image, one clinical image, three mandatory lesion data (i.e., definitive histopathological diagnosis, maximum diameter (mm), and precise body location), and two mandatory patient data (i.e., sex (F/M) and age (years). Histologic diagnosis could be (a) nevus with mild atypia, (b) nevus with severe atypia, (c) dysplastic nevus, or (d) melanoma in situ or stage Ia/Ib/IIa (pathologic TNM classification pTis/pT1a/pT1b/pT2a). Additional histological data were required for MM cases only: thickness, mitosis number, regression (%), and presence of lymphocytic infiltrate. Patients were required to be aged at least 18 years; there was no upper range limit. According to anatomical and morphologic criteria, a classification into 17 subareas was adopted (Figure 1), including 8 plantar areas (i.e., *anterior lateral eminence of the sole, anterior medial eminence of the sole, central eminence of the sole, heel, interdigital spaces, lateral surface of the fingers, and plantar region*) and 9 volar palmar areas (i.e., *plantar surface of the fingers of the sole, central metacarpal, fingertips, interdigital spaces, hypothenar surface, lateral surface of the fingers, metacarpal surface, thenar surface* and *volar surface of the fingers, and proximal phalangeal surface*).

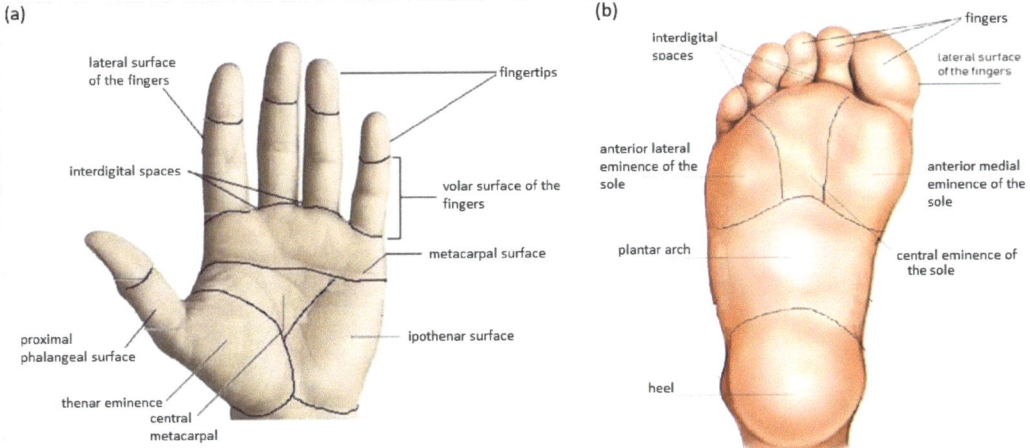

Figure 1. Schematic representation of the classification used in the *iDScore-PalmoPlantar* database into 17 areas: 9 palmar (**a**) and 8 plantar (**b**).

Patients' additional data. Details concerning 4 anamnestic data and 5 phenotypic traits were strongly recommended (Table 1). Four types of anamnestic data were strongly recommended, though not mandatory, namely personal or family history of melanoma (i.e., in a 1st-degree relative), history of sunburns (>3) in childhood below the age of 14 years, history of chronic traumatism on the soles for work, and chronic traumatism on the palms for work. Five types of patient clinical data were strongly recommended, though not mandatory, namely presence of multiple common nevi (>100) or dysplastic nevi (>10) on the body, phototype (I–IV), pheomelanin phototype [35–37], presence of green/light blue/blue eyes, and presence of blond hair. In order to avoid repetition of clinical/anamnestic data and thus bias affecting the analysis, each lesion should be derived from one patient only.

Table 1. Characteristics of the case study of 542 atypical melanocytic palmoplantar lesions (aMPPLs) comprising the *iDScore-PalmoPlantar* dataset.

Lesion Data	n (%)/Mean ± SD		
Histological Diagnosis	542		
Nevus	429 (79.2%)		
Malignant melanoma	113 (20.8%)		
Maximum diameter	8.83 ± 7.85		
Four macro-areas of the sole	490 (90.6%)		
• Toe area *(fingers + interdigital spaces + lateral surface of the fingers)*	111 (22.7%)		
• Eminence of the sole area *(anterior lateral + central + anterior medial eminence of the sole)*	87 (17.8%)		
• Plantar arch area	229 (46.7%)		
• Heel area	63 (12.9%)		
Three macro-areas of the palm	51 (9.4%)		
• Palmar lateral area *(proximal phalangeal surface + thenar eminence)*	12 (23.5%)		
• Fingers *(lateral surface of the fingers + fingertips + interdigital spaces)*	17 (33.3%)		
• Palmar medial area *(hypothenar surface + metacarpal surface + central metacarpal)*	22 (43.1%)		
Patient Data			
Age	46.33 ± 19.07		
Male	195 (36.0%)		
Female	347 (64.0%)		
ANAMNESTIC DATA/RISK FACTORS	**YES**	**NO**	**NA**
Personal/family history of melanoma—1st-degree-relative	11 (2.0%)	79 (14.5%)	452 (83.4%)
History of sunburns (>3) in childhood below the age of 14 years	41 (7.5%)	75 (13.8%)	426 (78.5%)
Chronic traumatism of palms	0 (0.0%)	7 (12.9%)	44 (86.3%)
Chronic traumatism of soles	10 (1.8%)	138 (25.4%)	342 (63.0%)
PHENOTYPIC TRAITS			
Presence of >100 common nevi or >10 dysplastic nevi on the body	24 (4.4%)	67 (12.3%)	451 (83.2%)
Phototype	355 (65.5%)		187 (34.5%)
• II	94 (17.3%)		
• III	248 (45.7%)		
• IV	11 (2.0%)		
• V	2 (0.3%)		
Pheomelanin phenotype	35 (6.4%)	65 (11.9%)	442 (81%)
Presence of green/light blue/blue eyes	51 (9.4%)	76 (14%)	415 (76%)
Presence of blond hair	93 (17.1%)	69 (12.7%)	380 (70.1%)

Technical requirements. Each site investigator should also respect a series of technical requirements for the dermoscopic images (i.e., ≥1.5 Mpx, 15–20× enlargement, JPEG format, in-focus picture) and device type (e.g., videodermatoscope—Fotofinder system

Medcam1000, camera-based systems—Dermlite Photo System Pro/Dermlite Foto II Pro WITH Nikon D500, 3GEN Dermlite Foto Dermoscopy System, Heine DL 20 Canon/Nikon, smartphone-based system—Foto X Dermlite).

Exclusion criteria and quality check. Exclusion criteria for center contribution relied on the impossibility of reaching the adequate number and proportion of MMs and AN required. Exclusion criteria for pictures included blurred/out-of-focus dermoscopic pictures; clinical pictures with recognizable patient personal characteristics (e.g., tattoos, etc.); and nodular/ulcerated/inflamed/intensely traumatized MPPLs. Duplicate cases (e.g., multiple dermoscopic images of the same patient uploaded as separate cases or the same case entered 2 or 3 times) were rejected as well. Once uploaded onto the platform, each submission was examined; if judged suitable, the case was transferred to the *iDScore-PalmoPlantar* dataset itself. A review of all the cases received in the registry was performed weekly by LT, AC, GC, and SL from October 2020 to July 2023. This rapid review after each submission allowed all Site Investigators to be updated on their acceptance rate and allowed them to proceed with contributions until the minimum criteria were reached.

Statistical analysis. Descriptive statistics was carried out; continuous variables were summarized as mean ± standard deviation, with the qualitative ones recorded as absolute frequencies and percentages. The χ-squared test was performed to examine the association between qualitative variables and histological diagnosis. Student's t test was performed to compare age and maximum diameter between MMs and AN. A significance of $p < 0.05$ was assumed. All analyses were carried out using R version 4.0.0. For statistical purposes, the 17 subareas were further grouped into 7 macro-areas, namely 3 macro-areas on the palm and 4 macro-areas on the sole (Table 1).

3. Results

3.1. Participating Centers

A total of 21 dermatologic centers from 14 European Countries were invited; all of them had a second-level ambulatory clinic active in screening and research on skin cancer. Among them, 10 were able to meet the minimum contribution criteria, namely Siena (Italy), Thessaloniki (Greece), Meldola (Italy), Milan (Italy), Gothenburg (Sweden), L'Aquila (Italy), Turin (Italy), Vienna (Austria), St. Etienne (France), and Naples (Italy). Each country contributed 65 cases on average (range 50–80), for a total of 565 cases. After a quality check, a total of 545 cases were definitively included in the final dataset, that is, 54 cases on average per center (range 44–64).

3.2. Dataset Characteristics

The *iDScore-PalmoPlantar* dataset comprised 542 aMPPL cases with defined histopathological diagnosis and doubtful clinical and dermoscopic appearance, namely 113 (20.8%) melanomas and 429 (79.2%) nevi. Morphologic data of the 542 lesions and patient demographics, anamnestic, and phenotypic data are reported in Table 1, while characteristics of MMs and nevi are reported in Table 2 The analysis of clinical pictures reveals that 291 nevi (67.8%) were flat and 138 (32.1%) were palpable (Figures 2–4).

Table 2. Distribution of anamnestic and phenotypic data of 542 atypical melanocytic palmoplantar lesion (aMPPL) cases, grouped according to seven macro-areas (four on the sole and three on the palm).

Lesion Data	n (%)/Mean ± SD		p
	MMs (113)	Nevi (429)	
Maximum diameter	17.39 ± 12.47	6.58 ± 3.58	<0.001
Body site			0.285
Four macro-areas of the sole *	98 (87.5%)	392 (91.4%)	
• Toe area	21 (21.4%)	90 (23.0%)	

Table 2. Cont.

Lesion Data	n (%)/Mean ± SD		p
	MMs (113)	Nevi (429)	
• Eminence of the sole area	21 (21.4%)	66 (16.8%)	
• Plantar arch area	29 (29.6%)	200 (51.0%)	
• Heel area	27 (27.6%)	36 (9.2%)	
Three macro-areas of the palm #	14 (12.5%)	37 (8.6%)	
• Palmar medial area	3 (21.4%)	9 (24.3%)	
• Finger area	7 (50.0%)	10 (27.0%)	
• Palmar lateral area	4 (28.6%)	18 (41.6%)	
Patient Data			
Age	65.30 ± 14.79	41.33 ± 16.81	<0.001
Male	55 (48.6%)	140 (32.6%)	
Female	58 (51.3%)	289 (67.4%)	0.002
Anamnestic Data/Risk Factors			
Personal/family history of melanoma—1st-degree relative			0.520
No	9 (7.9%)	70 (16.3%)	
Yes	0 (0.0%)	11 (2.5%)	
History of sunburns (>3) in childhood below the age of 14 years			
No	25 (22.1%)	50 (11.6%)	
Yes	7 (0.6%)	34 (7.9%)	
Chronic traumatism on soles			
No	15 (13.2%)	129 (30.0%)	
Yes	0 (0%)	10 (23.3%)	
Chronic traumatism on palms			
No	10 (8.8%)	94 (21.9%)	
Yes	0 (%)	1 (0.2%)	
PHENOTYPIC TRAITS			
Presence of >100 common nevi or >10 dysplastic nevi			1.000
No	7 (6.1%)	60 (13.9%)	
Yes	3 (2.6%)	21 (4,8%)	
Phototype (%)	100%	100%	0.717
II	19 (29.7%)	75 (25.8%)	
III	44 (68.8%)	204 (70.1%)	
IV	1 (1.6%)	10 (3.4%)	
V	0 (0.0%)	2 (0.7%)	
Pheomelanin phenotype			
No	17 (15.0%)	48 (11.1%)	0.610
Yes	9 (7.9%)	26 (6.0%)	
Presence of green/light blue/blue eyes			
No	23 (20.3%)	53 (12.3%)	0.320
Yes	18 (15.9%)	33 (7.6%)	
Presence of blond hair			
No	14 (12.3%)	55 (12.8%)	0.430
Yes	26 (23%)	67 (15.6%)	

* SOLE SUBAREAS: Toe area (plantar surface of the fingers + lateral surface of the fingers + interdigital spaces); eminence of the sole area (anterior eminence + central eminence + antero-medial eminence); plantar arch area; and heel. # PALM SUBAREAS: Finger area (fingertips + lateral surface of the fingers + interdigital spaces + volar surface of the finger + proximal phalangeal surface); palmar lateral area (metacarpal area + hypotenar); and palmar medial (thenar + central metacarpal).

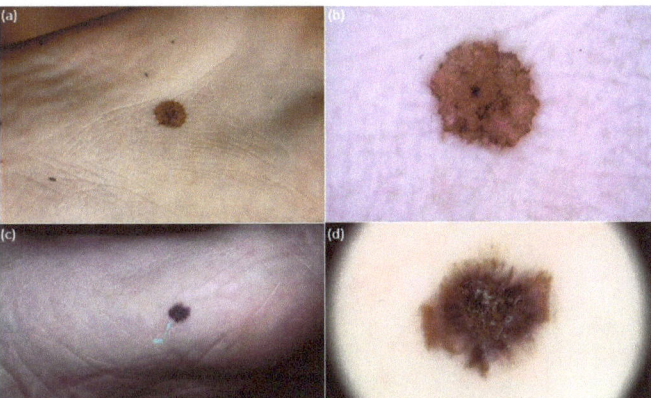

Figure 2. Clinical and dermoscopic (polarized light, 20×) appearance of 2 atypical melanocytic plantar lesions (aMPPLs) of the sole, localized at the central eminence (**a,b**) and anterior–medial eminence (**c,d**). Both lesions appear as brownish roundish pigmented macules with clear-cut borders and non-homogenous pigmentation, similar diameter and multiple colors, and irregular blotches observed under dermoscopy; however, the lesion of the central eminence was an atypical nevus of 12 mm in a 20-year-old female (**a,b**), while the lesion on the anterior–medial eminence was an early melanoma (pt1a) of 13.6 mm in a 63-year-old male (**c**), with additional dermoscopic features of a hyperkeratosic component/blue–white veil and irregular streaks.

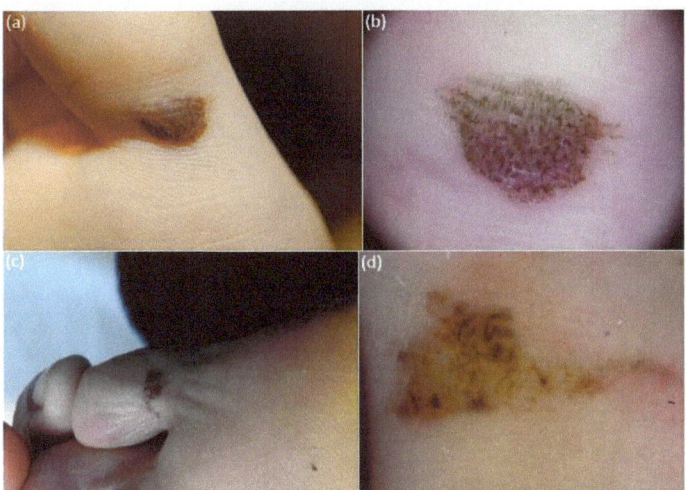

Figure 3. Clinical appearance of atypical melanocytic plantar lesions of the plantar surface of the fingers, namely first (**a**) and fifth (**c**) fingers, presenting as brownish elongated pigmented macules with clear-cut borders and irregular cobblestone-like pigmentation. Lesion one had a maximum diameter of 13 mm and belonged to an 18-year-old female (**a**). Lesion two had a maximum diameter of 11 mm and belonged to a 52-year-old male (**c**). Dermoscopic examination (polarized light, 20×) reveals an overall homogenous color arranged both in a parallel furrow and in a cobblestone (**b**) in case one, which was histologically classified as an acral nevus. Conversely, case two exhibits multiple colors (light brown, dark brown, gray, and reddish) arranged in a multicomponent pattern with streaks, globules, and irregular blotches (**d**); the lesion was histologically classified as an acral melanoma pt1a.

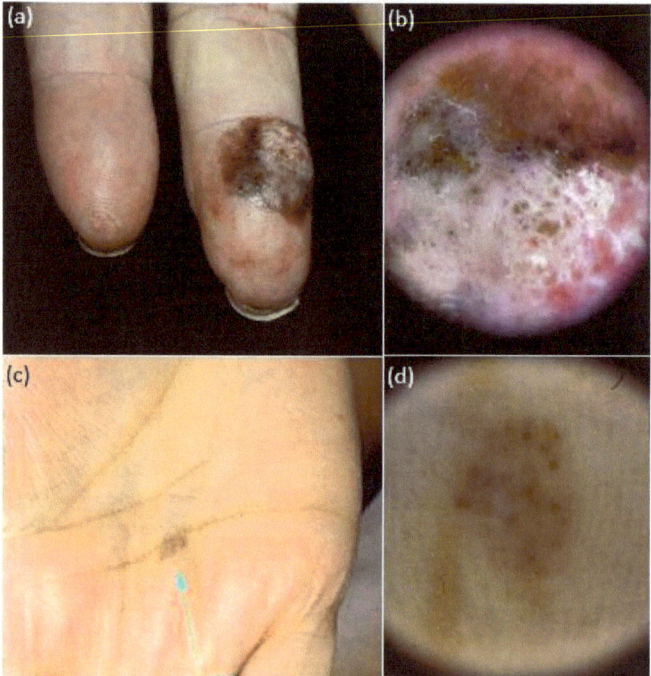

Figure 4. Clinical (**a,c**) and dermoscopic (**b,d**) appearance of two atypical melanocytic palmar lesions in two women aged 68: the lesion on the volar surface of the finger (**a**) is a multi-colored nodule, with irregular pigmentations and chaotic dermoscopic pattern (**b**), consistent with a histopathologic diagnosis of acral melanoma (pT3a); the lesion on the metacarpal surface appears as a multi-colored macule (**c**, *blue arrow*) with a quite regular dermoscopic pattern and a histopathologic report of acral nevus.

3.3. Lesion Morphological Features

The obtained maximum diameter range for all aMPPLs was 1–50 mm, the average value was 8.83 mm, and the standard deviation was ±7.85 mm (Figures 2–4). In melanoma cases, the average diameter was 17.39 (±12.47 standard deviation), range 6–50 mm; in nevi cases, the average diameter was 6.58 (±3.58 standard deviation), range 1–20 mm. The difference between the average diameter of the melanomas and that of the nevi was statistically significant ($p < 0.001$) (Table 2 and Figures 2–4).

3.4. Lesion Location
3.4.1. All aMPPLs

Among 542 aMPPL cases, 490 (90.6%) were located on the sole; of them, 98 (87.5%) were MMs and 392 (91.4%) were nevi. A total of 51 out of 542 aMPPL cases (9.4%) were located on the palm, including 14 (12.5%) melanomas and 37 (8.6%) nevi. According to the classification into five macro-areas, aMPPL cases of the sole were predominantly localized on the plantar arch with 229 (46.7%) cases, then on the toes with 111 (22.7%) cases, on the eminence of the sole with 87 (17.8%) cases, and on the heel with 63 (12.9%) cases. On the palm, aMPPL cases were more homogeneously distributed, namely 22 (43.1%) on the palmar medial area, 17 (33.3%) on the finger area, and 12 (23.5%) on the palmar lateral area (Table 1).

3.4.2. Malignant aMPPLs

On soles, melanomas were prevalent on the plantar arch (29.6%) and heel (27.6%), while on palms, skin distribution was homogeneous among nine subareas (Table 3). Regrouping determined similar proportions of melanomas among four plantar macro-areas and a predominance of malignant cases on the finger area of the palms (Table 2).

Table 3. Distribution of 542 atypical melanocytic palmoplantar lesions (aMPPLs) of the *iDScore-PalmoPlantar* dataset according to histologic diagnosis and detailed body location to 8 plantar and 8 palmar subareas.

Lesion Data	aMPPLs n = 542	MMs n = 113	Nevi n = 429
Eight Subareas of the sole	490	98 (87.5)	392 (91.4)
Anterior lateral eminence of the sole	21 (3.18%)	3 (3.1%)	18 (4.6%)
Anterior medial eminence of the sole	45 (7.85%)	15 (15.3%)	30 (7.7%)
Central eminence of the sole	21 (4.46%)	3 (3.1%)	18 (4.6%)
Heel	63 (1.21%)	27 (27.6%)	36 (9.2%)
Interdigital spaces (foot)	34 (5.73%)	4 (4.1%)	30 (7.7%)
Lateral surface of the fingers (foot)	36 (7.21%)	8 (8.2%)	28 (7.1%)
Plantar arch	229 (43.9%)	29 (29.6%)	200 (51.0%)
Plantar surface of the fingers	41 (7.85%)	9 (9.2%)	32 (8.2%)
Nine Subareas of the palms	36	14 (12.5%)	37 (8.6%)
Central metacarpal	2 (5.6%)	0 (0.0%)	2 (5.4%)
Fingertips (hand)	2 (5.6%)	2 (14.3%)	0 (0.0%)
Interdigital spaces	3 (8.3%)	0 (0.0%)	3 (8.1%)
Ipothenar surface	11 (30.6%)	1 (7.1%)	10 (27.0%)
Lateral surface of the fingers (hand)	5 (13.9%)	3 (21.4%)	2 (5.4%)
Metacarpal surface	11 (30.6%)	3 (21.4%)	8 (21.6%)
Thenar surface	10 (27.8%)	3 (21.4%)	7 (18.9%)
Volar surface of the fingers	7 (19.4%)	2 (14.3%)	5 (13.5%)
Proximal phalangeal surface	0	0	0

3.4.3. Benign aMPPLs

On soles, half of the cases were on the plantar arch site (51%), with no significant differences in size to the other seven sites and an unmodified trend after regrouping (Tables 2 and 4). On palms, a slight predominance was found on the hypothenar surface (27% of cases) (Table 3), but the palmar lateral area (41% of cases) was the most involved after grouping (Table 2).

Table 4. Characterization of digital imaging acquisition of 542 atypical melanocytic palmoplantar lesion (aMPPL) cases of the *iDScore-PalmoPlantar* dataset: three different devices for dermoscopic imaging acquisition are reported, along with the distribution per histologic diagnosis.

Device Type Used for Image Acquisition/	aMPPLs	Melanomas	Nevi
n (%)	542 (100%)	113 (100%)	429 (100%)
Camera-based system	254 (46.8%)	31 (27.4%)	223 (51.9%)
Videodermatoscope	160 (29.5%)	51 (45.1%)	109 (25.4%)
Smartphone-based system	97 (17.8%)	20 (17.6%)	77 (17.9%)
Unknown/unspecified	31 (5.7%)	11 (9.7%)	20 (4.6%)

3.5. Patient Data

3.5.1. Age

Patients with aMPPLs had an age range of 18–92 years. Patients with acral melanoma had an age range from 39 to 92 years old. The difference between the average age of patients with melanomas (65.30 on average ($\pm$14.79 sd) and patients with nevi (46.33 on average $\pm$ 19.07 sd)) was statistically significant ($p < 0.001$) (Tables 1 and 2).

3.5.2. Sex

The majority (64%) of patients with aMPPLs were women (347 cases), while men accounted for 36% of cases (i.e., 195). Specifically, this female predominance was sustained by a relevant number (67.4%) of women exhibiting acral nevi (i.e., 289) compared with men (140, 32.6%). Differently, the distribution of acral melanomas was very similar (only a 2% difference) between the two sexes: 51.3% of cases in women, and 48.6% of cases in men. In addition, the difference between the rate of female patients with melanoma and that of female patients with nevi is statistically significant ($p = 0.002$); in males, the two subgroups did not differ significantly (55 melanomas versus 140 nevi) (Tables 1 and 2).

3.6. Patient Optional Data

A total of 148 cases out of 542 (27.3%) had optional risk factor data assessed (Tables 1 and 2). The results of distribution analysis according to the histologic diagnosis are reported in Table 2 for those cases in which the optional data regarding patients' anamnestic/phenotypic and risk factor data were available.

3.6.1. Anamnestic Data/Risk Factors

Among the available records, the majority of patients with aMPPLs had a negative personal or familial history of melanoma (i.e., melanoma affecting a first-degree relative), which is 14.5% negative versus 2% positive. History of sunburns (>3) in childhood below the age of 14 years was present only in 7.5% of patients, negative in 13.8%, and not assessed in 78.5% of cases. Chronic traumatism was overall not reported on the palms and rarely on the soles (10 patients). In patients with melanomas, no specific anamnestic risk factors reach statistical significance. In patients with nevi, a positive history of sunburns in childhood was reported in 7.9% of cases, and chronic traumatism of soles in 23.3% of cases (Tables 1 and 2).

3.6.2. Phenotypic Traits

Concerning all patients with aMPPLs, a small proportion (24 cases, 4.4%) had more than 100 common nevi on the body (or more than 10 dysplastic nevi), but the number of missed assessments was relevant (83% of cases) (Table 1). Of them, 21 patients fell in the nevi group (Table 2).

Phototype III was the prevalent one in this case study (45.7% of patients) (Table 1), as well as in melanoma (68%) and nevi (70%) subgroups (Table 2). The second most prevalent prototype was type II.

A small number of patients had pheomelanin phenotype, either in the whole case study (6.4%) or in subgroups (7.9% of melanoma patients, 6% of nevi patients).

Only 51 patients were reported to have green/light-blue/blue eyes, with a high rate of non-reporting (76%); of them, 18 had a melanoma and 33 a nevus.

Lastly, a total of 93 patients were reported to have blond hair: 26 with melanoma, and 67 with a nevus.

3.7. Device for Image Acquisition

Table 4 reports in detail how the clinical and dermoscopic pictures for each aMPPL case were obtained. In 31 cases it was not specified what device was used for imaging acquisition (11 melanomas and 20 nevi). Taking into account the whole case study of 542 aMPPL cases, the more frequently employed devices were camera-based systems

(46.8% of cases), followed by videodermatoscope (29.5% of cases) and smartphone-based systems (17.8%).

This trend was similar for the imaging of nevi, with 52% of cases imaged with a camera-based system, 25.4% with a dermatoscope, and 18% with a smartphone. On the contrary, the majority of melanoma cases were imaged with a videodermatoscope (45% of cases) versus 27% with a camera-based system and 17.6% with a smartphone-based system.

4. Discussion

The current knowledge on clinical and epidemiologic features of PP nevi delineates the profile of a small (usually under 6 mm) macule, symmetric in shape and with homogenous pigmentation [9,13,16,38], and mainly derive from Asiatic [4,39,40] or South American countries [4,41,42], with fewer reports from South European countries [2,7,9]. However, equivocal aMPPLs have been poorly or not investigated, especially in Europe [26]. In parallel, large series of acral melanoma in early stages from European populations are lacking, [3,26] due to both low incidence and delayed diagnosis [22,23]. Compared with body or head and neck melanomas, indeed, the diagnosis of PP melanoma is frequently late, with a reported misdiagnosis rate of 20% [3,11,19–23]. A series of factors can be hypothesized to explain this trend: (i) physicians' reticence to perform biopsies/excision on the sole, which often causes discomfort and painful scar, in addition to nail dystrophy in case of biopsy on the nail apparatus [1,11,19–23]; (ii) immunohistochemical studies and molecular testing that may help to differentiate malignant from benign aMPPLs [1,13,14,43,44] are available only in specific centers, are time-consuming, and require a surgical excision as well; (iii) reflectance confocal microscopy, which is helpful in the non-invasive diagnosis of dermoscopically doubtful cases of the body and face, is not effective on acral skin due to the low penetration [45]; and (iv) patients are sometimes unaware of the onset date of their lesions on the soles (even if they are long-lasting benign nevi). In those cases, the dermatologist should make decisions without the clinical history data, relying on morphological features only; this has a relevant impact on the dermatologist management decision as well, ending up in surgical excision in most cases [22,23,43,44]. From an epidemiological point of view, nevi with mild/moderate/severe atypia and early melanomas on palms and soles are very rare. For this reason, a dataset that collects only PP melanomas at early stages and PP atypical nevi has not previously been set up, to the best of our knowledge. Thus, a better understanding of the aMPPL spectrum is deserved to improve clinical and dermoscopic diagnosis and management [13,23,43,44]. For this purpose, the setting up of a large multicentric European registry dedicated to aMPPLs was needed. Moreover, no specific classification according to plantar and volar subareas has been carried out to date [3,7,9–11].

The *iDScore-PalmoPlantar* dataset—comprising 542 aMPPL cases coming from 10 different European Centers—is innovative according to several aspects. First, it was designed to provide representative scenarios of the general characteristics of difficult PP lesions that dermatologists have to manage in secondary referring centers. It was indeed balanced to have 20% melanoma and 80% nevi cases and this proportion was chosen in order to reach a compromise between an adequate representation of malignant cases and a reproduction of the epidemiologic in secondary referring centers. Second, the minimum age for inclusion was set at 18 years in order to both exclude pediatric cases a priori (and, consequently, the bias of having large congenital acral nevi in the dataset) and not miss benign lesions in young adults exhibiting chronic traumatism-related alterations. Third, a specifically created classification into 17 subareas was adopted according to anatomical and morphologic criteria (Figure 1) in order to obtain details otherwise missed in previous acral lesion databases. Then, some of the 17 subareas (Table 3) were further grouped into macro-areas following the anatomo-functional criteria of weight bearing, obtaining three macro-areas on the palm and four macro-areas on the sole (Tables 1 and 4). Fourth, all possible risk factors known or hypothesized for PP melanoma were investigated at contribution time.

Concerning lesion objective data, we found that the maximum diameter value was a significant discriminant (Table 4, $p < 0.001$) between benign and malignant aMPPLs. These data are of main importance as the photographs of benign lesions are homogenously small (6.58 mm on average ± sd3.58), with a number of very equivocal nevi measuring around 12 mm (Figure 2) and few congenital lesions measuring >12 mm (Figure 3), while malignant cases show a larger variation in diameter according to presentation time (17.39 on average ± sd12.47).

The study of lesion location revealed that the hot sites for melanoma of the soles are the plantar arch (29.6%) and heel (27.6%), while those of palmar melanoma are the finger surfaces (50%).

Benign aMPPLs, instead, were slightly prevalent at hypothenar–metacarpal surfaces of palms, and clearly prevalent on the plantar arch of soles. These data show that there is essentially no difference between weight-bearing/non-weight-bearing areas of the soles in terms of melanoma development, which is in line with recent literature data that excluded a causative role of walking barefoot [16–18,46–48]. As per palmar melanoma, reports of a trauma occurrence are too very few to derive conclusions. [49]

According to patient data analysis, age turned out to be a significant discriminant factor for malignancy (Table 4, $p < 0.001$), with patients with PP melanoma generally being older (65.3 years on average) than those with benign aMPPLs (41.33 yrs on average). These data are globally in line with those reported in acral melanoma patients diagnosed in Asia [12], France [3], United States [26], Spain [46], Italy [9], and Korea [47], aged between 59 and 65 years, and those reported from acral nevi patients diagnosed in the United States [4], Italy [26], and Greece [25].

We did not detect any difference in sex distribution for PP melanoma cases (51%F/49%M); this trend is, however, in line with some retrospective studies on acral melanoma patients, reporting distribution of 54%/46%M [46] and 49%/51% [48], while previous monocentric studies showed a slight female or male prevalence (e.g., M:F = 1:1.86 [3], M:F = 1:1.6, [25 M:F = 1:1.9,12 F:M = 1:1.08,26 and M:F = 1:1.712). Precisely, a similar sex distribution was found in patients with cases of early melanoma of the body, in the context of retrospective studies on atypical melanocytic lesions [30,49]. Interestingly, the nevi group of this case study comprised 289 female patients (67,4%F/32.6%M) (Table 4) and the same distribution has been reported in Greek (70%F/30%M) [7], Hispanic (69.5%F/30.5%M) [42], and Italian (63%F/37%M) [9] cohorts of patients screened in secondary referral centers. This repetitive trend may be explained by the fact that women are generally more assiduous in attending skin cancer visits than men. Notably, we previously documented this tendency in multicentric investigations on atypical pigmented lesions of the face [31,34] and trunk [30,49].

The descriptive and association analysis of patient anamnestic data, risk factors, and phenotypic traits showed that the aMPPL population was essentially homogeneous, with no significant difference between benign and malignant cases. This can be first explained by the high rate of non-assessment for the majority of patients, mostly ascribable to the retrospective collection performed by participating centers; then, by the difficulty in defining the entity of the traumatism or sunburn by patients themselves; and lastly, by the fact that recent meta-analysis failed to confirm the hypothesis on a clear causative role of injuries/trauma or history of sunburns in infancy in acral melanoma development [3,42,44,46,50–52]. Indeed, the current evidence from laboratory studies suggests that PP acral melanoma development seems to arise in a certain cancer susceptibility setting (which is, however, different from the renowned genetic signature of melanoma families) and does not follow the classic risk factors addressed for body and face melanomas [3,13,14,42,44,46,47].

At last, the results of the imaging device analysis showed that there was a slight tendency to use the camera-based devices to photograph benign aMPPL lesions, while the majority of malignant aMPL case images were acquired with a videodermatoscope. These frequencies of use essentially reflect the equipment of each center, but a series of considerations can be raised. It can be argued that camera-based/smartphone-based methods may be preferred to acquire pictures of potentially benign lesions of the soles because they are more handy/rapid to use, whereas fixed videodermatoscope devices may be a bit uncomfortable/time-consuming, especially in front of elderly patients in standing position, and are best reserved for the ugliest lesions, in which a larger screen is required [53–56].

Limitations of this study to take into account are the following: (i) since all cases have been histologically analyzed, there is an intrinsic selection bias based on the excisional criteria; (ii) the majority of patients were identified as phenotype III, generating a potential bias in phenotypic data analysis; and (iii) the sample size of palmar lesions was small due to the very low incidence of palmar melanoma in Europe.

5. Conclusions

The creation of the integrated PP dataset and the analyses carried out (descriptive and univariate) are devoted to a better understanding of aMPPLs in the European population where they are poorly investigated and represent phase I of the *iDScore PalmoPlantar* project. Indeed, by combining both the morphological features and the patient data, we aimed to delineate some recurrent patterns of Caucasian patients with aMPPLs frequently attending skin cancer screening centers. In general, in a patient aged >50 years exhibiting an aMPPL larger than 8 mm on the heel/plantar arch or fingers of the hand, the risk of melanoma is very high, independent of sex. If a patient older than 65.3 years presents with a lesion larger than 17 mm, palpable, immediate excision should be performed with large margins. Then, if a patient aged up to 49 years has a flat lesion of up to 7 mm in diameter localized to the palmar/hypothenar or thenar surface of the palms or the plantar arch of the sole, we can be quite confident that it is a benign aMPL. However, these preliminary data need to be confirmed on a larger dataset, especially for palmar melanoma cases, during the next decades. Moreover, further investigations for the *iDScore-PalmoPlantar* project will be carried out to combine and interpret these data according to the dermoscopic analysis and the detailed localization/distribution analysis. Briefly, phase II of the *iDScore-PalmoPlantar* project will consist of obtaining the average pattern analysis values of all the collected cases based on the consensus of two out of three dermoscopists variously skilled, for a total of 156 tele-dermoscopic investigations across Europe [32–34,36]. Finally, in phase III, the large amount of data obtained in the two previous phases will undergo multivariate analysis (i.e., forward–backward stepwise logistic regression) in order to select a pool of interdependent significant parameters useful to the setting up of a scoring system Bayesian classifier. This risk checklist, named the *iDScore-PalmoPlantar* model, will be able to provide an aMPPL score between 0 (no risk) and 15 (100% risk of malignancy). The management suggestions will be derived from the risk ranges estimate (i.e., mild, moderate, high, or very high), with the score threshold estimated by the leave-one-out technique using the variation in the area under the ROC curve [27–32]. The ultimate goal of the present dataset is the development of an integrated clinic–anamnestic–dermoscopic *iDScore-PalmoPlantar* model to help clinicians—in real time—in orienting their diagnostic suspects in front of difficult atypical PP lesions and to support them in management decisions of no/long/short follow-up or excision. In the next future, also a DCNN (deep convolutional neural network) [57] based model could be derived from the *iDScore-PalmoPlantar* dataset [58,59].

Author Contributions: Conceptualization, L.T., P.R. and A.C.; methodology, L.T., P.R., A.C. and G.C. (Gabriele Cevenini); software, G.C. (Gabriele Cevenini) and G.C. (Gennaro Cataldo); formal analysis, A.C. and S.L.C.; investigation, L.T., A.C. and L.S.; resources, A.L., I.S., G.N., J.P., M.C.F., P.B., H.K. and J.-L.P.; data curation, L.T., A.C. and L.S.; writing—original draft preparation, L.T. and A.C.; writing—review and editing, E.C. and P.R.; supervision, G.C. (Gabriele Cevenini), E.M. and P.R.; project administration, L.T. and A.C. All authors have read and agreed to the published version of the manuscript.

Funding: This research received no external funding.

Institutional Review Board Statement: This study was conducted in accordance with the Declaration of Helsinki, and approved by the Ethics Committee of Siena University, Azienda Ospedaliero-Universitaria Senese, Siena, Italy, (Study Protocol No. 16801) obtained in April 2018.

Informed Consent Statement: Informed consent was obtained from all subjects involved in the study.

Data Availability Statement: Data are available from the corresponding author upon reasonable request.

Acknowledgments: Teledermoscopy Working Group of the EADV teledermatology task force.

Conflicts of Interest: The authors declare no conflicts of interest.

References

1. Bernardes, S.S.; Ferreira, I.; Elder, D.E.; Nobre, A.B.; Martínez-Said, H.; Adams, D.J.; Robles-Espinoza, C.D.; Possik, P.A. More than just acral melanoma: The controversies of defining the disease. *J. Pathol. Clin. Res.* **2021**, *7*, 531–541. [CrossRef] [PubMed]
2. Saida, T. Heterogeneity of the site of origin of malignant melanoma in ungual areas: "subungual" malignant melanoma may be a misnomer. *Br. J. Dermatol.* **1992**, *126*, 529. [CrossRef] [PubMed]
3. Phan, A.; Touzet, S.; Dalle, S.; Ronger-Savlé, S.; Balme, B.; Thomas, L. Acral lentiginous melanoma: A clinicoprognostic study of 126 cases. *Br. J. Dermatol.* **2006**, *155*, 561–569. [CrossRef] [PubMed]
4. Madankumar, R.; Gumaste, P.V.; Martires, K.; Schaffer, P.R.; Choudhary, S.; Falto-Aizpurua, L.; Arora, H.; Kallis, P.J.; Patel, S.; Damanpour, S.; et al. Acral melanocytic lesions in the United States: Prevalence, awareness, and dermoscopic patterns in skin-of-color and non-Hispanic white patients. *J. Am. Acad. Dermatol.* **2016**, *74*, 724–730.e1. [CrossRef] [PubMed]
5. Park, S.; Yun, S.-J. Acral Melanocytic Neoplasms: A Comprehensive Review of Acral Nevus and Acral Melanoma in Asian Perspective. *Dermatopathology* **2022**, *9*, 292–303. [CrossRef] [PubMed]
6. Roncati, L.; Piscioli, F.; Pusiol, T. SAMPUS, MELTUMP and THIMUMP—Diagnostic Categories Characterized by Uncertain Biological Behavior. *Klin. Onkol.* **2017**, *30*, 221–223. [CrossRef] [PubMed]
7. Papageorgiou, C.; Kyrgidis, A.; Ilut, P.A.; Gkentsidi, T.; Manoli, S.-M.; Camela, E.; Apalla, Z.; Lallas, A. Acral Melanocytic Nevi in a High-Risk Population: Prevalence, Clinical Characteristics and Dermatoscopic Patterns. *Dermatology* **2023**, *239*, 753–759. [CrossRef] [PubMed]
8. Minagawa, A.; Koga, H.; Saida, T. Dermoscopic characteristics of congenital melanocytic nevi affecting acral volar skin. *Arch. Dermatol.* **2011**, *147*, 809–813. [CrossRef]
9. Gumaste, P.V.; Fleming, N.H.; Silva, I.; Shapiro, R.L.; Berman, R.S.; Zhong, J.; Osman, I.; Stein, J.A. Analysis of recurrence patterns in acral versus nonacral melanoma: Should histologic subtype influence treatment guidelines? *J. Natl. Compr. Cancer Netw. JNCCN* **2014**, *12*, 1706–1712. [CrossRef]
10. Saida, T.; Yoshida, N.; Ikegawa, S.; Ishihara, K.; Nakajima, T. Clinical guidelines for the early detection of plantar malignant melanoma. *J. Am. Acad. Dermatol.* **1990**, *23*, 37–40. [CrossRef]
11. Phan, A.; Dalle, S.; Touzet, S.; Ronger-Savlé, S.; Balme, B.; Thomas, L. Dermoscopic features of acral lentiginous melanoma in a large series of 110 cases in a white population. *Br. J. Dermatol.* **2010**, *162*, 765–771. [CrossRef] [PubMed]
12. Mun, J.-H.; Jo, G.; Darmawan, C.C.; Park, J.; Bae, J.M.; Jin, H.; Kim, W.-I.; Kim, H.-S.; Ko, H.-C.; Kim, B.-S.; et al. Association between Breslow thickness and dermoscopic findings in acral melanoma. *J. Am. Acad. Dermatol.* **2018**, *79*, 831–835. [CrossRef] [PubMed]
13. Darmawan, C.C.; Jo, G.; Montenegro, S.E.; Kwak, Y.; Cheol, L.; Cho, K.H.; Mun, J.-H. Early detection of acral melanoma: A review of clinical, dermoscopic, histopathologic, and molecular characteristics. *J. Am. Acad. Dermatol.* **2019**, *81*, 805–812. [CrossRef]
14. Moon, K.R.; Choi, Y.D.; Kim, J.M.; Jin, S.; Shin, M.-H.; Shim, H.-J.; Lee, J.-B.; Yun, S.J. Genetic Alterations in Primary Acral Melanoma and Acral Melanocytic Nevus in Korea: Common Mutated Genes Show Distinct Cytomorphological Features. *J. Investig. Dermatol.* **2018**, *138*, 933–945. [CrossRef] [PubMed]
15. Smalley, K.S.M.; Teer, J.K.; Chen, Y.A.; Wu, J.-Y.; Yao, J.; Koomen, J.M.; Chen, W.-S.; Rodriguez-Waitkus, P.; Karreth, F.A.; Messina, J.L. A Mutational Survey of Acral Nevi. *JAMA Dermatol.* **2021**, *157*, 831–835. [CrossRef] [PubMed]
16. Kim, N.H.; Choi, Y.D.; Seon, H.J.; Lee, J.-B.; Yun, S.J. Anatomic mapping and clinicopathologic analysis of benign acral melanocytic neoplasms: A comparison between adults and children. *J. Am. Acad. Dermatol.* **2017**, *77*, 735–745. [CrossRef] [PubMed]
17. Minagawa, A.; Omodaka, T.; Okuyama, R. Melanomas and Mechanical Stress Points on the Plantar Surface of the Foot. *N. Engl. J. Med.* **2016**, *374*, 2404–2406. [CrossRef]
18. Costello, C.M.; Pittelkow, M.R.; Mangold, A.R. Acral Melanoma and Mechanical Stress on the Plantar Surface of the Foot. *N. Engl. J. Med.* **2017**, *377*, 395–396. [CrossRef]
19. Thomas, L.; Phan, A.; Pralong, P.; Poulalhon, N.; Debarbieux, S.; Dalle, S. Special locations dermoscopy: Facial, acral, and nail. *Dermatol. Clin.* **2013**, *31*, 615–624. [CrossRef]
20. Yun, S.J.; Bastian, B.C. Melanocytic tumours in acral skin. In *WHO Classification of Skin Tumours*; Elder, D.E., Massi, D., Scolyer, R.A., Willemze, R., Eds.; World Health Organization Classification of Tumours; International Agency for Research on Cancer: Lyon, France, 2018; Chapter 2; ISBN 978-92-832-2440-2.
21. Saida, T.; Miyazaki, A.; Oguchi, S.; Ishihara, Y.; Yamazaki, Y.; Murase, S.; Yoshikawa, S.; Tsuchida, T.; Kawabata, Y.; Tamaki, K. Significance of Dermoscopic Patterns in Detecting Malignant Melanoma on Acral Volar Skin: Results of a Multicenter Study in Japan. *Arch. Dermatol.* **2004**, *140*, 1233–1238. [CrossRef]

22. Costello, C.M.; Ghanavatian, S.; Temkit, M.; Buras, M.R.; DiCaudo, D.J.; Swanson, D.L.; Mangold, A.R. Educational and practice gaps in the management of volar melanocytic lesions. *J. Eur. Acad. Dermatol. Venereol.* **2018**, *32*, 1450–1455. [CrossRef] [PubMed]
23. Criscito, M.C.; Stein, J.A. Improving the diagnosis and treatment of acral melanocytic lesions. *Melanoma Manag.* **2017**, *4*, 113–123. [CrossRef] [PubMed]
24. Saida, T.; Koga, H.; Uhara, H. Key points in dermoscopic differentiation between early acral melanoma and acral nevus. *J. Dermatol.* **2011**, *38*, 25–34. [CrossRef]
25. Ingrassia, J.P.; Stein, J.A.; Levine, A.; Liebman, T.N. Diagnosis and Management of Acral Pigmented Lesions. *Dermatol. Surg.* **2023**, *49*, 926–931. [CrossRef]
26. Huang, K.; Fan, J.; Misra, S. Acral lentiginous melanoma: Incidence and survival in the United States, 2006-2015, an analysis of the SEER registry. *J. Surg. Res.* **2020**, *251*, 329–339. [CrossRef] [PubMed]
27. Bhor, U.; Pande, S. Scoring systems in dermatology. *Indian J. Dermatol. Venereol. Leprol.* **2006**, *72*, 315–332. [CrossRef] [PubMed]
28. Tognetti, L.; Cevenini, G.; Moscarella, E.; Cinotti, E.; Farnetani, F.; Mahlvey, J.; Perrot, J.L.; Longo, C.; Pellacani, G.; Argenziano, G.; et al. An integrated clinical-dermoscopic risk scoring system for the differentiation between early melanoma and atypical nevi: The iDScore. *J. Eur. Acad. Dermatol. Venereol.* **2018**, *32*, 2162–2170. [CrossRef]
29. Tognetti, L.; Cartocci, A.; Bertello, M.; Giordani, M.; Cinotti, E.; Cevenini, G.; Rubegni, P. An updated algorithm integrated with patient data for the differentiation of atypical nevi from early melanomas: The idScore 2021. *Dermatol. Pract. Concept.* **2022**, *12*, e2022134. [CrossRef]
30. Rubegni, P.; Tognetti, L.; Argenziano, G.; Nami, N.; Brancaccio, G.; Cinotti, E.; Miracco, C.; Fimiani, M.; Cevenini, G. A risk scoring system for the differentiation between melanoma with regression and regressing nevi. *J. Dermatol. Sci.* **2016**, *83*, 138–144. [CrossRef]
31. Tognetti, L.; Cartocci, A.; Żychowska, M.; Savarese, I.; Cinotti, E.; Pizzichetta, M.A.; Moscarella, E.; Longo, C.; Farnetani, F.; Guida, S.; et al. A risk-scoring model for the differential diagnosis of lentigo maligna and other atypical pigmented facial lesions of the face: The facial iDScore. *Acad. Dermatol. Venereol.* **2023**, *37*, 2301–2310. [CrossRef]
32. Tognetti, L.; Cevenini, G.; Moscarella, E.; Cinotti, E.; Farnetani, F.; Lallas, A.; Tiodorovic, D.; Carrera, C.; Puig, S.; Perrot, J.L.; et al. Validation of an integrated dermoscopic scoring method in an European teledermoscopy web platform: The iDScore project for early detection of melanoma. *J. Eur. Acad. Dermatol. Venereol.* **2020**, *34*, 640–647. [CrossRef] [PubMed]
33. Tognetti, L.; Cinotti, E.; Farnetani, F.; Lallas, A.; Paoli, J.; Longo, C.; Pampena, R.; Moscarella, E.; Argenziano, G.; Tiodorovic, D.; et al. Development and Implementation of a Web-Based International Registry Dedicated to Atypical Pigmented Skin Lesions of the Face: Teledermatologic Investigation on Epidemiology and Risk Factors. *Telemed. J. E Health* **2023**, *29*, 1356–1365. [CrossRef] [PubMed]
34. EUR-Lex-32016R0679-EN-EUR-Lex Regulation—2016/679—EN—Gdpr—EUR-Lex. Available online: https://eur-lex.europa.eu/eli/reg/2016/679/oj (accessed on 16 January 2024).
35. Vallone, M.G.; Tell-Marti, G.; Potrony, M.; Rebollo-Morell, A.; Badenas, C.; Puig-Butille, J.A.; Gimenez-Xavier, P.; Carrera, C.; Malvehy, J.; Puig, S. Melanocortin 1 receptor (MC1R) polymorphisms' influence on size and dermoscopic features of nevi. *Pigment Cell Melanoma Res.* **2018**, *31*, 39–50. [CrossRef] [PubMed]
36. Zocchi, L.; Lontano, A.; Merli, M.; Dika, E.; Nagore, E.; Quaglino, P.; Puig, S.; Ribero, S. Familial Melanoma and Susceptibility Genes: A Review of the Most Common Clinical and Dermoscopic Phenotypic Aspect, Associated Malignancies and Practical Tips for Management. *J. Clin. Med.* **2021**, *10*, 3760. [CrossRef] [PubMed]
37. Quint, K.D.; van der Rhee, J.I.; Gruis, N.A.; Ter Huurne, J.A.; Wolterbeek, R.; van der Stoep, N.; Bergman, W.; Kukutsch, N.A. Melanocortin 1 receptor (MC1R) variants in high melanoma risk patients are associated with specific dermoscopic ABCD features. *Acta Derm.-Venereol.* **2012**, *92*, 587–592. [CrossRef] [PubMed]
38. Ghanavatian, S.; Costello, C.M.; Buras, M.R.; Cumsky, H.J.L.; Pittelkow, M.R.; Swanson, D.L.; Mangold, A.R. Density and distribution of acral melanocytic nevi and acral melanomas on the plantar surface of the foot. *J. Am. Acad. Dermatol.* **2019**, *80*, 790–792.e2. [CrossRef] [PubMed]
39. Nishiguchi, M.; Yamamoto, Y.; Hara, T.; Okuhira, H.; Inaba, Y.; Kunimoto, K.; Mikita, N.; Kaminaka, C.; Kanazawa, N.; Jinnin, M. Difference in distribution of malignant melanoma and melanocytic nevus in the palm and finger. *Biosci. Trends* **2019**, *13*, 361–363. [CrossRef]
40. Kawabata, Y.; Tamaki, K. Distinctive dermatoscopic features of acral lentiginous melanoma in situ from plantar melanocytic nevi and their histopathologic correlation. *J. Cutan. Med. Surg.* **1998**, *2*, 199–204. [CrossRef]
41. Tan, A.; Stein, J.A. Dermoscopic patterns of acral melanocytic lesions in skin of color. *Cutis* **2019**, *103*, 274–276.
42. González-Ramírez, R.A.; Guerra-Segovia, C.; Garza-Rodríguez, V.; Garza-Báez, P.; Gómez-Flores, M.; Ocampo-Candiani, J. Dermoscopic features of acral melanocytic nevi ina case series from Mexico. *Ann. Bras. Dermatol.* **2018**, *93*, 665–670. [CrossRef]
43. Durbec, F.; Martin, L.; Derancourt, C.; Grange, F. Melanoma of the hand and foot: Epidemiological, prognostic and genetic features. A systematic review. *Br. J. Dermatol.* **2012**, *166*, 727–739. [CrossRef] [PubMed]
44. Metzger, S.; Ellwanger, U.; Stroebel, W.; Schiebel, U.; Rassner, G.; Fierlbeck, G. Extent and consequences of physician delay in the diagnosis of acral melanoma. *Melanoma Res.* **1998**, *8*, 181–186. [CrossRef] [PubMed]
45. Kolm, I.; Kamarashev, J.; Kerl, K.; Hafner, J.; Läuchli, S.; French, L.E.; Braun, R.P. Acral melanoma with network pattern: A dermoscopy-reflectance confocal microscopy and histopathology correlation. *Dermatol. Surg. Off. Publ. Am. Soc. Dermatol. Surg.* **2010**, *36*, 701–703. [CrossRef] [PubMed]

46. Nagore, E.; Pereda, C.; Botella-Estrada, R.; Requena, C.; Guillén, C. Acral lentiginous melanoma presents distinct clinical profile with high cancer susceptibility. *Cancer Causes Control* **2009**, *20*, 115–119. [CrossRef] [PubMed]
47. Han, B.; Hur, K.; Ohn, J.; Lim, S.S.; Mun, J.-H. Acral lentiginous melanoma in situ: Dermoscopic features and management strategy. *Sci. Rep.* **2020**, *10*, 20503. [CrossRef] [PubMed]
48. Weitao, Y.; Jiaqiang, W.; Peng, Z.; Xin, W.; Xinhui, D.; Xiaohui, N. A Retrospective Study of Acral Melanoma That Happened on Foot. 2020. Available online: https://www.researchsquare.com/article/rs-16460/v1 (accessed on 18 January 2024).
49. Jaroonwanichkul, S.; Fan, E.; Matthews, S.; Ho, B.V.; Hall, J.C. Acral Nodular Melanoma at a Site of Trauma. *Kans. J. Med.* **2023**, *16*, 187–188. [CrossRef] [PubMed]
50. Mikoshiba, Y.; Minagawa, A.; Koga, H.; Yokokawa, Y.; Uhara, H.; Okuyama, R. Clinical and Histopathologic Characteristics of Melanocytic Lesions on the Volar Skin Without Typical Dermoscopic Patterns. *JAMA Dermatol.* **2019**, *155*, 578–584. [CrossRef]
51. Hao, X.; Yim, J.; Chang, S.; Schwartz, E.; Rubenstein, S.; Friske, C.; Shamim, S.; Masternick, E.; Mirkin, G. Acral Lentiginous Melanoma of Foot and Ankle: A Clinicopathological Study of 7 Cases. *Anticancer Res.* **2019**, *39*, 6175–6181. [CrossRef]
52. Saida, T. Malignant Melanoma on the Sole: How to Detect the Early Lesions Efficiently. *Pigment. Cell Res.* **2000**, *13*, 135–139. [CrossRef]
53. Tognetti, L.; Cartocci, A.; Balistreri, S.; Cataldo, G.; Cinotti, E.; Moscarella, E.; Farnetani, F.; Lallas, A.; Tiodorovic, D.; Carrera, C.; et al. The Comparative Use of Multiple Electronic Devices in the Teledermoscopic Diagnosis of Early Melanoma. *Telemed. J. e-Health* **2021**, *27*, 495–502. [CrossRef]
54. Ozdemir, F.; Karaarslan, I.K.; Akalin, T. Variations in the dermoscopic features of acquired acral melanocytic nevi. *Arch. Dermatol.* **2007**, *143*, 1378–1384. [CrossRef]
55. Barcaui, C.B.; Lima, P.M.O. Application of teledermoscopy in the diagnosis of pigmented lesions. *Int. J. Telemed. Appl.* **2018**, *2018*, 1624073. [CrossRef] [PubMed]
56. Emiroglu, N.; Cengiz, F.P.; Onsun, N. Age and Anatomical Location-Related Dermoscopic Patterns of 210 Acral Melanocytic Nevi in a Turkish Population. *J. Cutan. Med. Surg.* **2017**, *21*, 388–394. [CrossRef] [PubMed]
57. Yu, C.; Yang, S.; Kim, W.; Jung, J.; Chung, K.Y.; Lee, S.W.; Oh, B. Acral melanoma detection using a convolutional neural network for dermoscopy images. *PLoS ONE* **2018**, *13*, e0193321. [CrossRef]
58. Tognetti, L.; Bonechi, S.; Andreini, P.; Bianchini, M.; Scarselli, F.; Cevenini, G.; Moscarella, E.; Farnetani, F.; Longo, C.; Lallas, A.; et al. A new deep learning approach integrated with clinical data for the dermoscopic differentiation of early melanomas from atypical nevi. *J. Dermatol. Sci.* **2021**, *101*, 115–122. [CrossRef]
59. Rubegni, P.; Cevenini, G.; Nami, N.; Argenziano, G.; Saida, T.; Burroni, M.; Quaglino, P.; Bono, R.; Hofmann-Wellenhof, R.; Fimiani, M. A simple scoring system for the diagnosis of palmo-plantar pigmented skin lesions by digital dermoscopy analysis. *J. Eur. Acad. Dermatol. Venereol. JEADV* **2013**, *27*, e312–e319. [CrossRef] [PubMed]

Disclaimer/Publisher's Note: The statements, opinions and data contained in all publications are solely those of the individual author(s) and contributor(s) and not of MDPI and/or the editor(s). MDPI and/or the editor(s) disclaim responsibility for any injury to people or property resulting from any ideas, methods, instructions or products referred to in the content.

Interesting Images

Eruptive Syringoma—Clinical, Dermoscopic, and Reflectance Confocal Microscopy Features

Agnieszka Rydz [1], Jakub Żółkiewicz [2,*], Michał Kunc [3], Martyna Sławińska [2], Michał Sobjanek [2], Roman J. Nowicki [2] and Magdalena Lange [2]

1. Student's Scientific Circle Practical and Experimental Dermatology, Medical University of Gdańsk, 80-214 Gdańsk, Poland
2. Department of Dermatology, Venereology and Allergology, Medical University of Gdańsk, 80-214 Gdańsk, Poland
3. Department of Pathomorphology, Medical University of Gdańsk, 80-214 Gdańsk, Poland
* Correspondence: zolkiewicz@gumed.edu.pl

Abstract: We present an interesting image of eruptive syringoma confirmed by histopathological assessment in a 37-year-old male who was consulted due to numerous brownish small macules and papules resembling maculopapular cutaneous mastocytosis (MPCM). We show difficulties in diagnosing ES, given its rare occurrence and resemblance to other dermatological disorders. Moreover, we discuss the role of dermoscopy and reflectance confocal microscopy in the differential diagnosis of syringoma.

Keywords: eruptive syringoma; syringoma; cutaneous mastocytosis; dermoscopy; dermatoscopy; reflectance confocal microscopy; histology

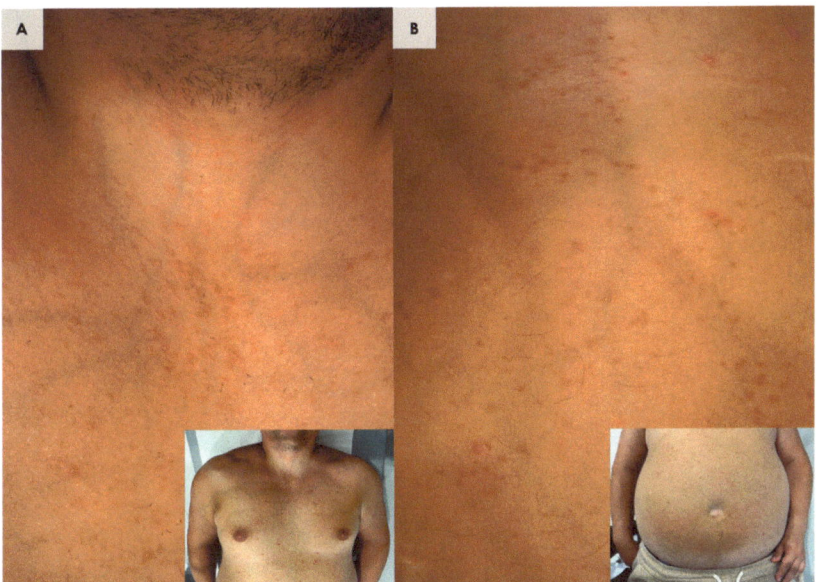

Figure 1. (**A**,**B**). We present a 37-year-old overweight male who presented with numerous small, monomorphic, brownish macules and papules scattered across the trunk, neck, and thighs (**A**,**B**). The patient exhibited multiple flat-topped, firm, hyperpigmented brown macules and papules, varying in

size from 1 to 3 mm, distributed across the neck, chest, abdomen, back, and lower extremities. The lesions were predominantly located on the anterior aspect of the body. According to the patient, skin lesions have been present since elementary school and remained stable without progression to other areas of the body. The patient was referred to our department under suspicion for maculopapular cutaneous mastocytosis (MPCM). Nevertheless, Darier's sign, which is pathognomonic for cutaneous mastocytosis, was negative [1]. Moreover, he had no cutaneous and systemic mast cell mediator-related symptoms typical for mastocytosis [1]. There was no history of an anaphylactic shock, allergic reactions, or a chronic illness. Complete blood count with differential, biochemistry, and serum tryptase level (3.35 ng/mL, range up to 11.4 ng/mL) were in normal ranges. Due to an unclear clinical presentation, dermoscopy (Figure 2A,B) and reflectance confocal microscopy (RCM) (Figures 3 and 4) were performed. Two skin biopsies from the skin of the trunk were performed, and histopathological examination indicated a diagnosis of syringoma in both samples (Figure 5). Due to the disseminated distribution of skin lesions, a final diagnosis of eruptive syringoma (ES) was established. Our patient was informed that syringoma is a benign tumor that usually remains unchanged over time and does not pose significant health risks. Moreover, various treatment modalities were offered to the patient, including surgical removal, dermabrasion, electrocautery, cryosurgery, chemical peels, topical atropine, botulinum toxin A, and oral medications, such as isotretinoin [2,3]. However, the patient was not interested in treatment for solely aesthetic reasons. Syringoma is a benign skin neoplasm characterized by the overgrowth or hyperplasia of eccrine sweat ducts, leading to the formation of small, flat, skin-colored, or brownish papules [4,5]. Syringomas are typically located in the periorbital region; however, they have also been found in other locations, such as the trunk, extremities, vulva, penis, scalp, and underarms [6]. There are four variants of syringoma: the localized form, the familial form, a form associated with Down syndrome (DS), and the generalized variant [7]. Eruptive syringoma, a rare form of the generalized variant, is characterized by the sudden appearance of multiple lesions that spread across two or more anatomical regions [2]. The exact etiology of ES remains unclear, but it is believed to result from reactive hyperplasia of the eccrine ducts, potentially triggered by chronic inflammation, hormonal changes, or other unknown factors [8]. The condition is more prevalent in females and often manifests during puberty or adolescence, indicating a possible hormonal influence, but ES has also been reported in children and the elderly [2,9]. This case report indicates that ES poses a diagnostic challenge because its clinical presentation can be easily mistaken for other dermatological conditions, such as eruptive xanthomas, disseminated granuloma annulare, MPCM, lichen planus, flat warts, or eruptive vellus hair cysts [10]. Therefore, using dermoscopy and RCM may provide useful clues in the diagnostic process (Supplementary Table S1). However, histopathological examination remains the gold standard in the diagnosis of syringomas, as clinical presentation and non-invasive skin imaging techniques alone are not sufficient to distinguish ES from other skin lesions considered in the differential diagnosis.

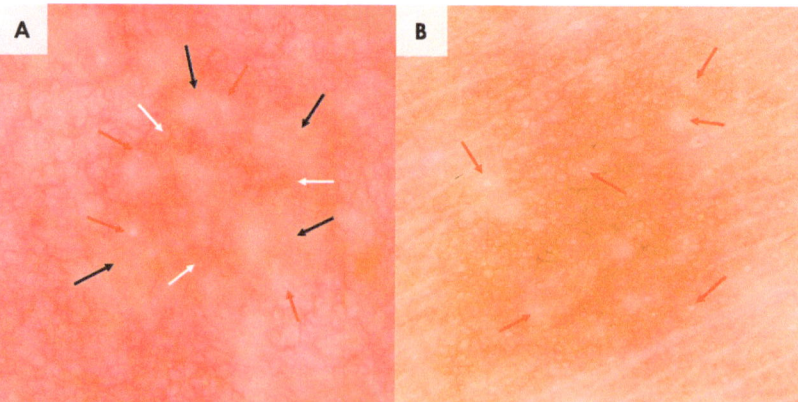

Figure 2. (**A**,**B**). Dermoscopy of syringomas located on the neck (**A**) and trunk (**B**). Dermoscopy of a syringoma located on the neck (**A**) showed linear vessels in reticular distribution (white arrows) and

light-brown structureless areas (black arrows) with small whitish globules (red arrows). Dermoscopy of the lesion located on the trunk (**B**) revealed brown reticular lines (pigment network) and white dots/globules (red arrows). Dermoscopic manifestations of ES differed according to the anatomical region. In the neck area, vascular pattern was observed, whereas pigment network prevailed in the abdominal region. In both instances, white dots/globules scattered across the lesion were identified. A similar location-dependent dermoscopic presentation was described in a case report by Botsali et al. [11]. Pigment network was identified in syringoma cases reported by Sakiyama et al. and Hayashi et al. [12,13]. The latter group also described multifocal hypopigmented areas under dermoscopy, as described in the reported patient.

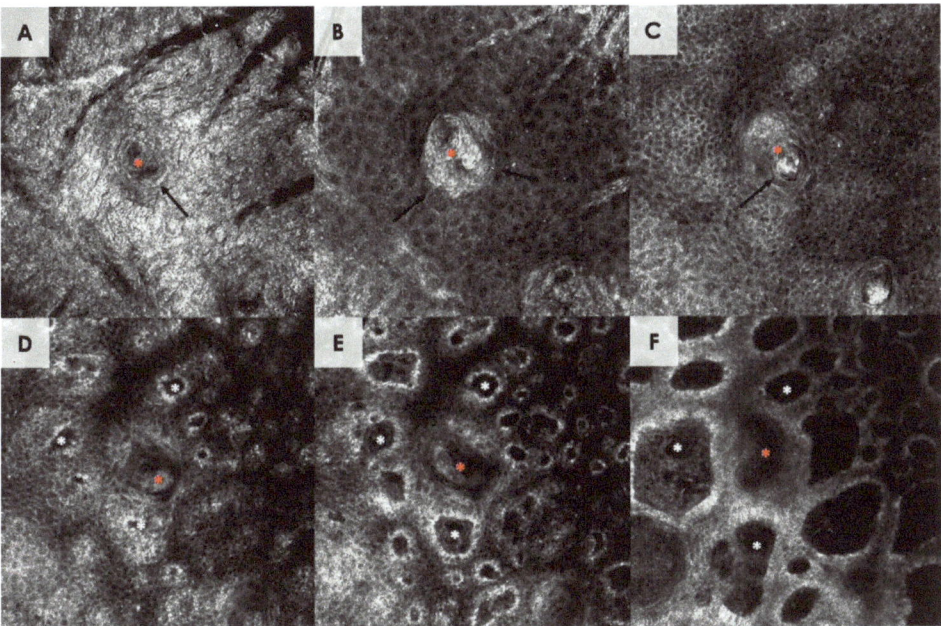

(Canfield D200 EVO; Canfield Scientific GmbH, Bielefeld, Germany; ×15 magnification; immersion ultrasound gel)

Figure 3. Reflectance confocal microscopy of syringoma. Dark hole (red asterisk) surrounded by bright, highly reflective layers of cells (black arrows), which correspond to acrosyringium, are seen within the stratum corneum (**A**), stratum granulosum (**B**), and stratum spinosum (**C**). A highly reflective layer, composed of densely packed, anucleated keratinocytes, constitutes the stratum corneum, whereas stratum granulosum and spinosum exhibit a typical honeycombed pattern. On the deeper sections (**D–F**), a dark, coiled tubular structure is visible (red asterisk). Moreover, bright cells around dermal papillae, which form edged dermal papillae (white asterisks), are seen at the entire level of the dermo–epidermal junction.

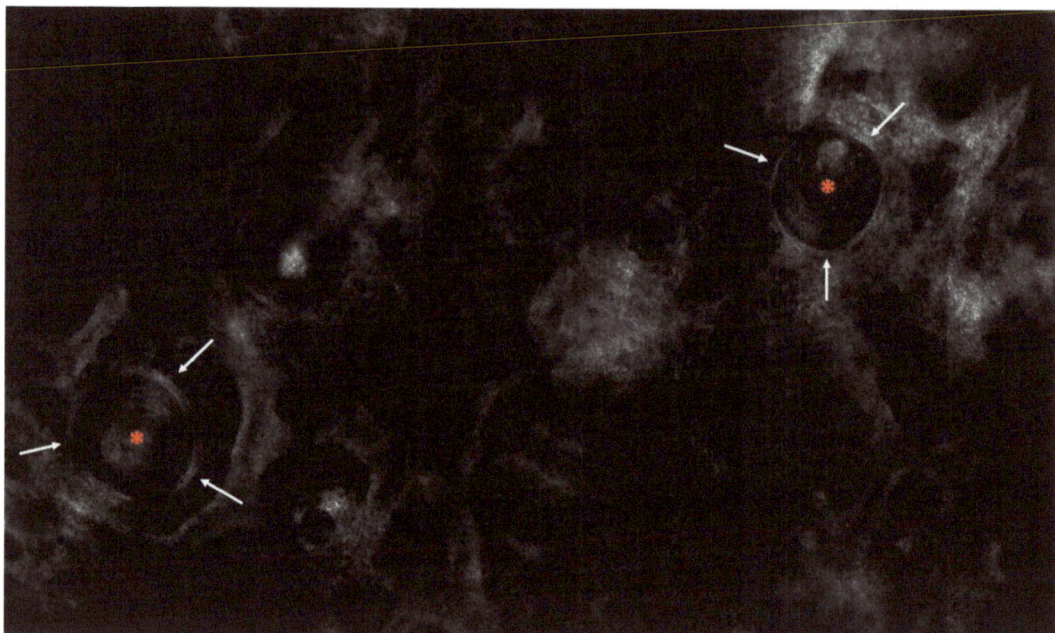

(VivaScope® 1500; Caliber Imaging and Diagnostics, Rochester, NY, USA)

Figure 4. Reflectance confocal microscopy of syringoma. Epithelial cells (white arrows) forming ducts filled with a grey amorphous material (red asterisks) are visible in the dermis. Data on RCM features of syringoma is scarce, as only one report on RCM attributes of ES has been published so far. Jiménez et al [14]. reported RCM presentations of 2 syringomas located on the face and neck in patients diagnosed with ES; however, RCM images were not correlated with corresponding dermoscopy. Nevertheless, our RCM findings are in line with the observations of Jiménez et al. [14]. Similar to the Brazilian authors, we identified ducts surrounded by pigmented epithelial cells, some of which were filled with a grey amorphous material. Additionally, we identified acrosyringia in the epidermis in both of the presented instances, which seem to correspond to white pinpoint dots observed under dermoscopy. Although the utility of RCM in syringoma recognition is limited, as histopathological features of syringomas are confined to the upper dermis, identification of acrosyringia in the epidermis, along with ducts filled with amorphous material in the dermis, may narrow the differential diagnosis.

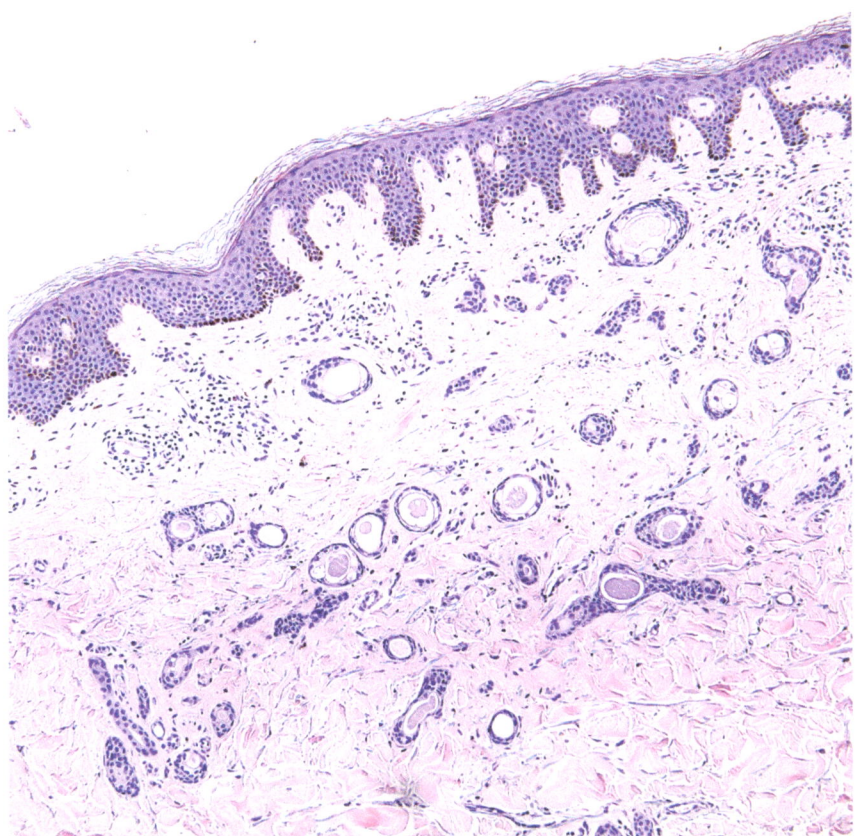

(VivaScope® 1500; Caliber Imaging and Diagnostics, Rochester, NY, USA) (hematoxylin & eosin staining; 40× magnification)

Figure 5. Syringoma displays multiple small ducts lined with cuboidal epithelial cells, some forming a characteristic 'tadpole' pattern, embedded in fibrous stroma within the dermis. Histology of syringoma typically reveals multiple small ducts and epithelial cords within the dermis, along with cystic eccrine ducts that often exhibit a characteristic comma-shaped tail [2,15].

Supplementary Materials: The following supporting information can be downloaded at: https://www.mdpi.com/article/10.3390/diagnostics15010110/s1, Table S1: Dermoscopic and reflectance confocal microscopy (RCM) features of the entities that may mimic eruptive syringoma. References [16–23] are cited in the Supplementary Materials.

Author Contributions: Conceptualization, M.L.; methodology, J.Ż. and M.K.; software, A.R.; validation, J.Ż. and M.K.; investigation, M.L., J.Ż. and M.K.; writing—original draft preparation, A.R.; writing—review and editing, J.Ż., A.R., M.S. (Martyna Sławińska) and M.S. (Michał Sobjanek); visualization, J.Ż. and M.K.; supervision, M.L.; project administration, R.J.N.; All authors have read and agreed to the published version of the manuscript.

Funding: The APC was funded by the Medical University of Gdańsk (GUM2024WUP09763).

Institutional Review Board Statement: Not applicable.

Informed Consent Statement: Written informed consent was obtained from the patient to publish this paper.

Data Availability Statement: The original contributions presented in this study are included in the article. Further inquiries can be directed to the corresponding author.

Acknowledgments: The authors would like to thank Karolina Lange for the linguistic proofreading of the article.

Conflicts of Interest: The authors declare no conflicts of interest.

References

1. Hartmann, K.; Escribano, L.; Grattan, C.; Brockow, K.; Carter, M.C.; Alvarez-Twose, I.; Matito, A.; Broesby-Olsen, S.; Siebenhaar, F.; Lange, M.; et al. Cutaneous Manifestations in Patients with Mastocytosis: Consensus Report of the European Competence Network on Mastocytosis; The American Academy of Allergy, Asthma & Immunology; And the European Academy of Allergology and Clinical Immunology. *J. Allergy Clin. Immunol.* **2016**, *137*, 35–45. [CrossRef]
2. Lei, H.; Wang, Z.; Ma, X.; Zhang, Z.; Feng, Y.; Zheng, Y. Eruptive Syringomas: Summary of Ninety Cases and a Brief Literature Review. *J. Cosmet. Dermatol.* **2023**, *22*, 1128–1133. [CrossRef] [PubMed]
3. Papageorgiou, M.; Theodosiou, G.; Mandekou-Lefaki, I. Eruptive Syringomas: Unresponsiveness to Oral Isotretinoin. *Int. J. Dermatol.* **2017**, *56*, e38–e39. [CrossRef] [PubMed]
4. Marrogi, A.J.; Wick, M.R.; Dehner, L.P. Benign Cutaneous Adnexal Tumors in Childhood and Young Adults, Excluding Pilomatrixoma: Review of 28 Cases and Literature. *J. Cutan. Pathol.* **1991**, *18*, 20–27. [CrossRef]
5. Huang, Y.H.; Chuang, Y.H.; Kuo, T.T.; Yang, L.C.; Hong, H.S. Vulvar Syringoma: A Clinicopathologic and Immunohistologic Study of 18 Patients and Results of Treatment. *J. Am. Acad. Dermatol.* **2003**, *48*, 735–739. [CrossRef] [PubMed]
6. Williams, K.; Shinkai, K. Evaluation and Management of the Patient with Multiple Syringomas: A Systematic Review of the Literature. *J. Am. Acad. Dermatol.* **2016**, *74*, 1234–1240.e9. [CrossRef] [PubMed]
7. Friedman, S.J.; Butler, D.F. Syringoma Presenting as Milia. *J. Am. Acad. Dermatol.* **1987**, *16*, 310–314. [CrossRef]
8. Hassab-El-Naby, H.M.M.; Nouh, A.H. Syringomatous Dermatitis: A Myth or an Existing Entity? *Arch. Dermatol. Res.* **2023**, *315*, 1649–1654. [CrossRef] [PubMed]
9. Wallace, M.L.; Smoller, B.R. Progesterone Receptor Positivity Supports Hormonal Control of Syringomas. *J. Cutan. Pathol.* **1995**, *22*, 442–445. [CrossRef] [PubMed]
10. Bolognia, J.; Schaffer, J.V.; Cerroni, L.; Callen, J.P. *Dermatology*; Elsevier: Amsterdam, The Netherlands, 2025; Volume 75.
11. Botsali, A.; Caliskan, E.; Coskun, A.; Tunca, M. Eruptive Syringoma: Two Cases with Dermoscopic Features. *Skin. Appendage Disord.* **2020**, *6*, 319–322. [CrossRef]
12. Sakiyama, M.; Maeda, M.; Fujimoto, N.; Satoh, T. Eruptive Syringoma Localized in Intertriginous Areas. *J. Dtsch. Dermatol. Ges.* **2014**, *12*, 72–73. [CrossRef] [PubMed]
13. Hayashi, Y.; Tanaka, M.; Nakajima, S.; Ozeki, M.; Inoue, T.; Ishizaki, S.; Fujibayashi, M. Unilateral Linear Syringoma in a Japanese Female: Dermoscopic Differentiation from Lichen Planus Linearis. *Dermatol. Rep.* **2011**, *3*, e42. [CrossRef]
14. Jiménez, M.R.; Rocchetto, H.; Ferreira, P.S.; Sangueza, M.; Lourenço, S.V.; Nico, M.M.S. Evaluation of Syringomas by in Vivo Reflectance Confocal Microscopy: A Report of Two Cases. *Am. J. Dermatopathol.* **2017**, *39*, 845–848. [CrossRef] [PubMed]
15. Aleissa, M.; Aljarbou, O.; Aljasser, M.I. Dermoscopy of Eruptive Syringoma. *Skin Appendage Disord.* **2021**, *7*, 401–403. [CrossRef]
16. Yan, Q.; Wang, X. Dermoscopic and reflectance confocal microscopy features of eruptive xanthoma. *Skin Res. Technol.* **2021**, *27*, 639–640. [CrossRef] [PubMed]
17. Pogorzelska-Antkowiak, A.; Corneli, P.; Zalaudek, I.; Szepietowski, J.C.; Agozzino, M. Characteristics of granuloma annulare in reflectance confocal microscopy. *Dermatol. Ther.* **2021**, *34*, e15021. [CrossRef] [PubMed]
18. Zhang, G.; Chen, J.; Liu, X.; Wang, X. Concordance of reflectance confocal microscopy with histopathology in the diagnosis of mastocytosis: A prospective study. *Skin Res. Technol.* **2020**, *26*, 319–321. [CrossRef] [PubMed]
19. Slawinska, M.; Kaszuba, A.; Lange, M.; Nowicki, R.J.; Sobjanek, M.; Errichetti, E. Dermoscopic Features of Different Forms of Cutaneous Mastocytosis: A Systematic Review. *J. Clin. Med.* **2022**, *11*, 4649. [CrossRef]
20. Lacarrubba, F.; Ardigo, M.; Di Stefani, A.; Verzi, A.E.; Micali, G. Dermatoscopy and Reflectance Confocal Microscopy Correlations in Nonmelanocytic Disorders. *Dermatol. Clin.* **2018**, *36*, 487–501. [CrossRef] [PubMed]
21. Chen, L.; Wang, Y.; Gao, X.; Qin, B.; Lian, J.; Ren, M.; Zhang, W.; Wei, R.; Li, Q. In vivo evaluation of facial papule dermatoses with reflectance confocal microscopy in children. *Skin Res. Technol.* **2022**, *28*, 703–707. [CrossRef]
22. Chen, L.X.; Wang, Y.; Qin, B.; Gao, X.B.; Li, Q.F. Features of hypopigmented verruca plana in reflectance confocal microscopy and comparative analysis of hypopigmented and classic verruca plana in children. *Skin Res. Technol.* **2021**, *27*, 993–996. [CrossRef]
23. Panchaprateep, R.; Tanus, A.; Tosti, A. Clinical, dermoscopic, and histopathologic features of body hair disorders. *J. Am. Acad. Dermatol.* **2015**, *72*, 890–900. [CrossRef] [PubMed]

Disclaimer/Publisher's Note: The statements, opinions and data contained in all publications are solely those of the individual author(s) and contributor(s) and not of MDPI and/or the editor(s). MDPI and/or the editor(s) disclaim responsibility for any injury to people or property resulting from any ideas, methods, instructions or products referred to in the content.

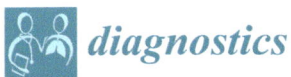 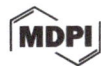

Case Report

Metastatic Nodular Melanoma with Angiosarcomatous Transdifferentiation—A Case Report and Review of the Literature

Adrian Vasile Dumitru [1,2], Dana Antonia Țăpoi [1,2,*], Mariana Costache [1,2], Ana Maria Ciongariu [1,2], Andreea Iuliana Ionescu [3,4], Horia Dan Liscu [3,5], Catalin Alius [6,7], Mircea Tampa [8,9], Andrei Marin [10] and Andreea Roxana Furtunescu [8,9]

1. Department of Pathology, Carol Davila University of Medicine and Pharmacy, 020021 Bucharest, Romania; vasile.dumitru@umfcd.ro (A.V.D.); mariana.costache@umfcd.ro (M.C.); ana-maria.ciongariu@drd.umfcd.ro (A.M.C.)
2. Department of Pathology, University Emergency Hospital, 050098 Bucharest, Romania
3. Department of Oncological Radiotherapy and Medical Imaging, Carol Davila University of Medicine and Pharmacy, 020021 Bucharest, Romania; andreea-iuliana.miron@drd.umfcd.ro (A.I.I.); horia-dan.liscu@drd.umfcd.ro (H.D.L.)
4. Department of Medical Oncology, Colțea Clinical Hospital, 030167 Bucharest, Romania
5. Department of Radiotherapy, Colțea Clinical Hospital, 030167 Bucharest, Romania
6. Faculty of Medicine, Carol Davila University of Medicine and Pharmacy Bucharest, 020021 Bucharest, Romania; catalin.alius@umfcd.ro
7. Fourth Department of General Surgery, Emergency University Hospital Bucharest, 050098 Bucharest, Romania
8. Department of Dermatology, Carol Davila University of Medicine and Pharmacy, 020021 Bucharest, Romania; mircea.tampa@umfcd.ro (M.T.); andreea-roxana.furtunescu@drd.umfcd.ro (A.R.F.)
9. Department of Dermatology, "Victor Babes" Clinical Hospital for Infectious Diseases, 030303 Bucharest, Romania
10. Department of Plastic Surgery, Carol Davila University of Medicine and Pharmacy, 020021 Bucharest, Romania; andrei.marin@umfcd.ro
* Correspondence: dana-antonia.tapoi@drd.umfcd.ro

Abstract: Diagnosing cutaneous melanomas relies mainly on histopathological analysis, which, in selected cases, can be aided by immunohistochemical evaluation of conventional melanocytic markers. Nevertheless, these malignancies, particularly in metastatic settings, may display divergent differentiation with unusual histological and immunohistochemical features. In this context, we present the case of a 65-year-old male diagnosed with typical superficial spreading melanoma who developed recurrence and metastatic lesions featuring angiosarcomatous differentiation. The diagnosis of the initial tumour and the subsequently dedifferentiated lesions was confirmed by ample immunohistochemical analysis, which included several melanocytic markers, as well as mesenchymal and vascular markers. The recurrent tumour and lymph nodes metastases were completely negative for Melan-A and PRAME, and focally positive for SOX10. Additionally, they also displayed diffuse, intense positivity for CD10 and WT1 and focal positivity for CD99, ERB, and CD31. Thus, the diagnosis of primary cutaneous melanoma with recurrent and metastatic divergent angiosarcomatous differentiation was established. This occurrence is particularly rare and can pose important diagnostic challenges. Therefore, in addition to presenting this highly unusual case, we also performed a comprehensive review of the literature on divergent differentiation in melanomas.

Keywords: cutaneous melanoma; angiosarcomatous; differentiation

1. Introduction

Cutaneous melanoma is the most aggressive form of skin cancer, in which survival is highly dependent on early and correct diagnosis [1]. Nevertheless, diagnosing primary and metastatic cutaneous melanomas is not always straightforward, as these tumours may display extraordinarily heterogenous histopathological and immunohistochemical features, including divergent differentiation, resembling various other neoplasms [2].

This is especially true of nodular melanoma (NM), which often lacks the clinical features of classic melanoma such as asymmetry, irregular borders, multiple colours, and dimensions greater than 0.6 cm. On dermatoscopy, atypical pigment network, regression structures, and irregular streaks are usually absent [3,4]. The diagnosis is further complicated by the fact that 20–30% of NMs are hypo- or amelanotic [3,5]. NM usually arises in previously normal skin, often in male patients over 50 years of age who do not have a personal or family history of skin cancer or other risk factors for melanoma development, such as freckles or numerous melanocytic naevi [5]. Moreover, NM is a fast-growing tumour with a high mitotic rate and the diagnosis is often made at advanced stages when the Breslow thickness of the tumour is already more than 2 mm [6–9]. Usually, the tumour is detected by the patient, and so far, the contribution of screening campaigns in the early detection of NM seems limited. Therefore, NM has a particularly poor prognosis and is associated with a disproportionately high mortality rate when compared with other melanoma subtypes [7].

Dermatoscopy can help raise the suspicion of NM and provide an earlier diagnosis of this aggressive tumour. NMs with a Breslow thickness of less than 2 mm are most often brown in colour and exhibit irregular brown dots or globules, irregular blue structureless areas, irregular eccentric black blotches, shiny white streaks, and dotted vessels. In more advanced NMs, asymmetry, blue colour, ulceration, and serpentine and corkscrew vessels become more common. There are three main features that can help in the diagnosis of thin NM: dotted vessels, shiny white streaks, and irregular blue structureless areas [3].

Some algorithms have been developed to aid in the diagnosis of NM. They can be used together with the ABCDE criteria in order to increase the specificity and sensitivity of NM diagnosis. The EFG rule refers to lesions that are elevated, firm, and growing [10], while the 3 Cs criteria evaluate colour, contour, and change [11]. The blue-black rule raises suspicion of melanoma in lesions that exhibit blue and black pigmentation in more than 10% of their surface [12].

The differential diagnosis of NM includes basal cell carcinoma; squamous cell carcinoma; Merkel cell carcinoma; melanocytic naevi, especially blue naevi and Spitz tumours; pyogenic granuloma; and atypical fibroxanthoma [6,13].

From a histopathological point of view, primary dedifferentiated cutaneous melanomas can be defined as biphasic tumours lacking conventional morphological and immunohistochemical characteristics while displaying non-melanocytic features [14]. Divergent differentiation, however, is more frequently noted in metastatic settings [15–18]. These tumours can present with widely variable morphologies and immune profiles and can be misdiagnosed as undifferentiated pleomorphic sarcoma, leiomyosarcoma, rhabdomyosarcoma, Ewing sarcoma, malignant peripheral nerve sheath tumour, poorly differentiated carcinoma, or, exceptionally rarely, angiosarcoma [14,16,19].

This phenomenon may represent a form of cancer plasticity aiding invasiveness and resistance to treatment [20,21]. Due to the presumed increased aggressiveness of dedifferentiated metastatic melanoma, establishing the correct diagnosis is tremendously important, but also a tedious process requiring extensive sampling, comprehensive immunohistochemical analysis, and even molecular tests for detecting genetic mutations typically associated with melanomas [14,22].

Given the rarity of dedifferentiated angiosarcomatous metastatic melanomas and their inherent diagnostic and management difficulties, we present the case of a superficial spreading melanoma with divergent angiosarcomatous differentiation in both locally recurrent and metastatic tumours. Furthermore, we performed an extensive review of previous published cases.

2. Materials and Methods

The tissue samples used for histopathological and immunohistochemical analyses were obtained after surgical removal of the primary cutaneous tumour and the recurrent cutaneous lesion, and lymphadenopathy. The tissue samples were fixed in 10% buffered formalin, paraffin-embedded, sectioned, and stained with Hematoxylin–Eosin (H&E) according to conventional histology protocols.

The sections used for immunohistochemistry were deparaffinised using toluene and alcohol, washed in phosphate saline buffer, incubated with normal serum, and later incubated with primary antibodies overnight. The secondary antibodies used were HMB45 (Biocare, mouse monoclonal, clone HMB45), PRAME (Biocare, rabbit monoclonal, clone EPR20330), SOX10 (Biocare, mouse monoclonal, clone BC34), Ki67 (Biocare, mouse monoclonal, clone MIB-1), desmin (Biocare, mouse monoclonal, clone D33), WT1 (Zeta, mouse monoclonal, clone 6F-H2), CD10 (Biocare, mouse monoclonal, clone 56C6), CD99 (Biocare, rabbit monoclonal, clone EP8), ERG (Biocare, mouse monoclonal, clone 9FY), CD31 (Biocare, mouse monoclonal, clone JC/70A), and BRAF V600E (Biocare, mouse monoclonal, clone VE1). The sections were developed using 3,3′-diaminobenzidine hydrochloride/hydrogen peroxide as a chromogen and counterstained with Meyer's Haematoxylin.

Finally, we provided an extensive review of the literature by including complete-length English papers published until 2024 in PubMed-indexed journals discussing dedifferentiated melanomas, focusing on angiosarcomatous differentiation. All types of articles were included: reviews, original studies, and case reports. The research keywords were undifferentiated melanoma, dedifferentiated melanoma, transdifferentiated melanoma, and angiosarcomatous melanoma.

3. Case Presentation

We present the case of a 65-year-old male who presented to our hospital in August 2021 with a pigmentary nodule on the upper posterior thorax. The tumour reportedly arose on previously normal skin about a year before, had been growing ever since, and had recently started to bleed. Clinical examination revealed an asymmetric pigmentary nodule of 1.2 × 0.9 cm, with well-demarcated borders and an uneven tumour surface. No on-transit or satellite metastases were seen, and palpation of the lymph nodes did not reveal any masses. A dermatoscopic examination revealed a blue colour, shiny white structures, and ulceration. The patient was otherwise well and did not have a personal or family history of melanoma or non-melanoma skin cancer. It was decided to excise the lesion, given its history of rapid growth and the clinical features.

On gross examination of the resection specimen, we noted the presence of a pigmented, nodular tumour with surface ulceration. Based on these findings, the clinical suspicion of a cutaneous melanoma was raised (Figure 1).

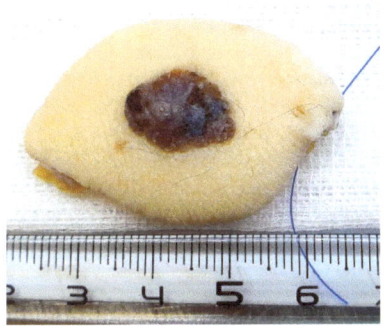

Figure 1. Post-excision photograph of a hyperpigmentary nodular melanoma, showing asymmetry, uneven surface, and ulceration.

Microscopically, the tumour was composed of nests and solid areas of atypical epithelioid cells with focal intracytoplasmic melanin, enlarged nuclei with conspicuous nucleoli, and frequent mitotic figures (5/mm^2). The tumour displayed a pagetoid growth pattern, ulcerating the epidermis, and was deeply invasive into the reticular dermis. The Breslow depth of invasion was 3.51 mm. No lympho-vascular invasion, perineural invasion, microsatellites, or necrotic areas were noted. Consequently, the diagnosis of pT3b nodular melanoma was established (Figure 2).

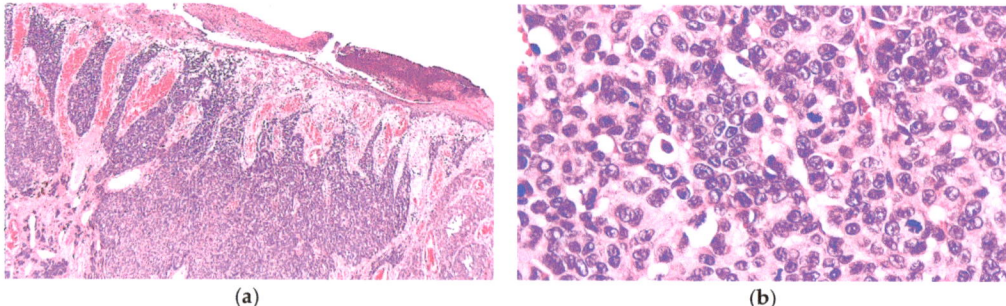

Figure 2. (a) Nodular melanoma composed of a solid growth pattern and epidermal ulceration (H&E, 40×). (b) Nests of epithelioid melanocytes with round nuclei displaying conspicuous nucleoli and frequent mitotic figures (H&E, 400×).

The diagnosis was also confirmed immunohistochemically. The tumour cells were diffusely and intensely positive for multiple melanocytic markers: MelanA, S100, SOX10, and PRAME. Additionally, the Ki67 proliferation index was 15% (Figure 3).

Due to the depth of the tumour, a re-excision with 2 cm safety margins was performed. Later, the patient underwent a sentinel lymph node biopsy and contrast-enhanced computed tomography (CT) examination of the head and neck, and thoracic and abdominopelvic regions, but no regional or distant metastases were detected at that time. Therefore, no other treatment was initiated at this stage and the patient was called back for follow-up visits every 3 months. Unfortunately, at the 9-month visit in May 2022, suprascapular lymphadenopathy was detected. After surgical removal of the suprascapular mass, histopathological examination confirmed the presence of 11 lymph nodes, out of which 2 showed features of a sarcomatoid tumour proliferation with a fascicular growth pattern, encompassing ill-defined vascular spaces. The neoplastic cells were spindle-shaped, with no intracytoplasmic melanin and very frequent mitotic figures (Figure 4).

Immunohistochemical analysis revealed that the tumour cells completely lacked expression of MelanA and PRAME, and focally expressed SOX10. On the other hand, CD10 was diffusely positive, and WT1 showed strong cytoplasmic expression. Desmin, CD99, and CD31 were negative, while ERG expression was noted in scattered tumour cells. Based on these findings, the diagnosis of metastatic melanoma with sarcomatoid features and areas of angiosarcomatous differentiation was established. Additionally, BRAF V600E immunohistochemistry was performed, but the test result was negative (Figure 5).

Even though immunohistochemical analysis for *BRAF* mutations rendered negative results, genetic testing for *BRAF* mutations was also performed using an Idylla™ *BRAF* Mutation Assay cartridge (Biocartis, Mechelen, Belgium), revealing a wild-type phenotype. No other metastases were detected at the time. The patient was therefore started on treatment with pembrolizumab 200 mg every 3 weeks.

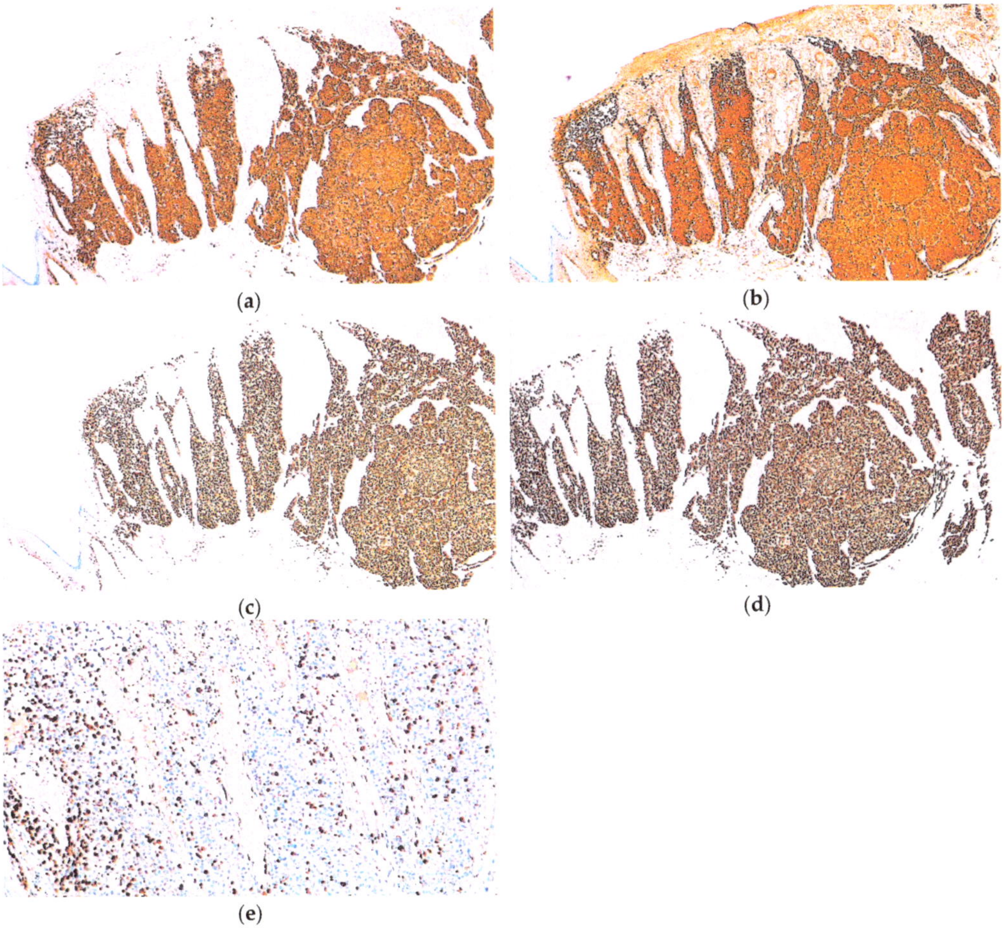

Figure 3. Immunohistochemical analysis of the cutaneous melanoma acknowledged diffuse positivity for (**a**) MelanA, (**b**) S100, (**c**) SOX10, and (**d**) PRAME. (**e**) The Ki67 immunoexpression was noted in 15% of the neoplastic cells.

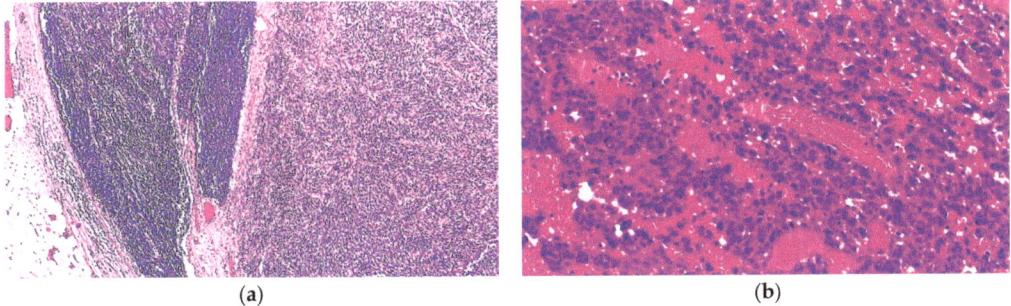

Figure 4. Histopathological analysis of the lymph node metastases revealed (**a**) the presence of a malignant spindle cell proliferation with a fascicular growth pattern (H&E, 40×) and (**b**) numerous ill-defined, branching vascular spaces (H&E, 400×).

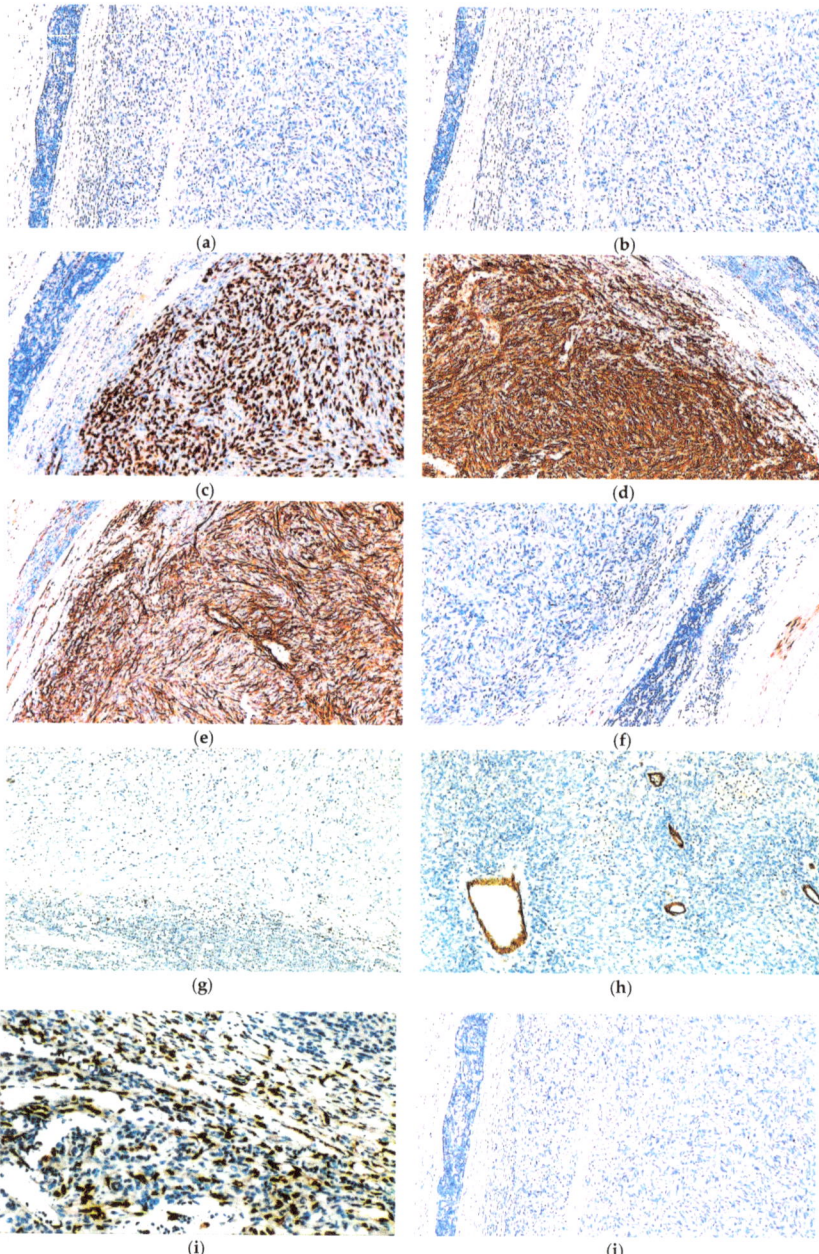

Figure 5. Immunohistochemical analysis of the lymph node revealed that the tumour cells were negative for (**a**) MelanA and (**b**) PRAME. However, the tumour cells displayed (**c**) strong positivity for SOX10 and showed strong and diffuse immunopositivity for (**d**) CD10 and (**e**) WT1, while (**f**) desmin, (**g**) CD99, and (**h**) CD31 were negative. (**i**) Positive ERG immunoreaction was noted in scattered tumour cells. (**j**) BRAF V600E was negative in the tumour cells.

In April 2023, the patient presented again with a tumour recurrence at the site of the initial lesion. The tumour was once again removed and on histopathological examination this neoplasm also displayed sarcomatoid features, with solid sheets of highly pleomorphic spindle cells with amphophilic cytoplasm and numerous mitotic figures (22/HPF) and no intracytoplasmic pigment. Additionally, there were frequent blood lakes with haemorrhagic areas and ill-defined vascular channels (Figure 6).

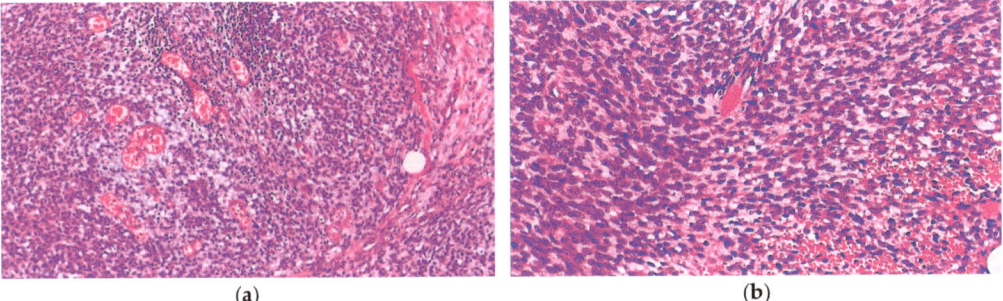

(a) (b)

Figure 6. Histopathological examination of the skin lesion acknowledged (**a**) the presence of a solid sarcomatoid proliferation with extensive haemorrhage and (**b**) pleomorphic spindle cells surrounding anastomosing vascular spaces.

Immunohistochemical analysis revealed a similar profile to the lymph node metastasis. The tumour cells were completely negative for MelanA and PRAME while showing only focal SOX10 positivity. CD10 and WT1 were both diffusely positive, and CD99 was weakly positive in scattered tumour cells. Additionally, this time, the vascular marker CD31 was strongly and diffusely positive and ERG was strongly positive in scattered cells. These histopathological and immunohistochemical profiles are consistent with the diagnosis of recurrent sarcomatoid melanoma with genuine angiosarcomatous dedifferentiation (Figure 7).

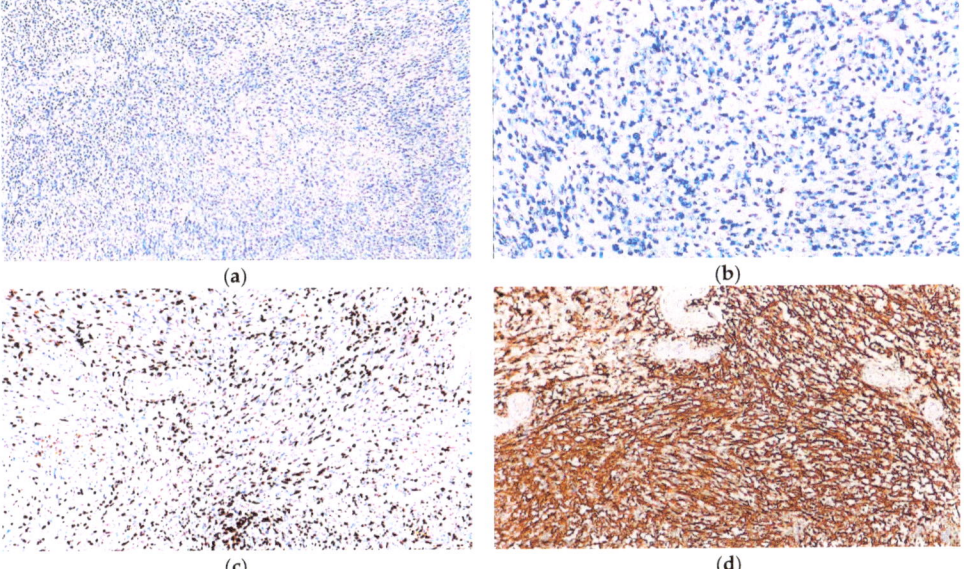

(a) (b)

(c) (d)

Figure 7. *Cont.*

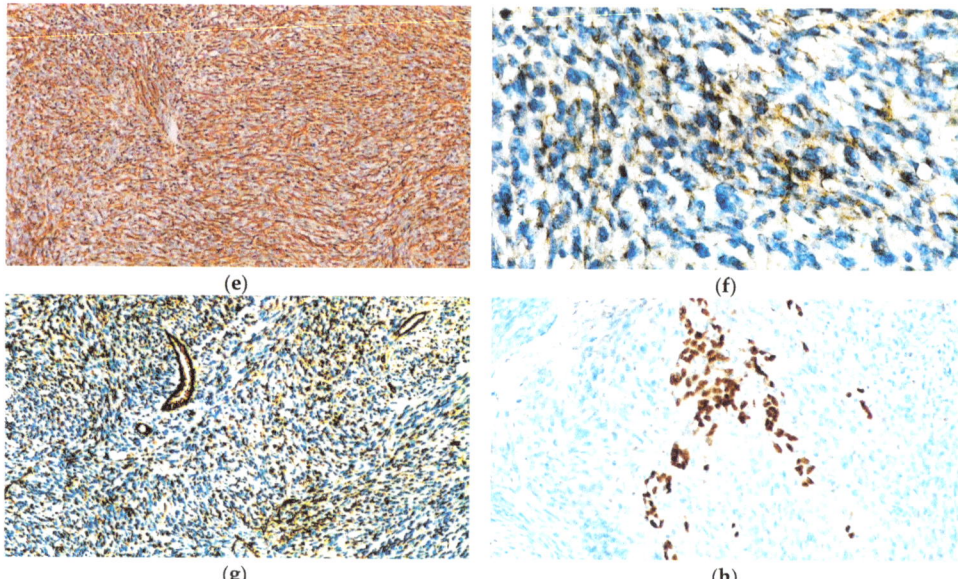

Figure 7. Immunohistochemical evaluation of the recurrent skin lesion proved that the tumour cells were not reactive for (**a**) MelanA and (**b**) PRAME. However, the tumour cells displayed moderate immunopositivity for (**c**) SOX10. Additionally, (**d**) CD10 and (**e**) WT1 were strongly and diffusely positive, while (**f**) CD99 was weakly positive in several areas. (**g**) CD31 was strongly positive in most of the neoplastic proliferation and (**h**) ERG was strongly positive in scattered tumour cells.

Due to tumour progression, treatment with pembrolizumab was deemed inefficient and the patient was switched to chemotherapy with dacarbazine but succumbed to widespread metastatic disease in February 2024.

4. Discussion

Angiomatoid morphology in melanomas is exceptionally rare. To the best of our knowledge, there are only four cases reported in primary cutaneous melanomas, and three of metastatic melanomas. However, to this date, genuine angiosarcomatous dedifferentiation was noted in only one of the metastatic tumours [16,23–28]. The clinical, histopathological, and immunohistochemical features of these neoplasms are presented in Table 1.

By analysing the data presented in Table 1, it can be noted that the mean age of patients with angiomatoid melanomas is 65,375 years (SD = 13.04), and the male–female ratio is 3:1. These findings are highly concordant with our newly reported case, as the patient was a 65-year-old male.

As mentioned above, the case presented in this paper is only the second reported melanoma with angiosarcomatoid dedifferentiation highlighted by immunohistochemical expression of ERG and CD31, while lacking expression of MelanA and PRAME. In this context, the diagnosis of metastatic and recurrent melanoma was established due to the retained expression of SOX10. Similarly, Ambrogio F. et al. also concluded that SOX10 is the most reliable marker for diagnosing angiomatoid melanomas [24]. Furthermore, the metastatic tumour also expressed WT1, and Mehta A. et al. noted cytoplasmatic WT1 staining in a dedifferentiated metastatic melanoma, arguing that this pattern of expression may be useful for establishing the final diagnosis [29]. Therefore, in the right clinical context, ample immunohistochemical analysis for multiple melanocytic markers should be performed so as not to miss a diagnosis of dedifferentiated melanoma.

Table 1. Clinical, immunohistochemical, and molecular features of angiomatoid melanomas.

Author	Age	Gender	Tumour Location	Immunohistochemistry	Genetics
Ramos-Rodríguez G. et al. [22]	59	Male	Thigh	Positive: S100, HMB45, MiTF1, D2-40 Negative: CD31, p63, AE1/AE3 Ki-67: 5–10%	N/A
Ambrogio F. et al. [23]	87	Male	Cutaneous	Differentiated component: • Positive: S100, MelanA, HMB45, SOX10 • KI67: 5–6% Dedifferentiated component: • Positive: SOX10 • Negative: S100, MelanA, HMB45, CD31, CD34, and ERG • KI67: 20%	*BRAF* V600E mutation
Fonda-Pascual P. et al. [24]	63	Female	Scapular region	Positive: S100, SOX9, HMB45 Negative: AE1/AE3, D2-40, CD31	*BRAF* V600E mutation
Baron J.A. et al. [25]	84	Male	Forehead	Positive: S100 Negative: HMB45	N/A
Adler M.J. et al. [26]	44	Male	Forehead metastases	Positive: S100, HMB 45, and vimentin	N/A
Zelger B.G. et al. [27]	56	Female	Subcutaneous metastases	Positive: S100, HMB45, MelanA, CD56	N/A
	61	Male	Axillary lymph node metastases	Positive: S100, CD56	N/A
Kilsdonk M.J. et al. [15]	69	Male	Inguinal lymph node metastases	Differentiated component: • Positive: S100, MelanA, SOX10 • Negative: ERG, CD31 Dedifferentiated component: • Positive: ERG, CD31 • Negative: S100, MelanA, SOX10	*NRAS* c.181_182delinsAGp mutation

N/A—not available.

Concerning the expression of vascular markers, the other reported angiomatoid melanoma with positivity for ERG and CD31 completely lacked expression of S100, MelanA, and SOX10 and required molecular tests for confirmation [16]. As angiomatoid features are exceptionally rare in melanomas, little is known about the mechanisms behind this phenomenon. One of the possible explanations is that "mechanical stress" during the biopsy induces the formation of vascular spaces [24]. However, this explanation cannot be applied to our current case, in which differentiation was noted in both lymph node metastases and local recurrence and it was also confirmed by immunohistochemical expression of ERG and CD31. Therefore, angiosarcomatoid dedifferentiation in melanomas may be explained by a real phenotype shifting towards mesenchymal cells, which can be a means of cancer resistance [22,24]. We also favour this hypothesis due to the fact that the tumour presented in this study was highly aggressive, with poor response to systemic therapy. The disease was rapidly progressive and fatal.

In addition to immunohistochemical positivity for endothelial markers, the neoplastic cells of both the lymph node metastases and the recurrent skin tumour diffusely expressed CD10. Similar results have been reported by various authors in dedifferentiated melanomas [30–33] and CD10 has also been linked to promoting tumour progression and resistance to therapy [34]. Therefore, CD10 should be evaluated in metastatic melanomas, particularly in poorly differentiated lesions, as its expression could be a sign of phenotype shifting towards a more aggressive neoplasm.

Unlike CD10 diffuse expression, CD99 positivity was only observed in scattered cells in the recurrent skin tumour, demonstrating the transdifferentiation pathway followed by melanomas in their progression. In this respect, rare cases of dedifferentiated metastatic melanomas with CD99 have also been reported [35,36], highlighting the extraordinary heterogeneity of these neoplasms.

In our patient, PRAME analysis was performed for the first time in an angiomatoid melanoma, with the primary tumour expressing PRAME while the metastatic and recurrent lesions were negative for this marker. These results may seem surprising, since PRAME is regarded as one of the most reliable immunohistochemical markers for diagnosing dedifferentiated melanomas, either primary or metastatic [2,37,38]. However, the accuracy of these findings may be limited due to the low number of dedifferentiated melanomas with PRAME assessment. Further studies are required in order to fully define the utility of PRAME analysis in dedifferentiated melanomas, and in tumours with angiomatoid features in particular.

Dedifferentiated melanomas, especially in a metastatic context, may benefit from molecular analysis, not only for choosing the proper treatment but also for establishing the correct diagnosis [2,31,39,40]. In this respect, dedifferentiated melanomas usually retain melanoma-specific mutations even in metastatic settings, but such cases may also present epigenetic abnormalities characteristic of mesenchymal malignancies, thus matching the histopathological and immunohistochemical profile. Nevertheless, these modifications seem to be confined to the methylation signature, while specific copy number profiling appears to be retained in metastatic melanomas [41]. These observations are significant, as they highlight both the risk of misdiagnosing a metastatic melanoma based solely on methylation profile and the prospect of adapting treatment according to genetic abnormalities of the metastatic lesions. However, at present, the only genetic mutation that can benefit from target therapy is *BRAF* [2]. For this reason, our patient was tested for *BRAF* mutations, and following the negative results, no further molecular tests were performed.

Lastly, despite the valuable role of molecular analysis in dedifferentiated melanomas, such tests are expensive and still not readily available. Consequently, surrogate immunohistochemical markers for the most frequently encountered mutations, *BRAF* p.V600E and *NRAS* p.Q61, have been developed and are highly correlated with DNA analysis [42–47]. This correlation was also noted in the current case, with negative results in both immunohistochemical and molecular tests for *BRAF* mutations.

Regarding the current state of treatment, the most commonly used therapies for locally recurrent or metastasised melanoma are immune checkpoint inhibitors and targeted therapies. Immune checkpoint inhibition is achieved by the use of anti-PD-1 agents (pembrolizumab, nivolumab) or by a combination treatment with the CTLA-4 inhibitor ipilimumab and the PD-1 inhibitor nivolumab. Targeted therapy uses BRAF inhibitors in combination with MEK inhibitors. This latter type of treatment is associated with a more rapid response but can only be used in melanomas that harbour an activating *BRAF* V600E mutation, and, unfortunately, resistance to treatment installs rapidly, after a median duration of 11 months [48–53].

The mechanisms that lead to targeted therapy resistance involve additional genetic mutations that activate the MAPK pathway, as well as non-genetic mechanisms, such as the remodelling of the extracellular matrix and transcriptional reprogramming. Remodelling of the extracellular matrix impedes T-cell migration and is implicated in resistance to immune checkpoint inhibitors as well. Additional alterations which lead to immune checkpoint inhibitor resistance are TGFβ-mediated downregulation of the expression of MHC class I molecules, decreased T-cell infiltration in the tumour, and loss of expression of melanoma differentiation antigens. In the future, this could have therapeutic implications. Molecules that inhibit the TGFβ pathway or collagen receptors could be added to therapeutic regimens in order to improve the response to targeted therapies and checkpoint inhibitors [10–12]. Nintedanib, a multikinase inhibitor and anti-fibrotic drug, shows promise in inhibiting extracellular matrix remodelling and preventing tumour relapse [54].

In the case of our patient, dedifferentiation occurred before the use of systemic treatments. Even though dedifferentiated melanomas have a grim prognosis, there have been some case reports of favourable responses to various treatment modalities, such as nivolumab [16] or interferon-α in combination with dacarbazine [28]. As of yet, there are no specific treatment recommendations for the treatment of dedifferentiated melanoma. Therefore, our patient was first treated with a PD-1 inhibitor, followed by conventional chemotherapy, but sadly did not respond. In the future, we can hope for more personalised therapies targeting factors that are implicated in the differentiation and cell survival of dedifferentiated melanoma.

Advancing knowledge about the molecular mechanisms involved in melanoma tumourigenesis and in the development of resistance to treatment will hopefully lead to the development of new effective, more personalised treatment options for this type of cancer. New immune checkpoint inhibitors and targeted therapies are under development. Examples are the lymphocyte activation gene-3 (LAG-3) inhibitor relatlimab, RAF inhibitors (sorafenib, tovorafenib), CDK4/6 inhibitors (palbociclib), and inhibitors of the Met/HGF signalling pathway (crizotinib, tivantinib, quercetin) [55]. Talimogene laherperepvec is an already approved oncolytic viral therapy containing live herpes simplex virus 1 that can be used for the intralesional treatment of unresectable melanoma. It may also be useful as a neoadjuvant treatment [50–53,55]. Recently, lifileucel, an adoptive immune cell therapy with autologous ex vivo-expanded tumour-infiltrating lymphocytes, has been approved by the US Food and Drug Agency (FDA) for patients with advanced or unresectable melanoma progressing under other treatment modalities [56]. Other promising therapeutic modalities that are currently under development include chimeric antigen receptor T-cell (CAR T) therapy and cancer vaccines [55].

5. Conclusions

Divergent differentiation is a frequent yet poorly understood phenomenon in melanomas, posing real diagnostic and therapeutic challenges. Even though metastatic melanomas can exhibit various heterologous components, angiosarcomatous transdifferentiation is still extraordinarily rare. This case report documents the transition of a classic cutaneous melanoma to a highly aggressive sarcomatoid lesion as the disease progressed, highlighting the utility of ample histopathological, immunohistochemical, and molecular analysis, as well as discussing the prognostic meaning of phenotype shifting.

Author Contributions: Conceptualisation, D.A.Ț. and A.R.F.; methodology, M.C. and C.A.; software, H.D.L.; validation, M.T., A.V.D. and A.M.C.; formal analysis, A.V.D. and C.A.; investigation, A.I.I. and A.M.; resources, M.T. and A.M.; data curation, D.A.Ț.; writing—original draft preparation, A.V.D. and H.D.L.; writing—review and editing, D.A.Ț. and A.R.F.; visualisation, A.M.C.; supervision, A.I.I.; project administration, M.C. All authors have read and agreed to the published version of the manuscript.

Funding: This research received no external funding.

Institutional Review Board Statement: The study was conducted in accordance with the Declaration of Helsinki and approved by the Ethics Committee of University Emergency Hospital, Bucharest, Romania (no. 79362/21 December 2023).

Informed Consent Statement: Written informed consent was obtained from the patient involved in the study.

Data Availability Statement: This article does not include any additional primary data besides the information already presented in the case report section.

Acknowledgments: Publication of this paper was supported by the University of Medicine and Pharmacy Carol Davila, through the institutional program Publish not Perish.

Conflicts of Interest: The authors declare no conflicts of interest.

References

1. Davis, L.E.; Shalin, S.C.; Tackett, A.J. Current state of melanoma diagnosis and treatment. *Cancer Biol. Ther.* **2019**, *20*, 1366–1379. [CrossRef] [PubMed]
2. Țăpoi, D.A.; Gheorghișan-Gălățeanu, A.-A.; Dumitru, A.V.; Ciongariu, A.M.; Furtunescu, A.R.; Marin, A.; Costache, M. Primary Undifferentiated/Dedifferentiated Cutaneous Melanomas—A Review on Histological, Immunohistochemical, and Molecular Features with Emphasis on Prognosis and Treatment. *Int. J. Mol. Sci.* **2023**, *24*, 9985. [CrossRef] [PubMed]
3. Sgouros, D.; Lallas, A.; Kittler, H.; Zarras, A.; Kyrgidis, A.; Papageorgiou, C.; Puig, S.; Scope, A.; Argenziano, G.; Zalaudek, I.; et al. Dermatoscopic features of thin (≤2 mm Breslow thickness) vs. thick (>2 mm Breslow thickness) nodular melanoma and predictors of nodular melanoma versus nodular non-melanoma tumours: A multicentric collaborative study by the International Dermoscopy Society. *J. Eur. Acad. Dermatol. Venereol.* **2020**, *34*, 2541–2547. [CrossRef]
4. Kalkhoran, S.; Milne, O.; Zalaudek, I.; Puig, S.; Malvehy, J.; Kelly, J.W.; Marghoob, A.A. Historical, Clinical, and Dermoscopic Characteristics of Thin Nodular Melanoma. *Arch. Dermatol.* **2010**, *146*, 311–318. [CrossRef] [PubMed]
5. Liu, W.; Dowling, J.P.; Murray, W.K.; McArthur, G.A.; Thompson, J.F.; Wolfe, R.; Kelly, J.W. Rate of growth in melanomas: Characteristics and associations of rapidly growing melanomas. *Arch. Dermatol.* **2006**, *142*, 1551–1558. [CrossRef]
6. Corneli, P.; Zalaudek, I.; Rizzi, G.M.; di Meo, N. Improving the early diagnosis of early nodular melanoma: Can we do better? *Expert Rev. Anticancer. Ther.* **2018**, *18*, 1007–1012. [CrossRef] [PubMed]
7. Mar, V.; Roberts, H.; Wolfe, R.; English, D.R.; Kelly, J.W. Nodular melanoma: A distinct clinical entity and the largest contributor to melanoma deaths in Victoria, Australia. *J. Am. Acad. Dermatol.* **2013**, *68*, 568–575. [CrossRef]
8. Warycha, M.A.; Christos, P.J.; Mazumdar, M.; Darvishian, F.; Shapiro, R.L.; Berman, R.S.; Pavlick, A.C.; Kopf, A.W.; Polsky, D.; Osman, I. Changes in the presentation of nodular and superficial spreading melanomas over 35 years. *Cancer* **2008**, *113*, 3341–3348. [CrossRef]
9. Țăpoi, D.A.; Derewicz, D.; Gheorghișan-Gălățeanu, A.-A.; Dumitru, A.V.; Ciongariu, A.M.; Costache, M. The Impact of Clinical and Histopathological Factors on Disease Progression and Survival in Thick Cutaneous Melanomas. *Biomedicines* **2023**, *11*, 2616. [CrossRef] [PubMed]
10. Đorđević Brlek, Z.; Jurakić Tončić, R.; Radoš, J.; Marinović, B. Dermoscopy of Nodular Melanoma: Review of the Literature and Report of 3 Cases. *Acta Dermatovenerol. Croat.* **2016**, *24*, 203–208.
11. Moynihan, G.D. The 3 Cs of melanoma: Time for a change? *J. Am. Acad. Dermatol.* **1994**, *30*, 510–511. [CrossRef] [PubMed]
12. Argenziano, G.; Longo, C.; Cameron, A.; Cavicchini, S.; Gourhant, J.-Y.; Lallas, A.; McColl, I.; Rosendahl, C.; Thomas, L.; Tiodorovic-Zivkovic, D.; et al. Blue-black rule: A simple dermoscopic clue to recognize pigmented nodular melanoma. *Br. J. Dermatol.* **2011**, *165*, 1251–1255. [CrossRef] [PubMed]
13. Moscarella, E.; Piana, S.; Specchio, F.; Kyrgidis, A.; Nazzaro, G.; Eliceche, M.L.; Savoia, F.; Bugatti, L.; Filosa, G.; Zalaudek, I.; et al. Dermoscopy features of atypical fibroxanthoma: A multicenter study of the International Dermoscopy Society. *Australas. J. Dermatol.* **2018**, *59*, 309–314. [CrossRef] [PubMed]
14. Agaimy, A.; Specht, K.; Stoehr, R.; Lorey, T.; Märkl, B.; Niedobitek, G.; Straub, M.; Hager, T.; Reis, A.C.; Schilling, B.; et al. Metastatic Malignant Melanoma with Complete Loss of Differentiation Markers (Undifferentiated/Dedifferentiated Melanoma): Analysis of 14 Patients Emphasizing Phenotypic Plasticity and the Value of Molecular Testing as Surrogate Diagnostic Marker. *Am. J. Surg. Pathol.* **2016**, *40*, 181–191. [CrossRef] [PubMed]
15. Campbell, K.; Kumarapeli, A.R.; Gokden, N.; Cox, R.M.; Hutchins, L.; Gardner, J.M. Metastatic melanoma with dedifferentiation and extensive rhabdomyosarcomatous heterologous component. *J. Cutan. Pathol.* **2018**, *45*, 360–364. [CrossRef] [PubMed]
16. Kilsdonk, M.J.; Romeijn, T.R.; Kelder, W.; van Kempen, L.C.; Diercks, G.F. Angiosarcomatous transdifferentiation of metastatic melanoma. *J. Cutan. Pathol.* **2020**, *47*, 1211–1214. [CrossRef] [PubMed]
17. Berro, J.; Abdul Halim, N.; Khaled, C.; Assi, H.I. Malignant melanoma with metaplastic cartilaginous transdifferentiation: A case report. *J. Cutan. Pathol.* **2019**, *46*, 935–941. [CrossRef] [PubMed]
18. Yousef, S.; Joy, C.; Velaiutham, S.; Maclean, F.M.; Harraway, J.; Gill, A.J.; Vargas, A.C. Dedifferentiated melanoma with MDM2 gene amplification mimicking dedifferentiated liposarcoma. *Pathology* **2022**, *54*, 371–374. [CrossRef]
19. Agaimy, A.; Stoehr, R.; Hornung, A.; Popp, J.; Erdmann, M.; Heinzerling, L.; Hartmann, A. Dedifferentiated and Undifferentiated Melanomas: Report of 35 New Cases with Literature Review and Proposal of Diagnostic Criteria. *Am. J. Surg. Pathol.* **2021**, *45*, 240–254. [CrossRef]
20. Arozarena, I.; Wellbrock, C. Phenotype plasticity as enabler of melanoma progression and therapy resistance. *Nat. Rev. Cancer* **2019**, *19*, 377–391. [CrossRef]
21. Diazzi, S.; Tartare-Deckert, S.; Deckert, M. The mechanical phenotypic plasticity of melanoma cell: An emerging driver of therapy cross-resistance. *Oncogenesis* **2023**, *12*, 7. [CrossRef] [PubMed]
22. Massi, D.; Mihic-Probst, D.; Schadendorf, D.; Dummer, R.; Mandalà, M. Dedifferentiated melanomas: Morpho-phenotypic profile, genetic reprogramming and clinical implications. *Cancer Treat. Rev.* **2020**, *88*, 102060. [CrossRef] [PubMed]
23. Ramos-Rodríguez, G.; Ortiz-Hidalgo, C. Primary angiomatoid melanoma as an exceptional morphologic pattern in cutaneous melanoma. A case report and review of the literature. *Actas Dermo-Sifiliográficas* **2015**, *106*, e13–e17. [CrossRef] [PubMed]
24. Ambrogio, F.; Colagrande, A.; Cascardi, E.; Grandolfo, M.; Filotico, R.; Foti, C.; Lupo, C.; Casatta, N.; Ingravallo, G.; Cazzato, G. Partially Dedifferentiated Primitive Malignant Melanoma with Pseudo-Angiomatous Features: A Case Report with Review of the Literature. *Diagnostics* **2023**, *13*, 495. [CrossRef] [PubMed]

25. Fonda-Pascual, P.; Moreno-Arrones, O.M.; Alegre-Sanchez, A.; Garcia-Del Real, C.M.; Miguel-Gomez, L.; Martin-Gonzalez, M. Primary cutaneous angiomatoid melanoma. *J. Dtsch. Dermatol. Ges.* **2018**, *16*, 345–347. [CrossRef] [PubMed]
26. Baron, J.A.; Monzon, F.; Galaria, N.; Murphy, G.F. Angiomatoid melanoma: A novel pattern of differentiation in invasive periocular desmoplastic malignant melanoma. *Hum. Pathol.* **2000**, *31*, 1520–1522. [CrossRef] [PubMed]
27. Adler, M.J.; Beckstead, J.; White, C.R., Jr. Angiomatoid Melanoma: A Case of Metastatic Melanoma Mimicking a Vascular Malignancy. *Am. J. Dermatopathol.* **1997**, *19*, 606–609. [CrossRef] [PubMed]
28. Zelger, B.G.; Zelger, B. Angiomatoid Metastatic Melanoma. *Dermatol. Surg.* **2004**, *30*, 336–340. [PubMed]
29. Mehta, A.; Sharma, L.; Gupta, G. Rhabdoid melanoma: A diagnostic ordeal. *Indian J. Cancer* **2020**, *57*, 473–477. [CrossRef]
30. Ferreira, I.; Arends, M.J.; van der Weyden, L.; Adams, D.J.; Brenn, T. Primary de-differentiated, trans-differentiated and undifferentiated melanomas: Overview of the clinicopathological, immunohistochemical and molecular spectrum. *Histopathology* **2022**, *80*, 135–149. [CrossRef]
31. Lefferts, J.A.; Loehrer, A.P.; Yan, S.; Green, D.C.; Deharvengt, S.J.; LeBlanc, R.E. CD10 and p63 expression in a sarcomatoid undifferentiated melanoma: A cautionary (and molecularly annotated) tale. *J. Cutan. Pathol.* **2020**, *47*, 541–547. [CrossRef] [PubMed]
32. Valiga, A.A.; Fuller, C.G.; Doyle, J.A.; Lee, J.B. Sarcomatoid Dedifferentiated Melanoma: The Diagnostic Role of Next-Generation Sequencing. *Am. J. Dermatopathol.* **2022**, *44*, 282–286. [CrossRef] [PubMed]
33. Ferreira, I.; Droop, A.; Edwards, O.; Wong, K.; Harle, V.; Habeeb, O.; Gharpuray-Pandit, D.; Houghton, J.; Wiedemeyer, K.; Mentzel, T.; et al. The clinicopathologic spectrum and genomic landscape of de-/trans-differentiated melanoma. *Mod. Pathol.* **2021**, *34*, 2009–2019. [CrossRef] [PubMed]
34. Oba, J.; Nakahara, T.; Hashimoto-Hachiya, A.; Liu, M.; Abe, T.; Hagihara, A.; Yokomizo, T.; Furue, M. CD10-Equipped Melanoma Cells Acquire Highly Potent Tumorigenic Activity: A Plausible Explanation of Their Significance for a Poor Prognosis. *PLoS ONE* **2016**, *11*, e0149285. [CrossRef] [PubMed]
35. Ramos-Rodríguez, C.; García-Arpa, M.; Relea-Calatayud, M.F.; González-López, L.; Romero-Aguilera, G. Metastatic Melanoma Negative for 5 Melanocytic Markers, Complete Regressed Primary Cutaneous Melanoma, and Melanoma-Associated Leukoderma in the Same Patient. *Am. J. Dermatopathol.* **2020**, *42*, 956–960. [CrossRef] [PubMed]
36. Tran, T.A.N.; Linos, K.; de Abreu, F.B.; Carlson, J.A. Undifferentiated Sarcoma as Intermediate Step in the Progression of Malignant Melanoma to Rhabdomyosarcoma: Histologic, Immunohistochemical, and Molecular Studies of a New Case of Malignant Melanoma with Rhabdomyosarcomatous Differentiation. *Am. J. Dermatopathol.* **2019**, *41*, 221–229. [CrossRef] [PubMed]
37. Gosman, L.M.; Țăpoi, D.-A.; Costache, M. Cutaneous Melanoma: A Review of Multifactorial Pathogenesis, Immunohistochemistry, and Emerging Biomarkers for Early Detection and Management. *Int. J. Mol. Sci.* **2023**, *24*, 15881. [CrossRef] [PubMed]
38. Hornick, J.L.; Plaza, J.A.; Mentzel, T.; Gru, A.A.; Brenn, T. PRAME Expression Is a Useful Tool in the Diagnosis of Primary and Metastatic Dedifferentiated and Undifferentiated Melanoma. *Am. J. Surg. Pathol.* **2023**, *47*, 1390–1397. [CrossRef]
39. Wiedemeyer, K.; Brenn, T. Dedifferentiated and undifferentiated melanomas: A practical approach to a challenging diagnosis. *Hum. Pathol.* **2023**, *140*, 22–31. [CrossRef]
40. Cilento, M.A.; Kim, C.; Chang, S.; Farshid, G.; Brown, M.P. Three cases of *BRAF*-mutant melanoma with divergent differentiation masquerading as sarcoma. *Pathologica* **2022**, *114*, 217–220. [CrossRef]
41. Hench, J.; Mihic-Probst, D.; Agaimy, A.; Frank, S.; Meyer, P.; Hultschig, C.; Simi, S.; Alos, L.; Balamurugan, T.; Blokx, W.; et al. Clinical, histopathological and molecular features of dedifferentiated melanomas: An EORTC Melanoma Group Retrospective Analysis. *Eur. J. Cancer* **2023**, *187*, 7–14. [CrossRef] [PubMed]
42. Rothrock, A.T.; Hameed, N.; Cho, W.C.; Nagarajan, P.; Ivan, D.; Torres-Cabala, C.A.; Prieto, V.G.; Curry, J.L.; Aung, P.P. BRAF V600E immunohistochemistry as a useful tool in the diagnosis of melanomas with ambiguous morphologies and immunophenotypes. *J. Cutan. Pathol.* **2023**, *50*, 223–229. [CrossRef] [PubMed]
43. Meevassana, J.; Anothaisatapon, K.; Subbalekha, S.; Kamolratanakul, S.; Siritientong, T.; Ruangritchankul, K.; Pungrasami, P.; Hamill, K.J.; Angsapatt, A.; Kitkumthorn, N. BRAF V600E Immunohistochemistry Predicts Prognosis of Patients with Cutaneous Melanoma in Thai population. *Plast. Reconstr. Surg. Glob. Open* **2022**, *10*, 4605. [CrossRef] [PubMed]
44. Long-Mira, E.; Picard-Gauci, A.; Lassalle, S.; Hofman, V.; Lalvée, S.; Tanga, V.; Zahaf, K.; Bonnetaud, C.; Lespinet, V.; Camuzard, O.; et al. Comparison of Two Rapid Assays for the Detection of *BRAF* V600 Mutations in Metastatic Melanoma including Positive Sentinel Lymph Nodes. *Diagnostics* **2022**, *12*, 751. [CrossRef] [PubMed]
45. Vallée, A.; Denis-Musquer, M.; Herbreteau, G.; Théoleyre, S.; Bossard, C.; Denis, M.G. Prospective evaluation of two screening methods for molecular testing of metastatic melanoma: Diagnostic performance of BRAF V600E immunohistochemistry and of a NRAS-BRAF fully automated real-time PCR-based assay. *PLoS ONE* **2019**, *14*, 221123. [CrossRef]
46. Uguen, A.; Talagas, M.; Costa, S.; Samaison, L.; Paule, L.; Alavi, Z.; De Braekeleer, M.; Le Marechal, C.; Marcorelles, P. NRAS (Q61R), BRAF (V600E) immunohistochemistry: A concomitant tool for mutation screening in melanomas. *Diagn. Pathol.* **2015**, *10*, 121. [CrossRef]
47. Ilie, M.; Long-Mira, E.; Funck-Brentano, E.; Lassalle, S.; Butori, C.; Lespinet-Fabre, V.; Bordone, O.; Gay, A.; Zahaf, K.; Poissonnet, G.; et al. Immunohistochemistry as a potential tool for routine detection of the NRAS Q61R mutation in patients with metastatic melanoma. *J. Am. Acad. Dermatol.* **2015**, *72*, 786–793. [CrossRef]

48. Flaherty, K.T.; Infante, J.R.; Daud, A.; Gonzalez, R.; Kefford, R.F.; Sosman, J.; Hamid, O.; Schuchter, L.; Cebon, J.; Ibrahim, N.; et al. Combined BRAF and MEK inhibition in melanoma with BRAF V600 mutations. *N. Engl. J. Med.* **2012**, *367*, 1694–1703. [CrossRef] [PubMed]
49. Garbe, C.; Amaral, T.; Peris, K.; Hauschild, A.; Arenberger, P.; Basset-Seguin, N.; Bastholt, L.; Bataille, V.; del Marmol, V.; Dréno, B.; et al. European Dermatology Forum (EDF), the European Association of Dermato-Oncology (EADO), and the European Organization for Research and Treatment of Cancer (EORTC). European consensus-based interdisciplinary guideline for melanoma. Part 1: Diagnostics: Update 2022. *Eur. J. Cancer* **2022**, *170*, 236–255. [CrossRef]
50. Garbe, C.; Amaral, T.; Peris, K.; Hauschild, A.; Arenberger, P.; Basset-Seguin, N.; Bastholt, L.; Bataille, V.; del Marmol, V.; Dréno, B.; et al. European consensus-based interdisciplinary guideline for melanoma. Part 2: Treatment—Update 2022. *Eur. J. Cancer* **2022**, *170*, 256–284. [CrossRef]
51. Lakshmi, A.; Shah, R.; Begaj, A.; Jayarajan, R.; Ramachandran, S.; Morgan, B.; Faust, G.; Patel, N. NICE 2022 guidelines on the management of melanoma: Update and implications. *J. Plast. Reconstr. Aesthetic Surg.* **2023**, *85*, 401–413. [CrossRef]
52. Keilholz, U.; Ascierto, P.; Dummer, R.; Robert, C.; Lorigan, P.; van Akkooi, A.; Arance, A.; Blank, C.; Sileni, V.C.; Donia, M.; et al. ESMO consensus conference recommendations on the management of metastatic melanoma: Under the auspices of the ESMO Guidelines Committee. *Ann. Oncol.* **2020**, *31*, 1435–1448. [CrossRef]
53. Seth, R.; Agarwala, S.S.; Messersmith, H.; Alluri, K.C.; Ascierto, P.A.; Atkins, M.B.; Bollin, K.; Chacon, M.; Davis, N.; Faries, M.B.; et al. Systemic Therapy for Melanoma: ASCO Guideline Update. *J. Clin. Oncol.* **2023**, *41*, 4794–4820. [CrossRef]
54. Kato, R.; Haratani, K.; Hayashi, H.; Sakai, K.; Sakai, H.; Kawakami, H.; Tanaka, K.; Takeda, M.; Yonesaka, K.; Nishio, K.; et al. Nintedanib promotes antitumour immunity and shows antitumour activity in combination with PD-1 blockade in mice: Potential role of cancer-associated fibroblasts. *Br. J. Cancer* **2021**, *124*, 914–924. [CrossRef]
55. Isaak, A.J.; Clements, G.R.; Buenaventura, R.G.M.; Merlino, G.; Yu, Y. Development of Personalized Strategies for Precisely Battling Malignant Melanoma. *Int. J. Mol. Sci.* **2024**, *25*, 5023. [CrossRef]
56. Parums, D.V. Editorial: First Regulatory Approval for Adoptive Cell Therapy with Autologous Tumor-Infiltrating Lymphocytes (TILs)—Lifileucel (Amtagvi). *Med. Sci. Monit.* **2024**, *30*, e944927. [CrossRef]

Disclaimer/Publisher's Note: The statements, opinions and data contained in all publications are solely those of the individual author(s) and contributor(s) and not of MDPI and/or the editor(s). MDPI and/or the editor(s) disclaim responsibility for any injury to people or property resulting from any ideas, methods, instructions or products referred to in the content.

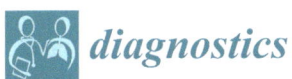

Systematic Review

T Cell Immunity in Human Papillomavirus-Related Cutaneous Squamous Cell Carcinoma—A Systematic Review

Shi Huan Tay [1] and Choon Chiat Oh [1,2,*]

[1] Duke-NUS Medical School, Singapore 169857, Singapore; tay_shi_huan@u.duke.nus.edu
[2] Department of Dermatology, Singapore General Hospital, Singapore 169608, Singapore
* Correspondence: oh.choon.chiat@singhealth.com.sg

Abstract: Cutaneous squamous cell carcinoma (cSCC) is an invasive malignancy that disproportionately afflicts immunosuppressed individuals. The close associations of cSCC with immunosuppression and human papillomavirus (HPV) infection beget the question of how these three entities are intertwined in carcinogenesis. By exploring the role of T cell immunity in HPV-related cSCC based on the existing literature, we found that the loss of T cell immunity in the background of β-HPV infection promotes cSCC initiation following exposure to environmental carcinogens or chronic trauma. This highlights the potential of developing T-cell centred therapeutic and preventive strategies for populations with increased cSCC risk.

Keywords: cutaneous squamous cell carcinoma; human papillomavirus; T cell; immunosuppression; animal model

1. Introduction

Cutaneous squamous cell carcinoma (cSCC) is an invasive malignancy that arises from keratinocytes. Its rising global incidence and its severe burden on immunosuppressed individuals put forth an urgent need to develop novel approaches for preventing and treating cSCC [1–4].

The human papillomavirus (HPV) has been implicated as a risk factor for cSCC. There is an increased HPV prevalence (in particular β-HPVs) in cSCC compared to normal skin [5,6]. However, the causal relationship between HPV and cSCC remains controversial. HPV may exhibit direct oncogenic effects, but it may also act as a co-carcinogen with other risk factors (e.g., UVB radiation) to amplify the risk of developing cSCC [6–9].

Immunosuppression profoundly elevates the risk of cancers associated with viral infection, including cSCC. Immunosuppressed patients have up to 100-fold higher cSCC rates compared with the general population [10–13]. Antiviral immunity is chiefly regulated by the adaptive immune system, where T cells orchestrate effective long-lived responses. Immunosuppression profoundly diminishes T cell function, metabolism, and proliferation. This results in compromised protection against HPV proliferation in the skin, which likely contributes to carcinogenesis.

In this study, we aimed to clarify the role of T cell immunity in HPV-related cSCC based on the current literature. We identified potential causal relationships among T cell immunity, HPV, and cSCC, which may guide future preventive and therapeutic approaches, particularly in high-risk populations.

2. Materials and Methods

A systematic search of research databases (PubMed, Embase, Scopus, Cochrane Library) was performed on 27 August 2023 in accordance with PRISMA guidelines (Figure 1; PROSPERO registry number CRD42023470491). Article screening and data extraction were performed in duplicate. Full-text studies (in vitro, in vivo, ex vivo, clinical) published in English that investigated T cell immunity in HPV-related cSCC were included.

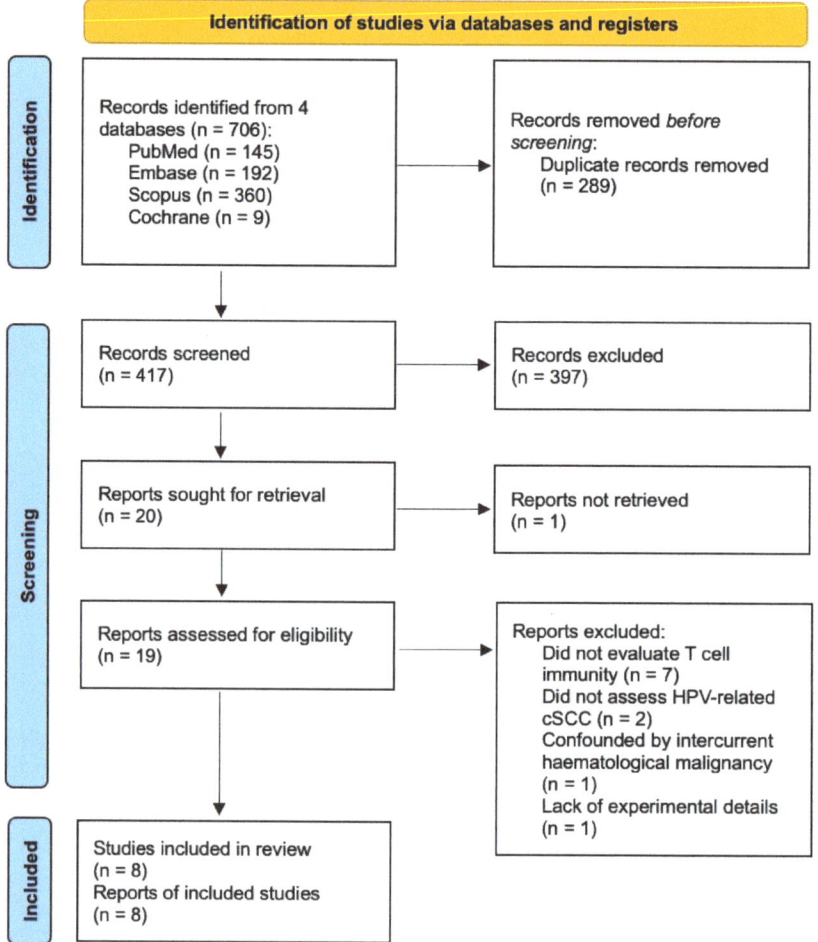

Figure 1. PRISMA flow diagram.

The retrieved sources were screened by two independent authors (SHT and CCO) using titles and abstracts for inclusion. In situations where article suitability was uncertain, full text assessment was conducted, and discrepancies were resolved by a vote of consensus. Articles were selected based on the following inclusion criteria: (1) written in the English language, (2) using validated in vitro and in vivo models of HPV-related cSCC, ex vivo studies on patients with HPV-related cSCC, or randomised control trials (RCTs) on patients with HPV-related cSCC, and (3) having an emphasis on T cell immunity. Articles were excluded for the following reasons: (1) not reporting original data, (2) not focusing on HPV-related cSCC, (3) not focusing on T cell immunity, (4) observational clinical studies, and (5) lacking available full text.

3. Results

Our literature search enabled us to retrieve 706 articles, from which 8 were included for the final qualitative analysis (Figure 1).

3.1. T Cell Immunity in HPV-Related cSCC Carcinogenesis

A total of six articles discussed T cell perturbations in HPV-related cSCC carcinogenesis (Tables 1 and 2). All articles employed cSCC mouse models and one of the six reported additional data from human cSCC samples. For the cSCC mouse models, five of the six studies focused on β-HPVs—HPV8 mice were used in two of the six studies and *Mus musculus* papillomavirus 1 (MmuPV1)-colonised mice in three of the six studies. Only one of the six studies investigated α-HPVs with HPV16 mice. For carcinogenesis protocols, four of the six studies utilised spontaneous tumorigenesis, four of the six looked into ultraviolet B (UVB) irradiation, while one of the six investigated 7,12-Dimethylbenz(a)anthracene-12-O-tetradecanoylphorbol-13-acetate (DMBA-TPA) chemical carcinogenesis.

Table 1. Key T cell perturbations in α-HPV-related cSCC carcinogenesis.

Author and Year	Study Population	Key T Cell Perturbations
De Visser et al. (2005) [14]	cSCC mouse models • $Rag1^{-/-}$:K14-HPV16 mice, $CD4^{-/-}$:K14-HPV16 mice, $CD8^{-/-}$:K14-HPV16 mice, $CD4^{-/-}CD8^{-/-}$:K14-HPV16 mice • Spontaneous tumorigenesis	• Genetic elimination of CD4$^+$ and/or CD8$^+$ T cells did not reduce mast cell and granulocyte recruitment into premalignant skin (vs. K14-HPV16 mice, p = n.s.)

cSCC, cutaneous squamous cell carcinoma; HPV, human papillomavirus; K14, keratin 14; n.s., non-significant.

3.1.1. T Cell Immunity in α-HPV-Related Epithelial Carcinogenesis

De Visser et al. (2005) hypothesised that an activated adaptive immunity promotes chronic inflammation in premalignant skin, thereby facilitating de novo epithelial carcinogenesis (Table 1) [14]. To address this, de Visser et al. used a transgenic mouse model of multistage epithelial carcinogenesis that expresses early region genes of HPV16 under the control of the human keratin 14 (K14) promoter/enhancer and is Recombination–Activating Gene-1 homozygous null ($Rag1^{-/-}$) [15,16]. HPV16 is one of the most common high-risk α-HPVs, responsible for most HPV-related anogenital and head and neck cancers [17]. $Rag1^{-/-}$ mice are deficient in mature B and T lymphocytes [16].

HPV16/$Rag1^{-/-}$ mice had reduced infiltration of innate immune cells and minimal inflammation in premalignant skin, which was associated with a decreased cSCC incidence. However, the lack of mature CD4$^+$ and/or CD8$^+$ T lymphocytes alone (using $CD4^{-/-}$:K14-HPV16, $CD8^{-/-}$:K14-HPV16, $CD4^{-/-}CD8^{-/-}$:K14-HPV16 mice) did not replicate the clinical phenotype (Table 1). On the contrary, the adoptive transfer of B lymphocytes and serum transfer from HPV16 mice into HPV16/$Rag1^{-/-}$ mice restored the characteristic chronic inflammation in premalignant skin and reinstated processes that are necessary for malignant progression. This study thus suggests a limited role for T cells in inflammation-associated α-HPV-driven, de novo epithelial carcinogenesis.

3.1.2. T Cell Immunity in β-HPV-Related Epithelial Carcinogenesis

Of the five major HPV genera, β-HPVs are the most implicated genus in cSCC. β-HPVs are commensal viruses of the skin that are usually associated with asymptomatic infection in healthy individuals. However, several studies have reported increased β-HPV replication in the skin and greater β-HPV seropositivity in cSCC patients, which suggest a potential role for viral oncogenesis [18]. More importantly, the increased incidence of cSCC with concomitantly higher rates of β-HPV amongst solid organ transplants suggests a role for anti-β-HPV immunity in carcinogenesis [10–13].

Borgogna et al. (2023) and Antsiferova et al. (2017) utilised transgenic mice that express early region genes (encoding E1, E2, E4, E6, and E7) of HPV8, the prototypical β-HPV that is studied in HPV-related cSCC [19–21]. Borgogna et al. demonstrated accelerated papilloma development and greater accumulation of UVB-induced epidermal DNA damage in $Rag2^{-/-}$:K14-HPV8 mice, which lack mature B and T lymphocytes (Table 2). They proposed that adaptive immune deficiency, such as that in solid organ transplant patients, sensitised β-HPV-infected skin to UVB-induced inflammation and promoted subsequent epithelial carcinogenesis.

Antsiferova et al. [20] reported more epidermal CD4$^+$ (including presumptive CD4$^+$CD25$^+$ regulatory T cells) and CD8$^+$ T cells in tumorous skin of activin A-overexpressing mice compared to that of age-matched wild-type mice (Table 2). Activin A, a member of the TGF-β superfamily, is a growth and differentiation factor that promotes wound healing and skin morphogenesis [22]. It has been shown to be upregulated in skin wounds and human non-melanoma skin cancers (including cSCC) [22,23]. The authors also observed fewer epidermal gamma delta T cells for the same comparison (Table 2). However, CD4$^+$ T cell depletion did not significantly reduce the tumour-promoting effect of activin A overexpression (Table 2). Hence, T cell perturbations alone appear to be insufficient for driving β-HPV-associated cSCC initiation, especially in the context of activin A overexpression.

Table 2. Key T cell perturbations in β-HPV-related cSCC carcinogenesis (HPV8 mice).

Author and Year	Study Population	Key T Cell Perturbations
Borgogna et al. (2023) [19]	cSCC mouse models • $Rag2^{-/-}$:K14-HPV8 mice • Spontaneous tumorigenesis, UVB	• Genetic elimination of T and B cells increased spontaneous tumour incidence in $Rag2^{-/-}$:K14-HPV8 mice (vs. $Rag2^{+/+}$:K14-HPV8 mice; week 10: $p < 0.05$; Week 25: $p < 0.0001$) • Genetic elimination of T and B cells increased percentage of spontaneously affected skin in $Rag2^{-/-}$:K14-HPV8 mice (vs. $Rag2^{+/+}$:K14-HPV8 mice; week 24: $p < 0.0001$) • Genetic elimination of T and B cells increased percentage of affected skin following UVB irradiation in $Rag2^{-/-}$:K14-HPV8 mice (vs. $Rag2^{+/+}$:K14-HPV8 mice and non-transgenic control mice; week 30: both $p < 0.01$) • Genetic elimination of T and B cells increased epidermal thickness following UVB irradiation in $Rag2^{-/-}$:K14-HPV8 mice (vs. $Rag2^{+/+}$:K14-HPV8 mice; $p < 0.0001$) • Genetic elimination of T and B cells increased epidermal DNA damage following UVB irradiation in $Rag2^{-/-}$:K14-HPV8 mice (vs. $Rag2^{+/+}$:K14-HPV8 mice; γH2AX-positive nuclei: $p < 0.001$, 53BP1-positive foci: $p < 0.001$) • Genetic elimination of T and B cells was associated with accumulation of epidermal DNA damage following UVB irradiation in $Rag2^{-/-}$:K14-HPV8 mice (vs. $Rag2^{-/-}$:K14-HPV8 mice without UVB irradiation; $p < 0.0001$)
Antsiferova et al. (2017) [20]	cSCC mouse models • HPV8-Act, HPV8-wt mice ± CD4KO • Spontaneous tumorigenesis	• Accumulation of epidermal and dermal CD4$^+$ and CD8$^+$ T cells in tumour-laden ear skin of 10-week-old HPV8-Act mice (vs. age-matched wt mice, CD4: $p < 0.0001$, CD8: $p = 0.0009$; vs. age-matched HPV8-wt mice, CD4: $p < 0.0001$, CD8: $p = 0.0022$) • Accumulation of epidermal CD4$^+$CD25$^+$ T cells in tumour-laden ear skin of 10-week-old HPV8-Act mice (vs. age-matched wt mice, $p = 0.0004$; vs. age-matched HPV8-wt mice, $p = 0.0007$) • Large increase in tumour incidence in HPV8-Act-CD4KO mice vs. HPV8-wt-CD4KO ($p < 0.0001$) • Slight but statistically insignificant increases in tumour incidence in HPV8-wt-CD4KO mice vs. HPV8-wt mice, and in HPV8-Act-CD4KO vs. HPV8-Act-wt ($p =$ n.s.) • Loss of epidermal gamma delta T cells in tumour-laden ear skin of 10-week-old HPV8-Act mice (vs. age-matched wt mice, $p < 0.0001$; vs. age-matched HPV8-wt mice, $p = 0.0007$)

Act, activin A-overexpressing; cSCC, cutaneous squamous cell carcinoma; HPV, human papillomavirus; KO, knockout; n.s., not significant; UVB, ultraviolet B; wt, wild-type.

Strickley et al. (2019), Johnson et al. (2022), and Dorfer et al. (2020) relied on another experimental model for studying commensal HPV interaction with human hosts: MmuPV1-colonised mice [24–26]. By doing so, these studies sought to interrogate T cell immunity through an infection-based system that models the natural history of HPV-related cSCC carcinogenesis [27].

Strickley et al. (2019) [24] observed that the adoptive transfer of T cells from MmuPV1-immune mice into wild-type FVB mice promoted wart rejection and protected against DMBA-TPA chemical carcinogenesis (Table 3). They also noticed an increased ratio of epidermal CD8$^+$ tissue–resident memory T (T$_{RM}$) cells to total T cells in the skin of MmuPV1-colonised mice compared to their sham-infected controls following chemical or UVB carcinogenesis (Table 3). Hence, the authors hypothesised that CD8$^+$ T cells mediate anti-tumour immunity that is induced by MmuPV1 skin colonisation. They showed that CD8$^+$ T cell depletion in MmuPV1-colonised mice increased the tumour incidence following chemical carcinogenesis (Table 3). Furthermore, they observed fewer CD8$^+$ T cells and CD8$^+$ T$_{RM}$ cells alongside a higher β-HPV load in cSCC samples from immunosuppressed patients than in those from immunocompetent individuals (Table 3). β-HPV E7 peptides activated CD8$^+$ T cells that were isolated from the normal facial skin of immunocompetent adults (Table 3). As such, the results showed that MmuPV1-immune mice were protected against epithelial carcinogenesis in a CD8$^+$ T cell-dependent fashion. This finding suggests a role for commensal β-HPV-specific adaptive immunity in eliminating virus-positive malignant keratinocytes, thereby achieving anti-tumour protection.

Table 3. Key T cell perturbations in β-HPV-related cSCC carcinogenesis (MmuPV1-colonised mice).

Author and Year	Study Population	Key T Cell Perturbations
Strickley et al. (2019) [24]	cSCC mouse models • MmuPV1-colonised FVB mice, MmuPV1-colonised SKH-1 mice • DMBA-TPA (FVB), DMBA-UVB (SKH-1) • Human cSCC patients (immunosuppressed, immunocompetent)	• Adoptive transfer of T cells from MmuPV1-immune mice into wild-type FVB mice with persistent warts reduced skin wart burden (vs. mice that received control T cells from spleen of uninfected wild-type FVB mice, n = 3 each group) • Adoptive transfer of T cells from MmuPV1-immune mice into wild-type FVB mice promoted wart rejection and protected against DMBA-TPA chemical carcinogenesis (vs. mice that received control T cells from spleen of uninfected wild-type FVB mice, n = 3 each group) • Increased ratio of epidermal CD8$^+$ T$_{RM}$ cells to total T cells in the skin of MmuPV1-colonised mice following DMBA-TPA chemical carcinogenesis (vs. sham-infected mice, p = 0.0287) and DMBA-UVB carcinogenesis (vs. sham-infected mice, p = 0.0054) • More tumour-infiltrating CD8$^+$ T cells in MmuPV1-colonised mice following DMBA-TPA chemical carcinogenesis (vs. sham-infected mice, p = 0.0208) • CD8$^+$ T cell depletion in MmuPV1-colonised mice increased tumour incidence following DMBA-TPA chemical carcinogenesis (vs. IgG-treated immunocompetent control mice, p = 0.0009) • Fewer tumour- and skin-infiltrating CD8$^+$ T cells and CD8$^+$ T$_{RM}$ cells in cSCC of immunosuppressed patients (vs. cSCC of immunocompetent patients; tumour-infiltrating CD8$^+$ T and CD8$^+$ T$_{RM}$: both p < 0.0001; skin CD8$^+$ T: p = 0.0001; skin CD8$^+$ T$_{RM}$: p = 0.0009) • CD8$^+$ T cells from normal facial skin of immunocompetent adults activated by β-HPV E7 peptides (vs. negative control; CD69$^+$: p < 0.01, CD137$^+$CD69$^+$: p < 0.01), but not by high-risk α-HPV HPV16 E7 peptides (vs. negative control; CD69$^+$: p = n.s., CD137$^+$CD69$^+$: p = n.s.)

Table 3. Cont.

Author and Year	Study Population	Key T Cell Perturbations
Johnson et al. (2022) [25]	cSCC mouse model • MmuPV1-colonised SKH-1 mice • DMBA-UVB	• CD8$^+$ T cell depletion increased MmuPV1 DNA levels in virus-colonised mouse skin following DMBA-UVB carcinogenesis (vs. IgG-treated immunocompetent control mice; p = 0.0229) • CD8$^+$ T cell depletion resulted in higher antibody titres to MmuPV1 E6, E7, and L1 antigens following DMBA-UVB carcinogenesis (vs. IgG-treated immunocompetent control mice; E6: p = 0.0030, E7: p = 0.0220, L1: p = 0.0041)
Dorfer et al. (2020) [26]	cSCC mouse models • MmuPV1-colonised FVB mice ± CsA immunosuppression • NMRI-Foxn1$^{nu/nu}$ mice • Spontaneous tumorigenesis, UVB	• MmuPV1 infection of back skin resulted in cSCC development in CsA-immunosuppressed mice (non-UVB-treated: n = 7/10; UVB-treated: n = 9/20), but not in immunocompetent mice (non-UVB-treated: n = 0/10; UVB-treated: n = 0/5) • MmuPV1 infection increased mean CD4$^+$ T cell numbers in back skin tissue of CsA-immunosuppressed/non-UVB-treated mice (vs. non-infected, equally treated controls; p < 0.05) • Non-tumorous back skin in MmuPV1-infected, CsA-immunosuppressed/UVB-treated mice had higher CD8$^+$ T cell numbers (vs. non-tumorous back skin in CsA-immunosuppressed/non-UVB-treated mice; p < 0.05) • Higher FoxP3$^+$ T cell numbers in tumorous back skin of MmuPV1-infected, CsA-immunosuppressed/non-UVB-treated mice (vs. non-tumorous back skin of same mice; p < 0.05) • Intradermal administration of primary cSCC cells of passage 11 (MmuPV1 DNA undetectable) to athymic NMRI-Foxn1$^{nu/nu}$ mice gave rise to secondary tumours at 30 days post-inoculation (n = 2)

CsA, cyclosporine A; cSCC, cutaneous squamous cell carcinoma; DMBA, 7,12-Dimethylbenz(a)anthracene; HPV, human papillomavirus; MmuPV1, *Mus musculus* papillomavirus 1; n.s., not significant; TPA, 12-O-tetradecanoylphorbol-13-acetate; T$_{RM}$, tissue-resident memory T; UVB, ultraviolet B; wt, wild-type.

Following up on Strickley et al. (2019) [24], Johnson et al. (2022) [25] investigated if a compromised T cell immunity could explain the increased β-HPV replication and seropositivity that is found in patients with an increased cSCC risk, such as those under immunosuppression. The authors demonstrated that CD8$^+$ T cell depletion did increase the MmuPV-1 DNA levels in virus-colonised mouse skin and resulted in higher antibody titres to MmuPV1 E6, E7, and L1 antigens (Table 3). Interpreting both Strickley et al. (2019) and Johnson et al. (2022) in conjunction, it appears that the loss of T cell immunity against commensal β-HPVs confers an increased cSCC risk and higher viral load in immunosuppressed patients.

Dorfer et al. (2020) [26] also looked into how MmuPV1 infection can induce cSCC development in the context of immunosuppression. For this study, they treated mice with cyclosporine A (CsA), which inhibits calcineurin and preferentially suppresses T cell activation. The authors reported that MmuPV1 infection of back skin caused cSCC development in CsA-immunosuppressed mice but not in immunocompetent mice. Additionally, athymic NMRI-Foxn1$^{nu/nu}$ mice developed secondary tumours after receiving intradermal administration of primary cSCC cells that were isolated from a cSCC of a MmuPV1-infected, CsA-immunosuppressed/UVB-treated mouse (Table 3). These primary cSCC cells were multiply passaged and lacked MmuPV1 DNA. Thus, this study concurs with the prior two articles that a deficient T cell immunity in the presence of β-HPV infection predisposes to cSCC initiation. It also implicates β-HPVs as non-essential in cSCC maintenance.

3.2. T Cell Immunity in Potential Vaccination Strategies against β-HPV-Related cSCC Carcinogenesis

Marcuzzi et al. (2014) and Hufbauer et al. (2022) assessed potential vaccination strategies against β-HPV-related epithelial carcinogenesis by relying on the preclinical keratin-14 (K14)-HPV8 transgenic mouse model [28,29]. This model preferentially expresses all early genes (E1, E2, E4, E6, and E7) of HPV8 in the epidermis and developing hair follicles [21,30,31]. Viral gene expression is controlled by the human K14 promoter. At baseline, the viral antigens are synthesised at a subthreshold level that does not induce carcinogenesis, which is comparable to asymptomatic colonisation in immunocompetent individuals. Mechanical skin irritation from tattooing and/or tape-stripping induces epithelial carcinogenesis by activating high levels of HPV8 early gene expression.

Marcuzzi et al. (2014) [28] first showed that tattooing HPV8 E6 DNA onto the skin could prevent papilloma formation, which depends on anti-HPV8-E6-specific T cell immunity (Table 4). The HPV8 transgenic skin grafts of 6/15 tattooed (i.e., HPV-E6-immunised) mice did not develop papillomas after mechanical wounding. Following a HPV8 E6 epitope aa76-90 challenge and subsequent ELISpot assaying, splenocytes that were isolated from these six mice yielded a higher median number of spots (reflecting IFN-γ-producing cells per 100,000 splenocytes) than splenocytes from mice with papillomas (Table 4). Hence, a cytotoxic T cell response induced by skin tattooing of HPV E6 DNA may offer protection against HPV8-related epithelial carcinogenesis, albeit unreliably.

Table 4. Key T cell perturbations in potential vaccination strategies against HPV-related cSCC carcinogenesis.

Author and Year	Study Population	Vaccination Strategy	Key T Cell Perturbations
Marcuzzi et al. (2014) [28]	cSCC mouse model • K14-HPV8-CER mice • Mechanical wounding	HPV8 E6 DNA tattooing onto skin	• Higher median number of spots reflecting IFN-γ-producing cells per 100,000 splenocytes (via IFN-γ ELISpot) following HPV8 E6 epitope aa76-90 challenge in splenocytes of DNA-immunised mice without papilloma (vs. with papilloma, $p < 0.00001$)
Hufbauer et al. (2022) [29]	cSCC mouse model • K14-HPV8-CER mice • Mechanical wounding	Poly(I:C) tattooing onto skin	• More total and activated CD4$^+$ T cells detected in poly(I:C)-treated non-tumorigenic sites (vs. untreated skin, total CD4: $p < 0.001$, activated CD4: $p < 0.01$) • More activated CD8$^+$ T cells detected in poly(I:C)-treated non-tumorigenic sites (vs. untreated skin, $p < 0.01$) • CD4$^+$ T cell depletion resulted in tumour formation in poly(I:C)-treated sites ($n = 5/6$ mice) • CD8$^+$ T cell depletion resulted in tumour formation in poly(I:C)-treated sites, but to a smaller extent ($n = 2/6$ mice) • CD4$^+$ T cell depletion resulted in larger tumour sizes in poly(I:C)-treated sites (vs. CD8$^+$ T cell depletion)

aa, amino acid; CER, complete early genome region; cSCC, cutaneous squamous cell carcinoma; ELISpot, enzyme-linked immunosorbent spot; HPV, human papillomavirus; IFN, interferon; K14, keratin-14; poly(I:C), polyinosinic-polycytidylic acid.

Hufbauer et al. (2022) [29] explored if innate immunity-driven in situ autovaccination against the patients' own commensal β-HPV types in the skin could induce T cell immunity against β-HPV-related epithelial carcinogenesis in high-risk groups. Tattooing polyinosinic–

polycytidylic acid (poly[I:C]) prevented tumour formation in eight out of eight treated mice. Poly(I:C) is a synthetic analogue of double-stranded RNA, a known ligand for the innate immune receptors TLR3 and MDA5 [32]. In poly(I:C)-treated non-tumorigenic sites, there were more activated $CD4^+$ and $CD8^+$ T cells than in untreated skin (Table 4). $CD4^+$ T cell depletion and, to a smaller extent, $CD8^+$ T cell depletion resulted in tumour formation in poly(I:C)-treated sites (Table 4). $CD4^+$ T cell depletion also resulted in larger tumour sizes in poly(I:C)-treated sites compared to $CD8^+$ T cell depletion (Table 4). As such, $CD4^+$ T cells are likely the main effectors of poly(I:C)-mediated protection against HPV8-related epithelial carcinogenesis.

4. Discussion

The coexistence of impaired T cell immunity, β-HPV infection, and carcinogen exposure (such as UVB irradiation and DMBA) or chronic trauma promote cSCC initiation (Figure 2). An impaired T cell immunity exists in certain populations, such as organ transplant recipients on chronic immunosuppression, atypical epidermodysplasia verruciformis (EV), and EV-like phenotypes [10–13,33–35]. Consequently, these individuals possess markedly weakened anti-β-HPV defences, which are primarily orchestrated by T cells. The compromised β-HPV-specific T cell immunity reduces the clearance of β-HPVs and virus-positive malignant keratinocytes that have spawned following carcinogen exposure or chronic trauma, thereby potentiating cSCC initiation.

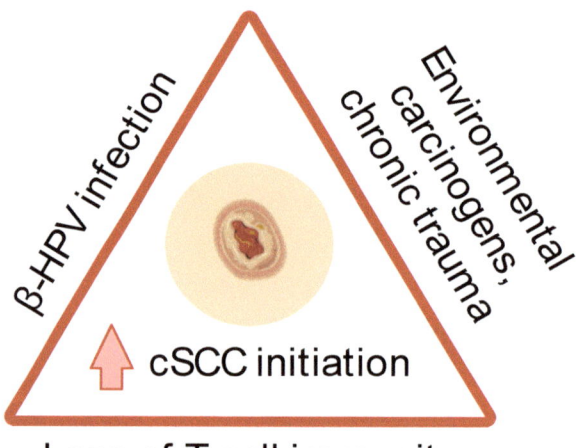

Figure 2. Loss of T cell immunity in the background of β-HPV infection promotes cSCC initiation following exposure to environmental carcinogens or chronic trauma. β-HPV, beta human papillomavirus; cSCC, cutaneous squamous cell carcinoma. Created with BioRender.com (accessed on 31 December 2023).

The host specificity of HPV has restricted the translatability of preclinical models when studying HPV-related cSCC [36]. An HPV transgenic mouse or animal papillomavirus-based infection model does not fully replicate the complex skin microbiome of human skin, is limited by inherent discrepancies in both innate and adaptive immunity, and may be affected by variations in experimental conditions. Nevertheless, the multitude of cSCC mouse model studies that were reviewed in this article have proved invaluable in revealing the anti-tumour effects of β-HPV-specific T cells in a tractable manner, which is otherwise not possible to conduct in human studies.

There is a significant lack of granularity regarding the specific T cell perturbations in HPV-related cSCC carcinogenesis. The included studies primarily relied on the enumeration of total T cell counts in affected skin and the depletion of total $CD4^+$ and/or $CD8^+$ T cells. Given that T cell diversity is wide-ranging, ranging from effector to regulatory, it is reasonable to hypothesise that specific T cell populations drive anti-tumour immunity. Addressing the β-HPV specificity of these populations is also pertinent, as the findings will provide crucial mechanistic evidence for whether the loss of β-HPV-specific T cell immunity or the de novo oncogenic effect of β-HPVs predominantly raises cSCC risk. Doing so will bridge key findings on T cell immunity in non-HPV-related cSCC models, where tumour-specific cytotoxic T cells (primarily Th1 and $CD8^+$ T cells) inhibit UVB and/or chemical carcinogenesis, while tumour-infiltrating regulatory T cells (Tregs) likely suppress anti-tumour immunity [37].

Topical imiquimod has emerged as a potential treatment for actinic keratosis, the prototypical premalignant lesion of cSCC that often possesses high β-HPV loads [38]. Its promise has been highlighted in pre-invasive α-HPV-related neoplasms of the female lower tract, whereby imiquimod may be a valid, cost-effective first-line treatment to avoid surgical excision [39]. Imiquimod directly induces apoptosis of malignant keratinocytes and partially overcomes HPV E6/E7 activity to stimulate robust Th1-Th17 responses [39]. Thus, it would be interesting to explore if imiquimod is effective as a monotherapy or in combination with other modalities to impair HPV-related cSCC initiation by enhancing β-HPV-specific T cell immunity.

The advent of spatial omics technologies can address these issues by permitting in tumorous and non-tumorous skin the high-dimensional interrogation of immune perturbations extending beyond just T cells [40,41]. The in situ single cell-level profiling would greatly complement traditional reductionist approaches in resolving the complexities of the tumour microenvironment, by uncovering spatio-temporal relationships between T cells, malignant keratinocytes, and other contributors to carcinogenesis. Doing so will clarify the role of T cells and simultaneously assess other cellular players like macrophages in protecting against HPV-related cSCC. Another advantage of these technologies is their amenability to limited tissue samples, facilitating ex vivo human studies. Discoveries via these modalities can rapidly aid explorations and validation in animal models, thereby seeding the future for improved therapy and prevention in high-risk populations.

All in all, T cells are intimately involved in the defence against HPV-related cSCC (specifically β-HPV), as their deficiency potentiates carcinogenesis in high-risk populations. Studies integrating omics approaches and appropriate animal models are warranted to elucidate T cell-mediated immunosurveillance and inhibition of HPV-related cSCC initiation. In parallel, further characterisation of the skin virome in immunocompetent and immunosuppressed individuals will shed light on the immunogenicity of different β-HPV types and the viruses' differential contributions to carcinogenesis. Future work can build upon these mechanistic studies to focus on protecting high-risk individuals with the prospects of T cell-centred vaccines against commonly occurring β-HPVs, β-HPV-specific T cell immunotherapy, and prognostication with β-HPV-specific T cells.

Author Contributions: Conceptualisation, S.H.T. and C.C.O.; data curation, S.H.T. and C.C.O.; formal analysis, S.H.T. and C.C.O.; methodology, S.H.T. and C.C.O.; investigation, S.H.T. and C.C.O.; writing—original draft preparation, S.H.T.; writing—review and editing, C.C.O. All authors have read and agreed to the published version of the manuscript.

Funding: This research received no external funding.

Institutional Review Board Statement: Not applicable.

Informed Consent Statement: Not applicable.

Data Availability Statement: No new data were created or analysed in this study. Data sharing is not applicable to this article.

Conflicts of Interest: The authors declare no conflicts of interest.

References

1. Alam, M.; Ratner, D. Cutaneous squamous-cell carcinoma. *N. Engl. J. Med.* **2001**, *344*, 975–983. [CrossRef] [PubMed]
2. Gloster, H.M.; Neal, K. Skin cancer in skin of color. *J. Am. Acad. Dermatol.* **2006**, *55*, 741–760; quiz 761–764. [CrossRef] [PubMed]
3. Tokez, S.; Hollestein, L.; Louwman, M.; Nijsten, T.; Wakkee, M. Incidence of Multiple vs First Cutaneous Squamous Cell Carcinoma on a Nationwide Scale and Estimation of Future Incidences of Cutaneous Squamous Cell Carcinoma. *JAMA Dermatol.* **2020**, *156*, 1300–1306. [CrossRef] [PubMed]
4. Oh, C.C.; Jin, A.; Koh, W.P. Trends of cutaneous basal cell carcinoma, squamous cell carcinoma, and melanoma among the Chinese, Malays, and Indians in Singapore from 1968–2016. *JAAD Int.* **2021**, *4*, 39–45. [CrossRef]
5. Chahoud, J.; Semaan, A.; Chen, Y.; Cao, M.; Rieber, A.G.; Rady, P.; Tyring, S.K. Association between β-Genus Human Papillomavirus and Cutaneous Squamous Cell Carcinoma in Immunocompetent Individuals-A Meta-analysis. *JAMA Dermatol.* **2016**, *152*, 1354–1364. [CrossRef] [PubMed]
6. Tampa, M.; Mitran, C.I.; Mitran, M.I.; Nicolae, I.; Dumitru, A.; Matei, C.; Manolescu, L.; Popa, G.L.; Caruntu, C.; Georgescu, S.R. The Role of Beta HPV Types and HPV-Associated Inflammatory Processes in Cutaneous Squamous Cell Carcinoma. *J. Immunol. Res.* **2020**, *2020*, 5701639. [CrossRef] [PubMed]
7. Howley, P.M.; Pfister, H.J. Beta genus papillomaviruses and skin cancer. *Virology* **2015**, *479–480*, 290–296. [CrossRef]
8. Tommasino, M. The biology of beta human papillomaviruses. *Virus Res.* **2017**, *231*, 128–138. [CrossRef]
9. Gheit, T. Mucosal and Cutaneous Human Papillomavirus Infections and Cancer Biology. *Front. Oncol.* **2019**, *9*, 355. [CrossRef]
10. Garrett, G.L.; Blanc, P.D.; Boscardin, J.; Lloyd, A.A.; Ahmed, R.L.; Anthony, T.; Bibee, K.; Breithaupt, A.; Cannon, J.; Chen, A.; et al. Incidence of and Risk Factors for Skin Cancer in Organ Transplant Recipients in the United States. *JAMA Dermatol.* **2017**, *153*, 296–303. [CrossRef]
11. Lanz, J.; Bouwes Bavinck, J.N.; Westhuis, M.; Quint, K.D.; Harwood, C.A.; Nasir, S.; Van-de-Velde, V.; Proby, C.M.; Ferrándiz, C.; Genders, R.E.; et al. Aggressive Squamous Cell Carcinoma in Organ Transplant Recipients. *JAMA Dermatol.* **2019**, *155*, 66–71. [CrossRef] [PubMed]
12. Urso, B.; Kelsey, A.; Bordelon, J.; Sheiner, P.; Finch, J.; Cohen, J.L. Risk factors and prevention strategies for cutaneous squamous cell carcinoma in transplant recipients. *Int. J. Dermatol.* **2022**, *61*, 1218–1224. [CrossRef] [PubMed]
13. Zavdy, O.; Coreanu, T.; Bar-On, D.Y.; Ritter, A.; Bachar, G.; Shpitzer, T.; Kurman, N.; Mansour, M.; Ad-El, D.; Rozovski, U.; et al. Cutaneous Squamous Cell Carcinoma in Immunocompromised Patients-A Comparison between Different Immunomodulating Conditions. *Cancers* **2023**, *15*, 1764. [CrossRef] [PubMed]
14. De Visser, K.E.; Korets, L.V.; Coussens, L.M. De novo carcinogenesis promoted by chronic inflammation is B lymphocyte dependent. *Cancer Cell* **2005**, *7*, 411–423. [CrossRef] [PubMed]
15. Arbeit, J.M.; Münger, K.; Howley, P.M.; Hanahan, D. Progressive squamous epithelial neoplasia in K14-human papillomavirus type 16 transgenic mice. *J. Virol.* **1994**, *68*, 4358–4368. [CrossRef] [PubMed]
16. Mombaerts, P.; Iacomini, J.; Johnson, R.S.; Herrup, K.; Tonegawa, S.; Papaioannou, V.E. RAG-1-deficient mice have no mature B and T lymphocytes. *Cell* **1992**, *68*, 869–877. [CrossRef]
17. Schiffman, M.; Doorbar, J.; Wentzensen, N.; de Sanjosé, S.; Fakhry, C.; Monk, B.J.; Stanley, M.A.; Franceschi, S. Carcinogenic human papillomavirus infection. *Nat. Rev. Dis. Primers* **2016**, *2*, 16086. [CrossRef] [PubMed]
18. Rollison, D.E.; Amorrortu, R.P.; Zhao, Y.; Messina, J.L.; Schell, M.J.; Fenske, N.A.; Cherpelis, B.S.; Giuliano, A.R.; Sondak, V.K.; Pawlita, M.; et al. Cutaneous Human Papillomaviruses and the Risk of Keratinocyte Carcinomas. *Cancer Res.* **2021**, *81*, 4628–4638. [CrossRef]
19. Borgogna, C.; Martuscelli, L.; Olivero, C.; Lo Cigno, I.; De Andrea, M.; Caneparo, V.; Boldorini, R.; Patel, G.; Gariglio, M. Enhanced Spontaneous Skin Tumorigenesis and Aberrant Inflammatory Response to UVB Exposure in Immunosuppressed Human Papillomavirus Type 8-Transgenic Mice. *J. Investig. Dermatol.* **2023**, *143*, 740–750.e744. [CrossRef]
20. Antsiferova, M.; Piwko-Czuchra, A.; Cangkrama, M.; Wietecha, M.; Sahin, D.; Birkner, K.; Amann, V.C.; Levesque, M.; Hohl, D.; Dummer, R.; et al. Activin promotes skin carcinogenesis by attraction and reprogramming of macrophages. *EMBO Mol. Med.* **2017**, *9*, 27–45. [CrossRef]
21. Schaper, I.D.; Marcuzzi, G.P.; Weissenborn, S.J.; Kasper, H.U.; Dries, V.; Smyth, N.; Fuchs, P.; Pfister, H. Development of skin tumors in mice transgenic for early genes of human papillomavirus type 8. *Cancer Res.* **2005**, *65*, 1394–1400. [CrossRef] [PubMed]
22. Namwanje, M.; Brown, C.W. Activins and Inhibins: Roles in Development, Physiology, and Disease. *Cold Spring Harb. Perspect. Biol.* **2016**, *8*, a021881. [CrossRef] [PubMed]
23. Antsiferova, M.; Huber, M.; Meyer, M.; Piwko-Czuchra, A.; Ramadan, T.; MacLeod, A.S.; Havran, W.L.; Dummer, R.; Hohl, D.; Werner, S. Activin enhances skin tumourigenesis and malignant progression by inducing a pro-tumourigenic immune cell response. *Nat. Commun.* **2011**, *2*, 576. [CrossRef] [PubMed]
24. Strickley, J.D.; Messerschmidt, J.L.; Awad, M.E.; Li, T.; Hasegawa, T.; Ha, D.T.; Nabeta, H.W.; Bevins, P.A.; Ngo, K.H.; Asgari, M.M.; et al. Immunity to commensal papillomaviruses protects against skin cancer. *Nature* **2019**, *575*, 519–522. [CrossRef] [PubMed]
25. Johnson, L.H.; Son, H.G.; Ha, D.T.; Strickley, J.D.; Joh, J.; Demehri, S. Compromised T Cell Immunity Links Increased Cutaneous Papillomavirus Activity to Squamous Cell Carcinoma Risk. *JID Innov.* **2022**, *3*, 100163. [CrossRef] [PubMed]

26. Dorfer, S.; Strasser, K.; Schröckenfuchs, G.; Bonelli, M.; Bauer, W.; Kittler, H.; Cataisson, C.; Fischer, M.B.; Lichtenberger, B.M.; Handisurya, A. Mus musculus papillomavirus 1 is a key driver of skin cancer development upon immunosuppression. *Am. J. Transplant.* **2020**, *21*, 525–539. [CrossRef]
27. Spurgeon, M.E.; Lambert, P.F. Mus musculus Papillomavirus 1: A New Frontier in Animal Models of Papillomavirus Pathogenesis. *J. Virol.* **2020**, *94*, 10–1128. [CrossRef]
28. Marcuzzi, G.P.; Awerkiew, S.; Hufbauer, M.; Schädlich, L.; Gissmann, L.; Eming, S.; Pfister, H. Tumor prevention in HPV8 transgenic mice by HPV8-E6 DNA vaccination. *Med. Microbiol. Immunol.* **2014**, *203*, 155–163. [CrossRef]
29. Hufbauer, M.; Rattay, S.; Hagen, C.; Quaas, A.; Pfister, H.; Hartmann, G.; Coch, C.; Akgül, B. Poly(I:C) Treatment Prevents Skin Tumor Formation in the Preclinical HPV8 Transgenic Mouse Model. *J. Investig. Dermatol.* **2022**, *143*, 1197–1207.e1193. [CrossRef]
30. Marcuzzi, G.P.; Hufbauer, M.; Kasper, H.U.; Weißenborn, S.J.; Smola, S.; Pfister, H. Spontaneous tumour development in human papillomavirus type 8 E6 transgenic mice and rapid induction by UV-light exposure and wounding. *J. Gen. Virol.* **2009**, *90*, 2855–2864. [CrossRef]
31. Pfefferle, R.; Marcuzzi, G.P.; Akgül, B.; Kasper, H.U.; Schulze, F.; Haase, I.; Wickenhauser, C.; Pfister, H. The human papillomavirus type 8 E2 protein induces skin tumors in transgenic mice. *J. Investig. Dermatol.* **2008**, *128*, 2310–2315. [CrossRef] [PubMed]
32. Cheng, Y.S.; Xu, F. Anticancer function of polyinosinic-polycytidylic acid. *Cancer Biol. Ther.* **2010**, *10*, 1219–1223. [CrossRef]
33. Landini, M.M.; Borgogna, C.; Peretti, A.; Colombo, E.; Zavattaro, E.; Boldorini, R.; Miglio, U.; Doorbar, J.; Ravanini, P.; Kumar, R.; et al. α- and β-Papillomavirus infection in a young patient with an unclassified primary T-cell immunodeficiency and multiple mucosal and cutaneous lesions. *J. Am. Acad. Dermatol.* **2014**, *71*, 108–115.e101. [CrossRef] [PubMed]
34. Saluzzo, S.; Pandey, R.V.; Gail, L.M.; Dingelmaier-Hovorka, R.; Kleissl, L.; Shaw, L.; Reininger, B.; Atzmüller, D.; Strobl, J.; Touzeau-Römer, V.; et al. Delayed antiretroviral therapy in HIV-infected individuals leads to irreversible depletion of skin- and mucosa-resident memory T cells. *Immunity* **2021**, *54*, 2842–2858.e2845. [CrossRef] [PubMed]
35. Uitto, J.; Saeidian, A.H.; Youssefian, L.; Saffarian, Z.; Casanova, J.L.; Béziat, V.; Jouanguy, E.; Vahidnezhad, H. Recalcitrant Warts, Epidermodysplasia Verruciformis, and the Tree-Man Syndrome: Phenotypic Spectrum of Cutaneous Human Papillomavirus Infections at the Intersection of Genetic Variability of Viral and Human Genomes. *J. Investig. Dermatol.* **2022**, *142*, 1265–1269. [CrossRef] [PubMed]
36. Doorbar, J. Model systems of human papillomavirus-associated disease. *J. Pathol.* **2016**, *238*, 166–179. [CrossRef] [PubMed]
37. Bottomley, M.J.; Thomson, J.; Harwood, C.; Leigh, I. The Role of the Immune System in Cutaneous Squamous Cell Carcinoma. *Int. J. Mol. Sci.* **2019**, *20*, 2009. [CrossRef]
38. Jansen, M.H.E.; Kessels, J.P.H.M.; Nelemans, P.J.; Kouloubis, N.; Arits, A.H.M.M.; van Pelt, H.P.A.; Quaedvlieg, P.J.F.; Essers, B.A.B.; Steijlen, P.M.; Kelleners-Smeets, N.W.J.; et al. Randomized Trial of Four Treatment Approaches for Actinic Keratosis. *N. Engl. J. Med.* **2019**, *380*, 935–946. [CrossRef]
39. Borella, F.; Gallio, N.; Mangherini, L.; Cassoni, P.; Bertero, L.; Benedetto, C.; Preti, M. Recent advances in treating female genital human papillomavirus related neoplasms with topical imiquimod. *J. Med. Virol.* **2023**, *95*, e29238. [CrossRef]
40. Lewis, S.M.; Asselin-Labat, M.L.; Nguyen, Q.; Berthelet, J.; Tan, X.; Wimmer, V.C.; Merino, D.; Rogers, K.L.; Naik, S.H. Spatial omics and multiplexed imaging to explore cancer biology. *Nat. Methods* **2021**, *18*, 997–1012. [CrossRef]
41. Hsieh, W.C.; Budiarto, B.R.; Wang, Y.F.; Lin, C.Y.; Gwo, M.C.; So, D.K.; Tzeng, Y.S.; Chen, S.Y. Spatial multi-omics analyses of the tumor immune microenvironment. *J. Biomed. Sci.* **2022**, *29*, 96. [CrossRef] [PubMed]

Disclaimer/Publisher's Note: The statements, opinions and data contained in all publications are solely those of the individual author(s) and contributor(s) and not of MDPI and/or the editor(s). MDPI and/or the editor(s) disclaim responsibility for any injury to people or property resulting from any ideas, methods, instructions or products referred to in the content.

MDPI AG
Grosspeteranlage 5
4052 Basel
Switzerland
Tel.: +41 61 683 77 34

Diagnostics Editorial Office
E-mail: diagnostics@mdpi.com
www.mdpi.com/journal/diagnostics

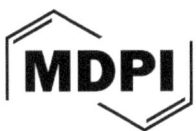

Disclaimer/Publisher's Note: The title and front matter of this reprint are at the discretion of the Guest Editor. The publisher is not responsible for their content or any associated concerns. The statements, opinions and data contained in all individual articles are solely those of the individual Editor and contributors and not of MDPI. MDPI disclaims responsibility for any injury to people or property resulting from any ideas, methods, instructions or products referred to in the content.

www.ingramcontent.com/pod-product-compliance
Lightning Source LLC
LaVergne TN
LVHW072356090526
838202LV00019B/2559